B. Hickey
Own copy.

CW01597320

A CASE STUDIES IN ABNORMAL PSYCHOLOGY

STEVEN SCHWARTZ
editor

JOHN WILEY AND SONS
BRISBANE • NEW YORK • CHICHESTER • TORONTO • SINGAPORE

First published 1992 by
JOHN WILEY & SONS
33 Park Road, Milton, Qld 4064

Offices also in Sydney, Melbourne and Auckland

Typeset in 11/12 pt English Times

© Jacaranda Wiley Ltd 1992

National Library of Australia
Cataloguing-in-Publication data

Case studies in abnormal psychology

Bibliography.
ISBN 0 471 33474 X.

1. Psychology, Pathological - Case studies. 2. Psychiatry - Case studies. I. Schwartz, Steven, 1946– .

616.8909

All rights reserved. No part of this publication may be reproduced, stored in a retrieval system, or transmitted in any form or by any means, electronic, mechanical, photocopying, recording, or otherwise, without the prior permission of the publisher.

The author and publisher would like to thank the following copyright holders for permission to reproduce material in this book: American Psychiatric Association, Washington D.C. (extracts on pp. 4, 5, 19, 20, 54-55, 75, 76,77, 132-33, 134, 160, 161, 162, 206, 225); American Medical Association (*Archives of General Psychiatry* (journal), pp. 23-27); Pergamon Press (*Behaviour Change* (journal), p. 41); Basic Books (quotations from Bruch, p. 53); Academic Press (fig. 8.1); The Royal College of Psychiatrists (fig. 8.2, reproduced by permission); quotation Monti et al., pp. 167-68 reprinted with permission from P.M. Monti, D.B. Abrams, R.M. Kadden and N.L. Cooney, *Treating Alcohol Dependence: A Coping Skills Training Guide*, 1992, New York, Guilford Press. Copyright 1989 by the Guilford Press; J. Bowlby, *Attachment and Loss* (Vol. 2), The Hogarth Press (quotations from Bowlby, pp. 211-12).

Every effort has been made to trace owners of copyright. If, however, any error or omission has been made, the publisher welcomes information that will assist in its rectification in subsequent reprints.

Printed in Singapore

10 9 8 7 6 5 4 3 2 1

Contents

Preface iv

1 Conduct disorders
S. Schwartz and L. R. Gaffney 1

2 Childhood autism
M. Prior 17

3 Obsessive compulsive disorder
M. R. Dadds and M. B. Powell 33

4 Overcoming anorexia nervosa
S. W. Touyz and P. Beumont 53

5 Sexual dysfunction
S. H. Spence 73

6 Mood disorder
M. J. Dyck 96

7 Born with a split brain: the 15-year development of a case of congenital absence of the corpus callosum
G. Geffen and P. Butterworth 113

8 Schizophrenia: understanding the processes underlying differences in symptoms and outcome
S. Andrews, P. B. Ward and S. V. Catts 128

9 Psychoactive substance dependence and associated states
R. P. Mattick 155

10 Psychophysiological disorders: hypertension and angina
P. C. Birrell 180

11 The nature and treatment of panic anxiety and agoraphobia
J. C. Clarke 192

12 Multiple personality disorder
J. T. Quinn 214

References 230

Preface

Abnormal psychology has made astonishing progress in the last century. One hundred years ago, mental hospitals were overcrowded, mainly custodial, institutions. Neuropsychology hardly existed. Psychoanalysis was being developed but there were no other psychological treatments, no personality or IQ tests and no antipsychotic drugs.

Abnormal psychology today is much more sophisticated than it was 100 years ago. The importance of carefully controlled research is widely acknowledged. Yet, it would be a serious distortion of reality to attribute all of the progress in abnormal and clinical psychology to controlled research. Clinical observations and case histories also played an important role. Conditions such as autism, anorexia nervosa and many others were first described in case histories. The controlled research studies which came later were often designed to test hypotheses derived from case studies.

All abnormal psychology textbooks acknowledge the importance of clinical observations and all contain case descriptions, but the traditional textbook format precludes an in-depth analysis of any single case. The result is that readers learn what clinicians do but not why. In contrast, this book is designed to give readers a look into the mind of experienced clinicians, to learn how they reason and how they go about planning and executing treatment programs.

The cases described in this book were deliberately chosen to represent a range of problems and treatments. For each case, the authors have tried to show how psychological theory and research can be applied to specific problems. Although the authors discuss research findings as well as clinical observations, they do not assume that readers have extensive prior knowledge. Thus, the book is suitable for undergraduates in psychology, social work, nursing and even medicine. General readers with an interest in abnormal psychology should also have no difficulty in following the discussions.

A book is always a group effort and this one is no exception. I am grateful to the chapter authors for sharing their expertise and for their cooperation in the editorial process. Nicole French deserves special thanks for her mastery of the intricacies of electronic word processing. I would also like to thank Anne Palmer, who assisted the entire process in numerous ways.

Steven Schwartz and Lisa Rosenthal Gaffney
University of Queensland

1 Conduct disorders

Mark was a 14-year-old boy when he came to our clinic via the Family Court. His parents had been preoccupied recently with their divorce and had little energy left to cope with their son's truancy, stealing and fighting.

Mark was the youngest of five children. All shared the same mother but only three had the same father. Mark's older brothers and sisters had left home before the age of 16, leaving Mark to bear the brunt of his alcoholic father's abuse. Mark's ineffectual mother was powerless to protect him from her husband's rages. Although Mark's mother was the object of the father's physical abuse, Mark was subjected to continuous mocking and criticism from his father.

Mark's father had had a series of small businesses which always lost money. He complained that were it not for his wife and children, he would have had more money to put back into the businesses and been a success. He worked long hours, stopped for a few drinks at the pub before coming home, and from time to time had a girlfriend 'who really appreciated him'. Mark's mother worked part-time as a waitress to try to make ends meet. She was worn out from having raised five children and bitter that her husband could not support the family properly. She knew about his periodic affairs and had threatened to leave him on numerous occasions, but had not done so. His request for a divorce, so that he could marry a younger woman with a bit of money, devastated Mark's mother. She had been loyal for so long, she thought his behaviour was totally unjust.

While Mark was growing up, his father would stay out late drinking several nights a week. Mark would never be able to sleep on these nights for fear of what his father might do when he returned home. On most of these occasions, the father would be belligerent and nasty, telling the mother how worthless she was, and if he could manage it, the father would physically strike out at his wife. Mark would be lying in bed in the next room, hearing everything. He would have to clench his hands together to stop himself from getting a knife and attacking his father. He felt like it, but he knew his father was bigger and would be the winner.

Often, both parents would be out during the evening, his mother working and his father drinking. Not one to sit still at home, he found companionship and excitement hanging around with older children. He started smoking cigarettes at 8 years of age, and had his first beer at 9. Because his father would complain every time he asked for money, Mark began to shoplift for the things he wanted.

From his very first day, Mark had problems at school. Although his IQ score was 'above average', Mark was a poor student. He seemed unable to concentrate and frequently disrupted the class. Mark received several medications during his primary school years. Although these drugs helped him concentrate, by the time he reached grade six, it became clear that Mark required a special class.

One year later, when Mark came to our clinic, he had still not adjusted to school. He was looking forward to leaving school as soon as he could, getting a job and moving to another city. Mark admitted that his behaviour had been less than exemplary but most of the blame, he felt, belonged to others — his father because of his drunkenness, his mother because of her weakness and the school for being 'useless'.

In the jargon of clinical psychology, Mark's behaviour is called 'acting out'. He behaves in 'antisocial' ways that transgress the standards of his society. In diagnostic terms, Mark has a 'conduct disorder', but this diagnostic label explains little. Indeed, at various stages of his life, Mark could just as easily have been diagnosed as having an 'attention-deficit hyperactivity disorder', or an 'oppositional-defiant substance abuse disorder'. Such a multitude of diagnoses is not at all unusual. These disorders often occur together, so often that it is rare to find one conduct problem without also finding others. In this chapter, we use Mark's story to show the relationship between attention-deficit disorder and conduct disorder. Throughout, we use Mark's history to illustrate the complications that arise when we generalise from the theoretical and research literature to an actual person.

Attention-deficit hyperactivity disorder: diagnosis and description

Attention-deficit hyperactivity disorder has been a controversial subject for almost 50 years. Debates about its symptoms, causes and even about whether the condition really exists have filled the professional literature, with most issues remaining unresolved. The controversies are illustrated by the many different labels used to refer to the same condition. At one time or another, the disorder has been known as 'Strauss' Syndrome', 'minimal brain dysfunction', 'hyperactivity', 'hyperkinesis' and 'attention-deficit disorder'. The current label, 'attention-deficit hyperactivity disorder' (ADHD), was introduced in 1987 when it appeared in the *Diagnostic and Statistical Manual of Mental Disorders,* third edition, revised (referred to as DSM-III-R). The fourth edition (DSM-IV) is due in 1993. Although the present plan for DSM-IV calls for the retention of the ADHD label, the diagnostic criteria are likely to change. The DSM-IV will explicitly recognise the close connection between ADHD and conduct disorder by grouping them together under the general category of Disruptive Behaviour Disorders (American Psychiatric Association, 1991).

The constantly changing names and diagnostic criteria suggest that ADHD is a somewhat elusive disorder. Everyone thinks it exists, but no one is sure exactly what it looks like or what it should be called.

ADHD children are usually described as impulsive, overactive and as having short attention spans (Barkley, 1987). Because attention spans lengthen with mental age (while impulsivity decreases), children are not considered to be in the ADHD category unless their attention spans are much shorter than those of other children their mental age. Impulsivity, too, must be judged according to a child's mental age; only those with developmentally inappropriate levels of impulsivity qualify as ADHD.

ADHD signs are said to become apparent before the age of 7 and last for months or, more commonly, years. The behavioural problems vary across settings with the worst problems reported by teachers (Prior & Griffin, 1985). The association between behaviour at school and the ADHD diagnosis probably explains why the diagnosis is often not made until the age of 6, the age when many children start first grade. Because of their overactivity, impulsivity and short attention spans, ADHD children do poorly at school; many also have trouble making friends.

The DSM-III-R (1987) criteria for diagnosing ADHD appear in table 1.1 (see page 4). Fourteen separate criteria are listed; a diagnosis requires that a child display at least eight at a level inappropriate for his or her age. The diagnosis also requires an onset of symptoms before the age of 7 and the absence of another disorder (Pervasive Developmental Disorder) which could also account for the child's problems.

Although the diagnostic criteria appear reasonable in theory, in practice they are difficult to implement. Few clinicians are qualified to judge whether a child's behaviour 'is considerably more frequent than that of most people at the same mental age'. Fewer still can make these judgements independent of context. Criterion 10, 'often talks excessively', for example, means one thing in the classroom and quite another in the school grounds after classes are done. The importance of context cannot be overstated. Indeed, context differences are why parents and teachers frequently disagree about whether a child belongs in the ADHD category (Sandberg, Wieselberg & Shaffer, 1980). That is, children may show their disorder at school but not at home. The changes proposed for the DSM-IV, which include dividing the various criteria into subgroups and the addition of such additional criteria as 'often acts before thinking', will not reduce the importance of context or make the diagnostician's task any easier.

The diagnostic picture is further complicated by the co-occurrence of ADHD and other disorders including 'learning disabilities', 'oppositional-defiant disorder' and, of course, 'conduct disorder'. Considerable effort has been expended trying to separate these problems, rarely with much success (see Share & Schwartz, 1988, for example). As a rough guide, ADHD is characterised by impulsivity and restlessness, oppositional-defiant disorder consists mainly of negativity, conduct disorders involve antisocial acts and learning disorders refer to significant delays in reading, mathematics or other skills despite adequate intelligence and adequate schooling (Barkley, 1987). The overlap among these diagnostic categories is substantial. Approximately 33 per cent of learning-disordered children may also be diagnosed as ADHD (Shaywitz & Shaywitz, 1989). The difficulty in separating overlapping diagnoses is most apparent when we try to differentiate ADHD from conduct disorder.

Table 1.1: Diagnostic criteria for Attention-Deficit Hyperactivity Disorder (ADHD)

Note: Consider a criterion met only if the behaviour is considerably more frequent than that of most people of the same mental age.

A. A disturbance of at least six months during which at least eight of the following are present:
  (1) often fidgets with hands or feet or squirms in seat (in adolescents, may be limited to subjective feelings of restlessness)
  (2) has difficulty remaining seated when required to do so
  (3) is easily distracted by extraneous stimuli
  (4) has difficulty awaiting turn in games or group situations
  (5) often blurts out answers to questions before they have been completed
  (6) has difficulty following through on instructions from others (not due to oppositional behaviour or failure of comprehension), e.g., fails to finish chores
  (7) has difficulty sustaining attention in tasks or play activities
  (8) often shifts from one uncompleted activity to another
  (9) has difficulty playing quietly
  (10) often talks excessively
  (11) often interrupts or intrudes on others, e.g., butts into other children's games
  (12) often does not seem to listen to what is being said to him or her
  (13) often loses things necessary for tasks or activities at school or at home (e.g., toys, pencils, books, assignments)
  (14) often engages in physically dangerous activities without considering possible consequences (not for the purpose of thrill-seeking), e.g., runs into street without looking.

Note: The above items are listed in descending order of discriminating power based on data from a national field trial of the DSM-III-R criteria for disruptive behaviour disorders.

B. Onset before the age of 7.

C. Does not meet the criteria for a Pervasive Developmental Disorder.

Conduct disorder diagnosis and description

Conduct disorder refers to a pattern of behaviour that has also been described as antisocial, acting out, aggressive and delinquent. The diagnosis of conduct disorder is given to children and teenagers who show a persistent pattern of antisocial behaviour. These youths are regarded as unmanageable by their parents and teachers and show impairment in their everyday functioning at home and at school. The DSM-III-R criteria for conduct disorder appear in table 1.2 (see page 5).

According to the DSM-III-R, approximately 9 per cent of males and 2 per cent of females under the age of 18 have a conduct disorder. While persistent patterns of antisocial behaviour in childhood correspond to the diagnosis of conduct disorder, these same characteristics in adulthood are linked to the diagnosis of antisocial personality disorder.

Children with conduct disorder often have other difficulties. Like ADHD, conduct disorder is associated with slightly depressed IQ scores, reading disabilities and, sometimes, neurological defects. Most importantly, conduct-disordered children show many symptoms of ADHD, including impulsivity, restlessness and inattentiveness (Rutter & Giller, 1983). Youth with antisocial behaviour are often deficient in many problem-solving and social skills (Kazdin, 1987). Robins (1981) emphasises that many of these children also suffer from psychological problems such as depression and anxiety, as well as from low self-esteem and a pervasive dissatisfaction with their lives.

Table 1.2: Diagnostic criteria for conduct disorder

A. A disturbance of conduct lasting at least six months, during which at least three of the following have been present:
   (1) has stolen without confrontation of a victim on more than one occasion (including forgery)
   (2) has run away from home overnight at least twice while living in parental or parental surrogate home (or once without returning)
   (3) often lies (other than to avoid physical or sexual abuse)
   (4) has deliberately engaged in fire-setting
   (5) is often truant from school (for older person, absent from work)
   (6) has broken into someone else's house, building or car
   (7) has deliberately destroyed others' property (other than by fire-setting)
   (8) has been physically cruel to animals
   (9) has forced someone into sexual activity with him or her
   (10) has used a weapon in more than one fight
   (11) often initiates physical fights
   (12) has stolen with confrontation of a victim (e.g., mugging, purse-snatching, extortion, armed robbery)
   (13) has been physically cruel to people.

Note: The above items are listed in descending order of discriminating power based on data from a national field trial of the DSM-III-R criteria for disruptive behaviour disorders.

B. If 18 or older, does not meet criteria for Antisocial Personality Disorder.

While there is considerable overlap in the behaviours which underpin conduct disorder, ADHD and delinquency, the terms are not synonymous. We have already noted that the term 'conduct disorder' is a diagnosis given to children who meet the DSM-III-R criteria summarised in table 1.2 and who have come to the attention of mental health professionals. Many of the behaviours which form the conduct disorder diagnosis can also result in a child's being labelled a juvenile delinquent if these same activities come to the attention of legal authorities. The legal term, 'delinquent', is given to youths who engage in behaviours which would be considered illegal if committed by adults (robbery or arson, for example) or in activities called 'status offences' which are activities considered illegal when engaged in by those under a certain age (drinking, not attending school and so on). Much of our understanding of conduct disorder comes from research involving juvenile delinquents. Because more boys than girls are identified as conduct-disordered and delinquent, and because the antisocial offences of boys more often involve physical aggression and threats to property, boys have been studied more often than girls.

According to some estimates, conduct problems and aggressive behaviour constitute between one-third and one-half of all child and adolescent referrals to mental health agencies (Robins, 1981). Conduct-disordered children have an enormous impact not only on their families and schools, but also on the wider society because their actions produce victims of theft, assault, arson and other criminal acts.

Mark, when young, could have been diagnosed as both ADHD (or 'hyperactive', as it was then called) and conduct disordered depending on which aspect of his behaviour was emphasised.

Mark's school folder, which eventually followed him to the clinic, bulged with psychological, social work and special education evaluations. In his first year at school, he was seen by a school psychologist, a special education expert and a social worker. By his second year, he had also seen a neurologist and a child psychiatrist.

His teachers described Mark as 'a constant problem'. He fidgeted, talked out of turn, never attended to stories or lessons, rarely cooperated with other children, took what did not belong to him and, perhaps most annoying to a teacher with a classroom full of students, he left his seat whenever he felt like it. Reprimands worked for only short periods; he needed constant supervision if he was to be kept from annoying the other children.

Psychological testing showed that Mark had a slightly above average IQ score of 102 with no obvious deficit on most subtests except those which required him to copy designs using blocks. The psychologist noted that Mark fidgeted frequently during testing and that he required considerable encouragement to complete the various tasks. Mark could identify letters and sounds but his reading comprehension was behind the class average in grade one and it fell even further behind in grades two and three. A special reading program was designed for Mark but progress was slow because Mark required close supervision (he needed a teacher all to himself) or he would not do his lessons.

A visit by a social worker to Mark's home revealed that he was 'a handful' there as well. He rarely sat still, not even when watching television. Indeed, he seemed unable to stick to any task or game for very long. Despite repeated requests, Mark often failed to complete household chores. He stayed out well past dinner time and often had to be 'fetched' home. If thwarted in any way, Mark would either have a temper tantrum or he would simply refuse to obey. At such times, his mother, who already had her 'hands full' dealing with her husband and her other children, often just 'gave up' and let Mark have his way. At the request of the school psychologist, a psychological measure designed to diagnose what was then known as 'hyperactivity' (Conners, 1973) was completed by Mark's mother and his teacher. Both placed Mark clearly in the 'hyperactive' range. The school psychologist told Mark's parents that their son suffered from attention-deficit hyperactivity disorder.

The social worker, on the other hand, was inclined to label Mark's behaviour as mainly a conduct disorder. Because he often refused to obey directions and because of his impulsive tendency to take whatever he wanted regardless of ownership, the social worker believed that Mark needed greater parental discipline if he was to avoid a life of petty crime.

As may be seen from this portrait of Mark at the age of 7, he was clearly a 'problem' child. But what, exactly, was his problem? He was retarded in reading and, despite his average IQ score and special tutoring, he fell even further behind as the years went by. This is a pattern often found in children diagnosed as 'learning disabled'. However, reading was not Mark's only problem. He frequently disobeyed adults acting in what could only be described as an 'oppositional' and, sometimes, an antisocial manner. But Mark was not only negative. He seemed also to have attentional difficulties and to be overactive, traits that would suggest ADHD. Such a confused diagnostic picture is the norm rather than the exception; pure ADHD is hard to find. This does not mean that ADHD is rare, however. Just the opposite, in fact. The diagnosis is actually used rather frequently. Approximately 3 per cent of elementary school children may be labelled ADHD (see Schwartz & Johnson, 1985), but the exact prevalence varies from place to place. Rutter (1982) estimated that American clinicians are 50 times more likely than their British counterparts to call children ADHD — British doctors prefer to label these children 'conduct-disordered'. In all cultures, however, the label ADHD is more often applied to boys than to girls. The sex ratio varies from a low of 3 to 1 to a high of 9 to 1 (Schwartz & Johnson, 1985).

Causes

First, we will look at the aetiology of ADHD; then, for a more complete understanding of Mark's problem, examine the causes of conduct disorder.

Aetiology of ADHD

The history of changing diagnostic labels (from minimal brain dysfunction to hyperactive, to hyperkinetic and so on) reflects the shifting consensus about the aetiology of ADHD (Douglas, 1988).

The original label, 'minimal brain dysfunction', was deliberately chosen to reflect the widely-held belief that a complex of behavioural and learning problems could be caused by mild brain damage. This notion was first put forward by Strauss and his colleagues (Strauss & Lehtinen, 1947, for example) who argued that a group of behaviours which included hyperactivity, aggressiveness, impulsivity and distractibility constituted a syndrome (a group of related symptoms). Strauss argued that this syndrome, by itself, is evidence of brain damage. Thus, rather than starting with known brain injury and looking for correlated symptoms, Strauss started with the symptoms and inferred that they reflect underlying brain damage. Over time, the occurrence of the behaviours, themselves, even without any history of brain damage or any physical signs of a neurological impairment, became sufficient for a diagnosis of minimal brain dysfunction.

Despite its popularity, minimal brain dysfunction was always controversial, mainly because no evidence was ever produced that such children were actually brain damaged. The arguments in favour of the diagnosis were almost entirely circular. Thus, a child is found to be impulsive, hyperactive and so on. This is taken to mean that the child has minimal brain dysfunction. Why is the child hyperactive? Because he or she suffers from minimal brain dysfunction. Reasoning such as this eventually led to the abandonment of the entire concept of minimal brain dysfunction (Rutter, 1989a, 1989b).

The demise of minimal brain dysfunction still left clinicians with a problem, what to call the children. Focusing on what was considered to be the most important aspect of the disorder, the children began to be called 'hyperactive' or 'hyperkinetic' (Ross & Ross, 1976). These terms became even more popular than minimal brain dysfunction but they brought their own problems. First, hyperactivity proved hard to define and even harder to identify or measure. Second, some children who were easily distractible showed few signs of excessive activity. Their main problem was attending at school.

Dissatisfaction with hyperactivity, both as a diagnostic label and as the unifying feature of the syndrome made up of impulsivity, distractibility and hyperactivity, led to the focus shifting to attention. This shift was formally acknowledged in the DSM-III (American Psychiatric Association, 1980) which renamed the syndrome 'Attention Deficit Disorder' which could occur with or without hyperactivity. The new name also reflected the interest of researchers who had conducted many studies of attention deficit in the 1970s (see Douglas & Peters, 1979, for a review). The inclusion of the word 'hyperactive' in the diagnosis in the DSM-III-R (1987) was an attempt to pull together the two historical strands — attention deficit and hyperactivity — into a single label.

As has often been the case with this elusive syndrome, satisfaction with the new diagnosis was short-lived. 'Attention deficit' turned out to be as vague a term as 'hyperactivity'. Aspects of attention which have been examined for deficits include selecting some aspects of the environment from others, 'concentrating hard' on a mental task and remaining alert over a prolonged period. Although any, or all, of these different types of attention could be disturbed in ADHD, investigators have made little attempt to separate them. Perhaps this is because the hypotheses about the origin of ADHD are too general to be tied to anything as specific as a deficit in selective attention as opposed to a deficit in alertness.

Current aetiological hypotheses fall into two categories: social and biological. Those who prefer social hypotheses point to the association between ADHD and parental psychopathology (Rutter & Quinton, 1984), marital conflict (Hetherington & Martin, 1986) and faulty child-rearing techniques (Williams & Forehand, 1984). Mark, our patient, certainly had his share of these social precursors in his background. But Mark may also have been the unfortunate victim of biological causes as well.

Studies of adopted children suggest that ADHD may be at least partly inherited (Cantwell, 1976). It seems particularly likely to occur in families, like Mark's, in which there is a history of alcoholism. Congenital problems, perhaps due to pregnancy complications, have also been implicated in ADHD (Gillberg, Carlstrom & Rasmussen, 1983). Environmental toxins can also produce 'hyperactivity' as has been shown in studies of lead poisoning (David, 1974).

At present, it is not possible to clearly identify any single cause of ADHD. While it seems fair to say that there is little evidence to indicate that ADHD children are brain damaged, minimal or otherwise, there is some suggestion that subtle biological factors play a role in the disorder's development. At the same time, social influences cannot be discounted. Like Mark, most ADHD children have a multitude of possible causes for their behaviour lurking in their backgrounds. Inconsistent parenting combined with an unstable home life when added to some biological disposition toward distractibility appear to produce ADHD. Several of these same factors have been implicated in the conduct disorders.

Aetiology of conduct disorders

Many theories have been developed to account for juvenile delinquency. A number of sociologists have argued that delinquency may result from feelings of alienation and rebellion in teenagers who do not feel part of the broader society. Many youths who do not feel accepted and valued by their families, teachers and prosocial peers may turn to a delinquent gang to meet these needs. Gang membership provides many young people with feelings of belonging, status and acceptance.

Other sociologists have highlighted the importance of social class in understanding delinquent behaviour. They argue that many people from the lower social classes have suffered economic and social disadvantages and may not be able to reach socially valued goals through legitimate means. These people may turn to criminal activities to achieve the material goods and status otherwise inaccessible to them. Numerous studies have shown that teens from all social classes report they have engaged in some forms of delinquent behaviour. However, higher rates and greater severity of offences are found more frequently in the lower classes. It is important to remember that, while there may be a relationship between social class and delinquent behaviour, not all youths from impoverished backgrounds engage in illegal activities (Rutter & Giller, 1983).

A number of psychologists have examined the possibility of a genetic component to delinquency. In a study conducted in Denmark, Schulsinger (1980) compared 57 psychopathic (antisocial) adoptees with 57 non-psychopathic adoptees matched for sex, age, social class, age at adoption, and geographical region. The biological parents of the adopted psychopaths, particularly the fathers, were more likely to have psychopathic characteristics than the biological parents of the controls. Since the biological parents had little contact with their children, the study supports the notion of a genetic predisposition to antisocial behaviour. Other researchers (for example, Zuckerman, 1974) have suggested that some delinquents may have a biologically determined arousal deficit. In order to increase their level of arousal to a more optimal level, they seek higher levels of stimulation through novel and unfamiliar activities, often engaging in thrilling and dangerous behaviours. Therefore, it is not a 'delinquent gene' per se which is inherited, but rather a tendency to seek out novelty and excitement.

Social learning theorists (Bandura & Walters, 1963) believe that delinquent behaviour is learned just as any other behaviour is, through modelling and reinforcement. According to the proponents of this theory, aggressive and delinquent behaviour is learned by watching parents, peers and others who model aggressive and illegal behaviour. It is also learned by having important people in the environment condone antisocial activities and ignore or belittle prosocial ones.

Support for the social learning theory explanation comes from a great body of research designed to examine family correlates of antisocial behaviour. Several longitudinal studies have been conducted in an attempt to understand the causes of conduct disorders. For example, McCord and McCord (1969) followed a group of several hundred boys living in poor neighbourhoods from their childhood in the 1930s through to adulthood in the 1960s. They found that the home atmosphere in which children were raised had a major impact on whether or not they became delinquent. Home environments described as quarrelsome and tense, in contrast to those described as cohesive, led to delinquency which began at a relatively early age. While consistent discipline was associated with low levels of criminal activity, either lax or inconsistent punitive discipline were closely related to criminal behaviour. The McCords pointed out that the home atmosphere and styles of discipline interacted in a complex fashion. For example, if the parents were not themselves psychologically disturbed and if the child's home was cohesive, then the effects of lax or inconsistent discipline were weakened. The McCords also found that paternal absence, cruelty or neglect tended to be associated with criminal activities in their sons.

Other researchers (West, 1982; West & Farrington, 1977) have identified parental psychopathology, alcohol abuse in one or both parents, large family size and poor socioeconomic status as also being related to the development of antisocial behaviour. The relationships among these factors are complicated and many authors have suggested that the greater the number of problem 'predictors' in a child's background, the greater the chance of delinquency.

Like ADHD, it is clear that not one cause can account for all cases of conduct disorder. Community and family influences, as well as biological factors may all play a role in the development of asocial behaviour. In fact, work by Quay (1979) has emphasised the notion that the term 'delinquent' does not refer to a homogenous group of teenagers, but rather there may exist subtypes of delinquency. Quay has identified four factors that represent dimensions of delinquent behaviour: socialised-subcultural delinquency, unsocialised-psychopathic delinquency, disturbed-neurotic delinquency and inadequate-immature delinquency.

A youth scoring high on socialised-subcultural delinquency has a strong allegiance to peers, often 'bad companions', yet shows little evidence of psychopathology. Juveniles scoring high on the unsocialised-psychopathic dimension have characteristics similar to the DSM-III-R conduct disorder diagnosis. The disturbed-neurotic delinquent is described as a timid and unhappy person who shows guilt and anxiety over his or her behaviour, and may be less likely to become repeat offenders. The inadequate-immature delinquent appears to be someone who is passive, easily frustrated, unable to cope with his or her surroundings and not accepted by delinquent peers. Quay cautions that important distinctions between delinquent and non-delinquent populations may be lost when delinquents are considered as a whole and subtypes ignored.

One of the major concerns about conduct-disordered children is their ability to affect the personal and property rights of others over extended periods of time. Because of the destructiveness of their actions, a great deal of research has been conducted to explore the stability of their behaviour and the predictors of serious and long-term offending.

Loeber (1982) reviewed studies examining the stability of antisocial and delinquent behaviour. His findings suggest that children who frequently displayed antisocial acts in more than one setting (say, both at home and at school) were at a higher risk of becoming chronic offenders than were those children who limited their antisocial activities to one setting. Robins (1966) reported that the age of onset of antisocial activities is also very important in predicting later behavioural problems. Robins followed 524 child guidance clinic patients and 100 normal school children from childhood to follow-up 30 years after the initial referral. She found that those children whose antisocial behaviour came to the attention of adults when the children were between 7 and 11 years of age had twice the risk of behaving antisocially in adulthood as those children whose antisocial acts only appeared after they were 11 years of age.

While not all conduct-disordered children go on to display severe antisocial behaviour as adults, childhood antisocial behaviour is the best predictor of severe antisocial behaviour in adulthood. At follow-up, 30 years after referral, Robins (1966) found that almost one-half the men referred for antisocial behaviour had been jailed, over one-quarter for one year or more. None of the male control subjects and only 13 per cent of the clinic subjects referred for problems other than antisocial behaviour had been jailed. A similar picture was found for the women. Twelve per cent of the women who were referred to the clinic because of antisocial behaviour as children were imprisoned as adults, while none of the other female clinic patients or controls were imprisoned. In a series of replications of the 1966 study which had used child guidance patients born around 1912, Robins (1978) investigated childhood predictors of antisocial behaviour in samples of black males born in 1933, Vietnam veterans born in 1951 and a group of matched non-veterans also born in 1951. She found that committing a variety of antisocial acts in childhood was a better predictor of adult antisocial behaviour than was any particular behaviour, and that adult antisocial behaviour was better predicted by childhood behaviour than by family background or social class. In fact, social class made little contribution to the prediction of serious adult antisocial behaviour.

Treatment

Mark's behaviour in school could not be tolerated. His constant interruptions and his refusal to cooperate annoyed his teacher and distracted the other children from their lessons. A special education teacher was consulted. She recommended a special class designed for 'children like Mark'.

For two hours per day, Mark was placed in a special class that met in a room with no windows, bulletin boards or pictures, and only the minimum of furniture. The walls, floors and ceiling were all painted the same drab colour. Cloth-covered partitions separated the students who could see the teacher but not one another.

Each child in the classroom received an individualised program including 'rewards' in the form of 'points' that could be traded for various prizes. Impulsive behaviour was discouraged but not actively punished. Attention to lessons as well as good performance earned points.

Mark initially did well in the special class, but his behaviour in his normal class remained much the same. The special program did not appear to produce changes that generalised to other situations.

Mark's mother was becoming increasingly concerned by the reports she received from his school. She had heard about special diets and decided to try her son on one that eliminated artificial food colourings and other ingredients. This diet required considerable supervision and time but it seemed to pay off. Mark seemed calmer and more amenable to suggestion both at home and at school. The improvement did not last, however, and the complaints from school soon resumed.

Just when she thought that all possible avenues had been exhausted, Mark's mother heard of a doctor who was treating 'hyperactive' children with special drugs. Within a week, Mark was taking the stimulant drug, Ritalin. According to his mother, the effect was dramatic. Mark was more attentive, less impulsive and generally happier. The effect of the drug was less pronounced at school, noticeable mainly in a lower level of activity. Mark stayed on the drug for almost two years. He then began to rebel at taking the medicine, denying strenuously that he was 'sick'. His mother tried to convince him to keep taking the drug even though it had little effect on his academic performance which was still poor. After a few months of struggling, Mark's mother finally gave up and the drug was discontinued.

Not only was Mark's in-class behaviour unsatisfactory, but there were many days when he was truant from school. Mark took the train to school each day with two friends. Sometimes they would decide to hang out at the local shoppingtown instead of attending school. In talking with Mark and his mother, the therapists discovered that Mark desperately wanted a new bicycle. The therapists tried to organise a system where if Mark would attend school daily and do at least 30 minutes of homework a night, he would be able to earn a new bicycle. This intervention failed. Mark's mother was not always at home to monitor his homework and the pulls for Mark to skip school with his friends were too great.

The therapists were also aware of the importance of parents showing their children they were interested in their daily lives, praising achievements and setting firm and consistent consequences for inappropriate behaviour. Over the time that Mark was seen in treatment at school and at the clinic, the therapists tried to engage Mark's parents in learning better parent management techniques. Although his father would rarely attend sessions and was highly critical of this technique, Mark's mother said she could see some value in the ideas of the system. However, her attendance at sessions was sporadic and she seemed to have little energy to devote to the system, being preoccupied with her own marital difficulties.

Treatment of ADHD

Many parents of ADHD children relate stories similar to Mark's. Numerous treatments are tried; all work initially but then the improvements begin to fade away. Curiously, treatments derived from conflicting theories seem equally effective. For example, the rationale for placing Mark in a bland classroom, devoid of windows, pictures and other stimuli, came directly from Strauss' early writing. Strauss believed that minimal brain damage rendered the children incapable of 'screening out' stimuli. These stimuli constantly bombard the child through all five senses, producing hyperactivity. The best way to reduce this hyperactivity is to reduce stimulation.

In contrast to stimulus reduction, stimulant medication treatment is designed to raise the child's 'arousal' level. The theory is that under-aroused children seek to increase their arousal by increasing their activity. According to this theory hyperactivity is the result of too little stimulation, not too much.

Because all treatments work for a while, it seems reasonable to suspect some sort of non-specific 'placebo' phenomenon is at work. Placebos are inert substances used in medical research to evaluate new drugs. Patients who receive the placebo are compared with those who receive the drug. Neither group of patients is told which they are getting — placebo or drug. Because those who receive the placebo alone often show signs of improvement, the drug is only considered effective if its benefits exceed those of the placebo alone.

Why should a placebo lead to improvement? There are several possibilities. First, because most conditions improve spontaneously, we would expect some improvement no matter what drug we administer. More important from a psychological viewpoint are the expectations people hold for treatment. Mark and his mother's faith in diet treatment could, by itself, lead to improvement in Mark's behaviour (or at least a readiness to see improvements whether or not they were actually present). Finally, placebos lead to improvement because of the extra attention their administration requires. Mark's mother had to devote considerable time to supervising Mark's diet therapy, time she might not otherwise have devoted to her son. It is possible that this extra attention, and not the diet itself, was responsible for any improvements.

At present, it seems that stimulant drugs remain the most common treatment offered to ADHD children. In some cases, this is augmented by behaviour modification and even with special diets. None of these treatments has been shown to produce long-term effects in school performance or in adult functioning (see Ross & Ross, 1976; Schwartz & Johnson, 1985).

Treatment of conduct disorders

Given the seriousness of the problem, it is not surprising to find that a vast amount of effort has also gone into designing, and to a lesser extent evaluating, treatment programs. Kazdin (1987) has reviewed the current treatments for conduct-disordered youth. There are some encouraging techniques which have been developed in the fields of 'functional family therapy', 'problem solving skills training', 'community based treatment' and 'parent management training'.

In Functional Family Therapy (FFT), the antisocial behaviour in the youth is conceptualised as the family's method of meeting interpersonal needs such as intimacy, distancing and support (Alexander & Parsons, 1982). For example, if parents have poor communication with one another and are unhappy in their marriage, a child forever misbehaving can serve as a common target for the parents to focus their attention on while putting aside troubling aspects of their own relationship. Therapy based on this orientation is focused on altering communication patterns in order to foster more adaptive functioning. Several therapy studies by Alexander and Parsons show promise in altering communication in families towards greater discussion and more equitable speaking, and in lowering recidivism rates among the youthful offenders. Replications by independent researchers are needed, however, before the full implications of this approach can be known.

Problem Solving Skills Training (PSST) is aimed at altering a youth's attributions, self-statements, and problem-solving skills. PSST is based on the idea that aggressive behaviour is not an automatic result of environmental events, but rather the result of the ways in which the individual perceives and thinks about events. Therefore, changes in behaviour can be brought about by teaching children and teenagers to question their automatic assumptions about other people's intentions, to stay calm before impulsively reacting and to think about consequences prior to acting. While there has been some research showing the effectiveness of this approach, the majority of studies have focused on laboratory tasks and not on deviant child behaviour. More work is needed in this area to demonstrate that PSST can assist conduct-disordered youth to make substantial gains in their problem solving abilities and to relate these gains to more adaptive behaviour overall (Kazdin, 1987).

Community based interventions, as the name implies, are treatment programs carried out in the community, rather than in institutions built for criminal offenders. One of the most widely researched community based interventions is Achievement Place, established in 1967 in Kansas. Eight boys live in a home run by two trained 'houseparents'. Boys attend the local school and take part in a token economy program where points are gained for engaging in appropriate behaviours and lost for showing unacceptable behaviours. Points can later be exchanged for reinforcers such as money and permission to watch television. They are taught new social skills and self-government procedures by their 'houseparents'.

Outcome evaluations have shown positive effects during treatment in terms of increasing social skills and reducing delinquent behaviour. However, follow-up studies show that while delinquent behaviour is reduced following treatment, the level of offending is still well above national norms (Wolf, Braukmann & Ramp, 1987).

Treatment effectiveness has been evaluated most thoroughly for parent management training. Much of the rationale for this approach is based on the analysis, by Patterson, Dishion and Bank (1984), of family functioning. Patterson and his colleagues have identified a number of features associated with the home environments of delinquent children. According to them, parents of antisocial boys are 'deficient' in one or more family management skills. These skills include: (1) adequately monitoring the child's whereabouts, (2) appropriately disciplining the child for antisocial behaviour, (3) negotiating and problem solving for resolution of family conflicts and (4) positively reinforcing socially appropriate academic, vocational and relationship skills.

The focus of parent management training is on changing the patterns of interaction in the family. Parents are taught to reward appropriate behaviours and to use mild forms of punishment to suppress antisocial behaviour. They are also instructed to provide clear rules, be consistent in their interactions and to negotiate compromises. This method of therapy essentially retrains parents to be better managers of their children's behaviour. While the treatment has been shown to be effective in the short term, long-term follow-up (more than one year) is needed. In addition, according to Kazdin (1987), the interaction of child (types of problem behaviours) and parent (motivational level, type of support system) characteristics need to be studied more systematically.

Part of the difficulty in treating conduct disorder is the range of behaviours involved. A given child might show temper tantrums, fire setting, aggressive behaviour, lying and stealing. All of these behaviours need to be addressed in treatment, and all can vary in frequency, intensity and lethality. Kazdin (1987) suggests that rather than target 'conduct disorder' for treatment, the focus of therapy should be on identifying and treating specific problem areas. As discussed above, conduct-disordered children may also have a range of problems other than antisocial behaviour, such as social skills and attention deficits, which may make them more or less responsive to treatment. These areas also need to be addressed in treatment programs.

Prognosis

Mark left school at the age of 16. He was unable to find any work other than as a stable hand at a country property not far from his home. He kept at this job for a few months but then left when he had a fight with the supervisor. He felt that he was being made to work more than the other stable hands and resented his ill-treatment. After leaving this job, Mark drifted from one short-term position to another, never staying long in any one place. He had a few minor run-ins with the law, once when he was accused of shoplifting and a second time when he went for a ride with several others in a stolen car. On both occasions, Mark was given warnings but not jailed.

Mark, who is now 20, has developed the habit of drifting from job to job and from place to place. His relationships — with employers and with friends — inevitably lead to tension and friction. He has avoided any serious legal difficulties and seems able to look after himself but his behaviour so far does not seem to have a plan, goal or purpose. He has lost touch with most of his family, only seeing a brother from time to time when he needs money.

Prognosis for ADHD children

A major question concerning children diagnosed ADHD is what happens to them as they grow older. Although clinical lore suggests that the problems (particularly hyperactivity) decrease with age, follow-up studies indicate that most children are not so lucky. Their problems persist, making the ultimate prognosis less than favourable (Loeber, 1991). For example, Weiss et al. (1971), in a five-year follow-up of children with a diagnosis of minimal brain dysfunction, found that although their hyperactivity decreased over time, the children continued to display serious problems in attention, concentration and under-achievement. Huessy and Cohen (1976) found that by adolescence, 50–70 per cent of hyperactives have failed at least one school grade and many have failed two. Hoy et al. (1978) reported that 'hyperkinetic' children upon reaching adolescence displayed problems in sustained attention, performed less well on visual-motor tasks, exhibited more reading problems and rated themselves lower in self-esteem than did a group of normal adolescents.

There have not been many follow-up studies of attention-disordered children through adulthood, but some writers have suggested (on the basis of retrospective studies) that antisocial adults may have been hyperactive as children (Robins, 1979).

One study of particular import was conducted by Borland and Heckman (1976), who compared male hyperactive children with their non-hyperactive brothers over a 25-year period. The hyperactive children were found to have poorer school records and to have a lower socioeconomic status in adulthood. Although no longer hyperactive, the formerly hyperactive children were described as nervous, restless adults who easily lost their tempers. These men were also found to change jobs more often than their brothers and to perceive their work as more boring. Psychiatric problems were also more common among the hyperactive group than among their brothers, although none were reported to be incapacitated by these problems.

Follow-up findings, taken as a whole, suggest that although motor activity levels may decline as the attention-disordered child grows older, many problems remain to affect their lives even as adults. The outlook for conduct-disordered children is much the same.

Prognosis for conduct disorder

Even if conduct-disordered children do not continue in criminal activities after their teenage years, research has shown that many still have a poor prognosis for satisfactory adjustment to adult life. Whereas emotional disorders in childhood rarely lead on to antisocial behaviour in adult life, conduct disorders frequently lead to a wide range of social, relationship and emotional problems. These problems include alcoholism and poor marital and occupational adjustment. Robins (1966) found that as adults, the antisocial children from her study showed much higher rates of arrests, alcoholism, divorce, poor job histories, child neglect, dependency on social agencies and psychiatric hospitalisation than either of the other two groups.

According to Wolf, Braukmann and Ramp (1987) it might be better to conceptualise conduct disorder as a complex developmental disability rather than a specific short-term problem of childhood. In fact, they raise the issue of referring to antisocial children as having a 'social disability', that is, a predisposition to engage their environments in antisocial and dysfunctional ways, and to be at risk for parental abuse and neglect. Certainly, studies by Robins (1966), West (1982), McCord and McCord (1969) and others point to the lifelong implications of conduct disorder.

In the same vein, Kazdin (1987) suggests thinking of conduct disorders in terms of a chronic disease model. He makes an interesting analogy to the treatment of diabetes. Just as one would not expect to give a diabetic a brief course of insulin therapy, then stop the insulin and expect the person to function in a healthy way, one should not expect to treat a youth with a lifelong pattern of antisocial behaviour with a limited term of therapy. If one considers conduct disorder to be a pervasive and entrenched way of operating in the world, the most promising therapy would be one in which continuous management and support is given. Several treatments for conduct-disordered youth have shown promising results during the course of treatment and immediately following therapy. Perhaps, then, the reason these interventions do not show lasting effects is not due to any deficiencies in the techniques themselves, but because, by its nature, conduct disorder requires continuous treatment.

Acknowledgement
The authors' research is supported by The Australian Research Council.

Margot Prior
La Trobe University

2 Childhood autism

Childhood autism was first specifically identified in the clinical literature by the noted American child psychiatrist Leo Kanner in 1943. In a paper entitled 'Autistic Disturbances of Affective Contact' Kanner described 11 children characterised by a collection of distinct and idiosyncratic behaviours including: aloneness from the beginning of life, an obsessive desire for the preservation of sameness in the environment, a good relationship with objects which were manipulated with considerable skill, evidence of good cognitive potentialities and failure to use language for the purposes of communication. These children seemed to have a very specific and unique disorder which was difficult to explain in the absence of any physical signs of maldevelopment and an apparently clear family history of mental disorder.

Kanner's diagnostic criteria were central to the exploration of autism in the 1950s and 1960s but accumulating research led to the questioning of his original criteria, especially the presumption of good cognitive potentialities. As the following discussion will show, almost 50 years of sustained research has modified the original conceptualisation in important ways.

The disorder aroused considerable interest and has continued to attract a vast quantity of clinical and research attention over the years. This is perhaps because the existence of such a severely handicapping disorder in a group of children who, for the most part, appear physically normal, and who are indeed often extremely attractive and appealing, is very mysterious. There is a challenge in trying to find the key which will unlock this puzzle.

Early writings about autism assumed that it was the earliest form of psychosis, possibly an infantile manifestation of schizophrenia. Diagnosis was uncertain, controversial and unsystematic, and early research into autism probably was based on a heterogeneous collection of severely disturbed children, only some of whom would have clearly met Kanner's criteria for the disorder.

However, a substantial body of clinical and research investigation concerned with diagnosis and classification, and greater understanding of the particular characteristics of autism which were reliably observed in a growing number of identified cases, led to a marked shift in the conceptualisation of this disorder. In 1980, with the publication of the *Diagnostic and Statistical Manual of Mental Disorders*, third edition (DSM–III) (American Psychiatric Association, 1980), autism was classified as a 'pervasive developmental disorder', with the term 'psychosis' eliminated from further discussion. The classification was prefaced in 1979 by a change in the name of the journal which publishes much of the research in this field. Formerly known as the *Journal of Autism and Childhood Schizophrenia*, the journal is now called *Autism and Developmental Disorders*. It has been argued that this change in thinking about autism came about to a considerable degree because of the developmental and clinical research which profited from methodological and theoretical advances in the 1970s, and which permitted more systematic assessment of the development and behaviour of autistic children by comparing them with normal children and other handicapped groups (Prior, 1984). In particular, developmental cognitive theory and research has been helpful in this regard.

There is now a general consensus that the basis of the autistic disorder is in severe cognitive disabilities which make the world a confusing, probably chaotic, puzzle which is extremely difficult for the autistic child to understand. Hence, the behavioural peculiarities such as bizarre responses to social and sensory stimuli, and the strong need to maintain 'sameness' or predictability in the environment are responses to the anxiety evoked by a lack of comprehension. There have been a number of summaries of the nature of the cognitive disabilities which are characteristic of autism (for example, Hermelin, 1976; Prior, 1979, 1984; Rutter, 1983; Waterhouse & Fein, 1984). Most reviews concur in noting that basic perceptual and memory processes in autistic children are delayed in their development but are consistent with their general mental age levels, rather than being deviant. Where specific deficits stand out is in higher levels of cognitive processing where stimuli must be filtered, encoded, recoded, transformed and interpreted. So many stimuli bombard the young child that a failure to filter and organise them leads to the child feeling overwhelmed and to the development of stereotyped and self-isolating behaviour. Failure to develop a capacity to abstract and to use symbols in thinking results in severely restricted information processing capacities. The most critical example of symbolic processing deficits, of course, is in the comprehension and use of language. In these areas, autistic children are specifically handicapped, since they operate in a concrete, rigid, often perseverative way (Prior & Hoffmann, 1990; Ozonoff, Pennington & Rogers, 1991; Schwartz, 1981), seeming to be unable to extract important from unimportant elements and to operate flexibly and adaptively on the multitude of stimuli in their environment. Hence rote learning is their most commonly used strategy, and this imposes limits on their ability to generalise what is learned. More than one-half of the autistic population do not acquire functional language at all and their non-verbal communication strategies are also severely impaired.

The research of the late 1980s and early 1990s has focused on understanding the social deficits in autism, again using advances in knowledge about the unfolding of social cognitive abilities in young children as they mature (Baron-Cohen, 1988; Shantz, 1983; Frith, 1989), to guide experimental and clinical investigations.

The starting point of this research has been the observation that autistic children lack the ability to perceive the mental and emotional states of other people, that their social behaviour is either primitive and minimal or that it lacks the reciprocity of interest, and the two-way communicative nature of that of normal children. Autistic children's communications are one-sided; they do not share interests in either objects or people with others in their environment, and, in what is seen as a reaction to their cognitive problems, they impose stereotyped and inflexible strategies on their social interactions. This is characteristic even of those autistic individuals who do seem connected with the environment and with other people to a useful extent and who try to make social contacts. They do not seem able to perceive and use social signals.

The burgeoning knowledge arising from research focused on autism has had a major influence in current conceptualisations of the disorder, and contemporary diagnostic and classification systems have tried to reflect this understanding.

The two major classification systems in current use — *Diagnostic and Statistical Manual of Mental Disorders*, third edition, revised (DSM-III-R) (American Psychiatric Association, 1987), and *International Classification of Diseases*, tenth edition (ICD-10) (World Health Organization, 1988 — see Rutter, 1989a) — both classify autism as a Pervasive Developmental Disorder (PDD), that is, a disorder which affects all or most aspects of development from very early in life. The category of PDD currently has a number of subtypes within each of these diagnostic systems, and the proposals for DSM-IV, to come in 1993, seem very much in line with the current ICD-10 subtypes.

Subtypes of the DSM-III-R Pervasive Developmental Disorders (PDD) — Autism and Allied disorders are: Infantile Autism, PDD-Childhood Onset, and Atypical PDD. Little is known about these latter two categories except that autistic behaviours may occur after a period of apparent normal development. Subtypes in ICD-10 are: Childhood Autism, Atypical Autism; Rett Syndrome, other childhood disintegrative disorders; overactive disorder associated with mental retardation and stereotyped movements; and Asperger Syndrome. The arguments for this somewhat disparate collection of types have been summarised by Rutter (1989a). In this chapter, only Childhood Autism and Asperger Syndrome will be further discussed on the grounds that they represent the core syndromes. Moreover, the DSM-III-R rather than the ICD-10 criteria for diagnosis will be emphasised here on the grounds that it is the most detailed in symptom specification and it is almost certainly the most commonly used system for those working with autism, as well as the most generally cited system in the research literature.

Table 2.1: Criteria for autism (ICD–10)

1. qualitative impairments in reciprocal social interaction
2. qualitative impairments in communication
3. restricted, repetitive and stereotyped patterns of behaviour, interests and activities
4. developmental abnormalities must have been present in the first three years for the diagnosis to be made.

Diagnostic criteria for autism (DSM-III-R) (American Psychiatric Association, 1987)

The criteria according to the DSM-III-R are listed in table 2.2 below.

Table 2.2: Diagnostic criteria for autism (DSM-III-R)
(adapted from Gillberg, 1990)

A. Qualitative impairment in reciprocal social interaction as manifested by at least two of the following:
  (1) marked lack of awareness of the existence of feelings of others
  (2) no or abnormal seeking of comfort at times of distress
  (3) no or impaired imitation
  (4) no or abnormal social play
  (5) gross impairment in ability to make peer friendships.

B. Qualitative impairment in verbal and non-verbal communication, and in imaginative activity, as manifested by at least one of the following:
  (1) no mode of communication, such as communicative babbling, facial expression, gesture, mime, or spoken language
  (2) markedly abnormal non-verbal communication, as in the use of eye-to-eye gaze, facial expression, body posture, or gestures to initiate or modulate social interaction
  (3) absence of imaginative activity, such as play-acting of adult roles, fantasy characters, or animals; lack of interest in stories about imaginary events
  (4) marked abnormalities in the production of speech, including volume, pitch, stress, rate, rhythm and intonation
  (5) marked abnormalities in the production of speech, including stereotyped and repetitive use of speech
  (6) marked impairment in the ability to initiate or sustain a conversation with others, despite adequate speech.

C. Markedly restricted repertoire of activities and interests, as manifested by at least one of the following:
  (1) stereotyped body movements, e.g.; hand-flicking, twisting, spinning, head-banging, complex whole-body movements
  (2) persistent preoccupation with parts of objects
  (3) marked distress over changes in trivial aspects of environments, e.g., when a vase is moved from usual position
  (4) unreasonable insistence on following routines in precise detail, e.g., insisting that exactly the same route always be followed when shopping
  (5) markedly restricted range of interests and a preoccupation with one narrow interest, e.g., interested only in lining up objects, in amassing facts about meteorology, or in taking the role of a fantasy character.

D. Onset during infancy or childhood.
  At least eight of 16 specified items above must be fulfilled.

It will be noted that, in the American Psychiatric Association system, an attempt has been made to systematically quantify the diagnosis by requiring a certain number of signs to be present in sections A, B and C; and an overall total of eight of the 16 specified items. Despite widespread acceptance of the syndrome of autism, it is true that there is great heterogeneity within the population, hence some systematic approach is highly desirable. While the requirement of a minimum number of signs does not solve the difficult diagnostic problems, it does represent an attempt at identifying a threshold for classification as autistic.

The spectrum notion

An alternative to the syndrome approach which is typified in DSM-III-R is the spectrum notion which sees autistic behaviours not as a distinct package but existing along a continuum from the most severe to the most mild (Gillberg, 1990). Wing and Gould (1979) studied a large group of handicapped children with autistic behaviours in an epidemiological study in London. They claimed that the most meaningful way to describe the characteristics of these children is in terms of a triad of impairments: in reciprocal social interaction, in verbal and non-verbal communication skills, and in imaginative activities (Wing, 1981). In their study, children varied along a continuum of severity from profoundly handicapped to normal on each of these factors. There was a consistent relationship between the extent of the cognitive and the social deficits. At the most severe end were children who were completely aloof and 'autistic' and who were severely handicapped cognitively. At the other extreme were individuals who were aware of their social environment but whose social behaviour was restricted and 'odd' and lacking in reciprocity and empathy. For this latter group, non-verbal intelligence was in the normal range (Shah & Wing, 1986).

The spectrum concept is useful in understanding the varying degrees or severity of autistic impairments which are seen in the population of children given the diagnosis. At the upper end of this spectrum may be those individuals thought to be cases of Asperger Syndrome. This syndrome is a subtype in both ICD-10 and DSM-IV. Whether this diagnosis should be a separate and independent one appropriate for a particular syndrome, or whether it is an alternative way of describing high-functioning cases of autism whose intelligence and language facility are in the normal or near normal range, remains unknown. A number of recent studies have attempted to document specific characteristics of Asperger cases without, however, succeeding in making clear distinctions between such cases and high-functioning autistic people (Frith, 1991; Gillberg, 1989; Gillberg, Steffenburg & Jakobssen 1987). However, at least in Australia, Asperger Syndrome is becoming a popular diagnosis and it is as well to be aware of its characteristics.

A recent comparison of the characteristics of autism and Asperger Syndrome provided by Wing (1991) emphasises the difficulties in distinguishing between the two disorders. At this point in research it appears that Asperger cases cannot be clearly discriminated from high-functioning cases of autism on any symptomatic, behavioural or ability grounds, and there are no systematic differences in their developmental histories. None of the early (Asperger, 1944; Van Krevelen, 1971) or the recent writings on this topic (Frith, 1991; Gillberg & Gillberg, 1989; Szatmari, Bartolucci & Bremner, 1983) provide a basis for differential diagnosis, when the cases themselves are subject to rigorous and detailed examination. The current diagnostic systems which do suggest subclassification are perhaps a sign of hope that further work will identify the means of separating the categories. At the moment, the most meaningful distinction within the autistic spectrum is probably according to level of functioning (Bartak & Rutter, 1976; Prior, 1979), since there are notable and measurable differences between high and low functioning children in cognitive and social areas. (Case histories of Asperger cases may be found in Frith, 1991.)

Epidemiology

Although the reliability and validity of the diagnosis of autism remains somewhat questionable, there is considerable consistency concerning its prevalence in the child population. A rate of about four in 10 000 is reported from a number of different countries (Prior & Werry, 1986). Children with autistic behaviours but not the complete syndrome are more common (see Wing & Gould, 1979). Thus, estimates vary according to the rigour of the diagnostic criteria used. The male-female ratio also varies from a figure of about 2:1 to about 10:1 males to females, with an average estimate of about 4:1. Whatever the exact statistic it is clear that, as with almost all developmental disorders, males greatly outnumber females.

The onset of the disorder before 30 months is usually required for a diagnosis of autism and this is specified in DSM-III-R. Nevertheless, there are reports of cases with later onset after apparently normal early development. Purists might maintain that in such cases the diagnosis of Childhood Onset Pervasive Developmental Disorder should be given. This remains an area where there is considerable uncertainty.

Authoritative data on the outcome of the disorder are in short supply, but the review by De Myer, Hingten and Jackson (1981) suggested that a 'good' outcome was found in a maximum of 20 per cent of cases. At least 50 per cent will have a poor outcome, with the remainder variable according to level of language and intellectual functioning. There is generally some behavioural improvement over time and many individuals do form some attachments and limited social relationships. A substantial proportion of cases (up to 25 per cent) are reported to develop seizures in adolescence (Deykin & McMahon, 1979).

The causes of autism remain unknown. There is a non-specific association between autism and a variety of genetic, neurological, biochemical and pathological factors. Some recent large-scale genetic studies support the notion of inherited problems although these seem to be related to general cognitive and language deficiencies rather than being specifically the autistic disorder. The mechanism of transmission has not been identified (Rutter et al., 1990). Autism is notably associated with a number of organic disorders affecting the central nervous system (see Gillberg, 1990). It is believed that autism is a biologically based disorder but, so far, more specific hypotheses concerning the nature of the organic influences have not been substantiated.

Case study

The case to be described here is a rare one in the literature. It is rare because the outcome for the subject was so good. It should be emphasised that for most autistic children the prognosis is poor, with lifelong shelter, care and supervision being required. Outcome is largely a function of the level of cognitive disabilities, and the majority of cases suffer from moderate to severe intellectual and language disability. Thus the need for care and supervision consequent upon these handicaps tends to overshadow the particular symptomatology of autism in its influence on the long-term outcome. Nevertheless, about one-fifth to one-quarter of cases recover to the extent that they may lead useful lives within the community even if many of them are odd, eccentric and somewhat socially impaired people. Recent advances in the treatment and education of autistic children may mean that this proportion of relatively well-functioning cases could increase in future. However, changes in outcome as a function of contemporary treatment methods remain to be properly documented and confirmed. It is also possible that a broadening of the diagnostic criteria to include high-functioning mildly-impaired cases could affect outcome statistics.

This case of A has been selected for study despite its atypicality because: development has been well documented from very early childhood into adulthood; diagnostic, neurological and psychometric test data are available from several life stages; and the particular circumstances of growing up suggest some useful possibilities for the optimal management of autistic people. Moreover, as I have argued elsewhere (Prior, 1979), it is important to study high-functioning cases of autism in order to be able to say something about autism as a distinct disorder which is not overwhelmed by the functional deficits consequent upon intellectual disability. Dealing with these deficits dominates the management and outcome of the majority of low-functioning cases. The first part of the case study is reproduced directly from a paper published in 1974 (Gajzago & Prior) and written when this child was 8 years of age and in the very early years of school. Following this early history, A's later developmental pathways will be described up until his present age of 26 years. It should be noted that A was studied in the early 1970s (that is, before the existence of DSM-III and ensuing diagnostic systems). However, as his history indicates, as a young boy he would undoubtedly have met criteria for a diagnosis of autism by any of our contemporary systems.

Early infancy and onset

It is noteworthy that much of the material on A is not retrospective but comes from records kept by his mother. A was adopted shortly after birth into a family that now includes four younger, natural-born siblings. No information is available on A's natural parents. His health was excellent during infancy and his mother believed he was normal up until the age of 6 months. At this time 'bouts of odd behaviour' appeared, he was said not to assume an anticipatory posture on being picked up, held himself stiff and was unresponsive to cuddling. By the time A was 12 months old, definite abnormal behaviour patterns had developed. These included screaming and severe temper tantrums, hyperactivity, refusal to sleep more than two to four hours daily, obsessive attachment to one particular play object, and odd play patterns. He also rocked in the cot and banged his head. His mother reports that A 'attacked' her as a baby, and showed extreme dislike of physical contact. Milestones such as crawling, walking and so on were normal and he also showed some imitative behaviour before the age of 18 months.

Presenting problems

During the 12- to 18-month period all progress ceased and behaviour problems such as extreme violence, destructiveness and obsessiveness worsened. A was described as a screaming, severely disturbed child who ran around in circles making high-pitched sounds for hours. He also liked to sit in boxes and under mats and blankets. He habitually piled up furniture and bedding in the centre of the room. At times he was thought deaf although he also showed extreme fear of loud noises. He refused all food except in a bottle, refused to wear clothes, chewed stones and paper, whirled himself, and spun objects. Although he had eye contact he did not seem to be 'with you' and was indifferent to, or rejected, attention. He varied between states of hyper- and low activity.

A showed intense preoccupation with sameness and was very ritualistic. He played repetitively with the same toy for months, lined things in rows, collected objects such as bottle tops, and insisted on having two of everything, one in each hand. He became extremely upset if interrupted and if the order or arrangement of things were altered. He refused to visit new places and showed some extreme fears (for example, of white coats). He was fascinated by light switches and power points.

A began to speak before the age of 12 months but stopped at 18 months and did not speak for almost two years. He began to speak again at 3 years 6 months after which speech continued to develop. There was echolalia, no use of 'I' or 'yes'; and although A could name objects he could not answer questions. He showed an excellent memory for routes and places, and his mother thought he showed above average intelligence. Drug treatment at various stages did not lead to any noticeable improvement. He attended kindergarten from the age of 3 years 8 months and began school a year later when psychological assessment indicated that he was in the dull to normal range. At 4 years 6 months A joined a travelling teacher scheme. The teacher found him 'hyperactive, aggressive, destructive, distractable, with poor concentration and attention, withdrawn and lacking in confidence'. Problems at this time were difficult behaviour at home, extreme anxiety about going to school, poor concentration in class, apparent failure to absorb lessons, constant bed-wetting, and resistance to the teaching of new skills. However, he had good eye contact, and social and self-help skills were developing well. A's physical coordination was good. He still occasionally engaged in toe-walking and hand-flapping; spun objects; was extremely preoccupied with maintaining sameness; and played perseveratively with a favourite object.

A score of 30 on the Rimland Checklist for Behaviour Disturbed Children Form E-2 (Rimland, 1971) and clear evidence of the presence of the essential features indicate that A was a classic case of early infantile autism. (The Rimland Checklist is a diagnostic form that is completed by parents. It includes multiple-choice questions covering physical, perceptual, intellectual, emotional, social and speech development.)

Environment in which the recovery progressed

A's mother is capable, intelligent and articulate, and is interested in reading, music and geology. The father is a skilled motor mechanic and is quiet, somewhat shy and conscientious. Both parents are devoted to the family and have made considerable adjustment in order to cope with A's problems. Having failed initially to receive help from their local doctor, and being convinced that there was something seriously wrong, they decided to try themselves to modify A's behaviour.

In an attempt to reduce violent and destructive behaviour, the house was cleared of all portable and breakable objects including all furniture except beds and a table. This had the effect of both reducing destructive behaviour and allowing the mother more time for direct interaction with A. The very serious sleeping problem was treated by insisting that A remain in bed during the night even if he was not asleep. One parent sat up with him every night, putting him back to bed if he got up, until the habit of remaining in bed from 11.00 p.m. until dawn was established. This training took about 18 months.

To overcome the problem of refusal to wear clothes, the mother bought clothes which seemed to attract A (he wore favourite garments continuously). By the time he began kindergarten, A seemed to have realised that it was necessary to wear clothes at least while 'out'. Wetting and soiling on the floor was overcome when the mother insisted that A clean up the mess himself.

Both parents tried to spend as much time with A as possible, like joining him in water play which he enjoyed particularly. At these times, when A was happy and responsive, his mother took advantage of his increased receptiveness to talk and play with him. Although initially, shopping and visiting were traumatic experiences, his mother persisted in such outings so that gradually A became accustomed to them and social behaviour improved. Behaviour at home also improved when A's mother, realising how much he hated change, began a systematic and frequent change of the furniture arrangement and of routine. Strong protests and tantrums gradually gave way to acceptance without fuss.

Since A's speech was not developing normally, his mother made a special effort to talk to A all the time. She kept up a running commentary on her activities, led him about touching and naming things and discussed subjects such as traffic on the road. She also showed him books and sang and recited nursery rhymes regardless of his apparent complete lack of interest. A's speech began to develop at 3 years 6 months and at the same time A began to engage in some constructive play. Contact with other children and with a younger brother (2 years 3 months) who was speaking well seemed to stimulate A. At 3 years 8 months A began kindergarten and a slight improvement in all areas was noticeable.

The development of speech appeared concurrent with an increased awareness of people and an interest in the activities of other children. Early speech was echolalic or limited to the expression of needs or desires and was not communicative. Pronunciation was good from the beginning. Neither 'I' nor 'yes' were used until A was about 5 years 6 months of age. He also used metaphorical language such as referring to his father's driving gloves, kept in the glove box of the car, as 'Bockies' (his word for 'box').

A had understood simple requests before speech began, although he did not always obey. His comprehension appeared to improve with the development of speech. However, complicated requests were poorly understood and he showed great distress if conversations continued for any length of time. He did not seem to be able to follow a story on the radio until about 6 years of age. He became less distressed by sounds after developing speech but still showed distress at some loud sounds such as sirens or telephones.

A rather peculiar feature of speech development was a period, between 4 and 5 years, of 'talking in numbers'. Anything A spoke of was given a number, for example, 'Look at that big truck, that's a 23'. Anything that appealed to him was a 7, 8, 9', and the highest praise was 'Wow that's a 39!'. During this phase almost all sentences used by A contained a number.

Travelling teacher

A began school at the age of 4 years 6 months and at the same time joined the travelling teacher scheme. This scheme provided a trained travelling teacher who lived with the families of severely disturbed children for short periods varying from one to three weeks. The teacher drew up a program of activities for each child as a guide for the parents, and provided remedial teaching.

The program for A emphasised participation in family and school activities and encouraged the development of more self-confidence. Problems of competition for parental attention and aggressive behaviour were approached by allowing a certain time each day when A could have the undivided attention of his mother. The program was designed to facilitate intellectual, physical, social and emotional development and was in essence similar to that provided in normal preparatory grades at primary school.

A showed much improvement by the second year of school. He showed more interaction with peers, was willing to go to school alone and to take his lunch, and seemed generally happier at school. He was less aggressive, although there were still outbursts of temper, and much sibling rivalry. Learning problems including short concentration span, particularly in a classroom situation, remained. He had learned many letters, numbers and words, but recall was still poor, and there was a problem with reversals in numbers and letters. Shyness persisted, though his play had become more imaginative and constructive.

Current adjustment (1974) (as described in Gajzago & Prior)

A's speech is now described as 'fairly normal for his age' although it is not really fluent. Hesitancy and poor comprehension are probably attributable to poor concentration. A still becomes very confused about messages given at school and is inclined to be upset if he has to relay messages.

Some behaviour problems still persist, particularly at home. He is very egocentric and inclined to tantrums if refused any of his desires. Thumb sucking is still a habit. Bed wetting has been virtually eliminated (with the assistance of a 'Stop-Wet' alarm device) and sleeping is fairly normal. A is much less anxious and confused and will readily accept new experiences such as spending a holiday with his grandmother. He seems to be learning how to behave like the other members of his family and appears to know how he is expected to behave. He will still swear and make embarrassing comments but his mother sees this as a form of attention-seeking.

A has the disadvantage of being in an extremely large class at school but, nevertheless, his progress is described as 'good'. He enjoys school and is mixing freely with peers. His reading has been slow and he is having remedial teaching both at school and at home. Both concentration and self-confidence have increased and he is beginning to enjoy school work. A is very good at drawing and at constructing things. He seems to have some grasp of abstract ideas but is still confused by time concepts such as 'tomorrow or yesterday'. He is good at sports and joins in football, running and swimming.

A continues to experience some difficulty in a group situation, at play and in the family group. Although he plays well with children his own age, he is better with one child than with a group. He has friends who call at the house to seek his company. He still hangs back when approached by a stranger but will respond if spoken to. He is still changeable in his relationships — affectionate occasionally, at other times rather aloof.

A appears to have developed some empathy and becomes involved and concerned with others in distress. He is coping well emotionally and has begun to express his feelings very eloquently, for example, 'I'm very sad that our little dog is dead', 'I'm happy at this barbecue'. His current most apparent problems are lack of self-confidence and poor concentration.

This was the end of the account of A's development as published in 1974. In the following section, A's progress from that time up until adulthood is described. The main sources of data were reports from A's parents and siblings and A himself. He was also assessed at our clinic on three occasions during his teenage years.

Later development

Although A began school at the normal age level, his early years were described as generally unhappy. He was rather isolated in a large primary school, was very poor at his school work and required special help. He was moved to a small rural school with only 15 pupils where his adjustment improved considerably and he was able to make friends. He was good at outdoor activities, was adventurous and well co-ordinated. He was considered exceptionally 'quiet' and 'deep' by family, siblings, and friends but was not labelled as abnormal or 'autistic' within his small country community at this stage of his development. His learning problems were persistent but he was 'good with his hands' and artistic. His siblings thought of him as someone who was not as bright as they were but had his own skills which were valued. He had a few quite close friends with shared interests, but his preference was to stay at home engaged in his own pursuits. His mother reports that he was always a very anxious child and had frequent nightmares.

At secondary technical school, A was given remedial Maths and English but always had difficulties, and these skills have remained weak. While A is now functionally literate he does not read or write except when this is essential, as for example when he sat for and passed his driver's licence test. While he did not get into trouble at school, he went through a period of truancy, was 'easily led' and was under the influence of 'bad company' in his early teens. This was firmly and effectively dealt with by his parents. He completed only three years of secondary school.

A was tested on a number of neuropsychological tests at the age of 14 when his non-verbal IQ was 76 (Hoffmann & Prior, 1982). On a battery of tests which are thought to reflect left hemisphere brain functioning and which depend on verbal and abstract thinking, A showed severe deficits, performing below the level predicted by his overall mental as well as his chronological age. Scaled scores on the Comprehension, Similarities, and Vocabulary subtests of the Wechsler Intelligence Scale for Children (WISC) were 6, 5 and 3 respectively. These tests measure understanding of common social situations and problems, conceptual and abstract thinking, and knowledge of word meanings which must be clearly defined. A's abstract thinking capacities were minimal.

However, on tests purporting to measure right hemisphere functioning such as visual perception and synthesis, A was performing in the normal range and was particularly strong on the Object Assembly and Block Design test from the WISC. These results are typical of the ability profiles of higher-functioning autistic children. At 14 years of age he was given a brain scan which showed no sign of any abnormality (Prior et al., 1984).

After leaving school, A developed a special interest in collecting antique bottles, and Chinese artefacts which were common in his local area. He amassed a substantial collection of bottles which he still keeps stored in his home. In addition, he was involved in much research about the history, origins and types of bottles and he became very knowledgeable. Whether this could be called an 'obsessive' interest is unclear. Certainly his family did not acknowledge it as having abnormal qualities.

A had several jobs during his teens, all of a relatively low level and repetitive quality, not requiring independence or flexibility. He had a few close friends but did not go out with girls, preferring to stay at home with his TV and record collection. Since there are no first-hand reports of A's friendships, it is not possible to judge the qualities of these relationships, that is, whether they were truly normal, or passive or odd as described by Wing (1987). No member of his family could recall any evidence of subtle use of language such as jokes, teasing, irony or sarcasm. He was seen as an extremely quiet but very nice person who always thought the best of people and noted their good points; and who was helpful to people in trouble. His life was very sheltered and took place primarily within a very close and supportive family system where his mother, in particular, was very much the manager of the family and the main spokesperson.

At the age of 17, A was tested again on a number of tests of planning and organisational skills (Prior & Hoffman, 1990). On a maze-solving task he was extremely quiet and deliberate in his approach, used a set pattern of responses and was unable to correct his mistakes. On a test of the abstraction of categories of objects and ideas, he developed a repetitive 'set' and showed poor memory and very little ability to correct his responses on the basis of feedback. His conceptual thinking was at a low level and he showed no reaction when he made mistakes on the tasks. However his copy and memory with the Rey Figure test, where he was asked to copy a complex, many-faceted figure in a limited time and then recall as much of it as possible a few moments later, was excellent. This task probably tapped his good visual perception and drawing skills.

In his late teens, A left the family home and began a job in a timber mill in a small rural community which was familiar to him through his extended family. Relatives arranged this job for him. He met a young woman, a few years older than himself who had a young son by a previous marriage. He described the woman as 'the best thing that ever happened to me'. He moved into her parents' home with her. For the last six years they have lived together in rented accommodation provided by the timber mill and they recently married after the birth of their son.

Although A is still very quiet, he is reported to have changed considerably during this relationship and is now much more at ease socially, can talk to people, mix more easily and stand up for his rights. He has developed confidence as he has become more competent. His wife is cheerful, easy going, extroverted, sociable and fun loving. A is good with the children, very attached to his home and to both his extended families. One brief sign of social tactlessness was observed when he told everybody, including his wife, that his new baby was very ugly. He appears happy in his work and his lifestyle, is materially comfortable, and does not see himself as different. Indeed, he would not be identified today, on normal acquaintance, even by experts, as any different from the average young working class Australian male, with culturally 'normative' interests in cars, motor bikes, fishing and socialising over a glass of beer. He is able to express his opinions, albeit in a concrete way, on local and immediate family and community issues such as the threat of unemployment.

A appears more like a young man in his late teens than one in his twenties, as somewhat immature, socially slightly awkward, and slow in conversation. His cognitive deficiencies are evident although, again, they are not notably outside the normative range in his community. A had great difficulty giving instructions to find his house, omitting essential details, mistaking right for left and he could not achieve an ordered sequence of clues (his house had no number).

He appears to remember almost nothing of his childhood and could only produce a few very concrete facts after considerable prompting. He expressed little emotion over any of his childhood history, and there was no verbal expression of feelings about his parents or siblings, although he is clearly very attached to his family. When asked for a description of himself that might be given by someone else who knew him, he was very much at a loss and could only note that he would be seen as quiet. His wife reported that he is easily led, impulsive, lacking in forethought, and that this sometimes gets him into trouble. A agreed with these contributions in a good-humoured way. He is 'a bit of a worrier' over small things, especially new experiences. He is well liked in his community and is seen as a caring person, well integrated into an extended family which provides considerable support in all facets of his life.

A's history, once he had passed through the first few years of his development, is not very typical of that of an autistic person. However, there are other accounts in the literature of cases who have 'done well' and who are integrated successfully into normal life, despite continuing idiosyncrasies or mildly eccentric behaviour (Bemporad, 1979; Happe, 1991). In addition, Lovaas (1987) has suggested recently that some of the children who completed his lengthy and intensive behaviour modification program were not identified by their teachers as autistic in their normal school setting. Hence a notable degree of recovery is possible for some cases. A's mother suggested that he was most disturbed up to the age of 5 or 6, when he was hyperactive, ritualistic and obsessive. However, he 'slowed right down and burnt himself out'.

There are some useful lessons to be learned from the history of A even though these lessons could not be taken as recipes for recovery. As noted earlier, A's mother was not able to find much help for his autism when he was young. She therefore accepted the challenge herself to socialise and manage this very difficult child. She is exceptionally competent, determined, insightful and persistent, and decided that A was to become normal. As far as she is concerned she succeeded in this task. Her persistence, energy and dedication were remarkable. A's father is loyal, calm and very supportive. It is significant that A grew up in a large family network with plenty of social support for himself and his parents. There was frequent close contact with extended family and considerable socialising in which no concessions were made for A. He was accepted, and expected to be normal. His warm, competent and supportive family managed his problems with great skill and care. His young siblings provided stimulus for cognitive growth and language development and this was of considerable benefit throughout his development. His good points were always appreciated. Tantam (1991) has also reported improvement in some cases where these factors were helpful. A grew up within a secure, protective rural lifestyle where his peculiarities were little remarked upon. He was just summed up as 'quiet'. It is worth noting that in a follow-up study of 100 autistic children in the state of Victoria in 1978 (Prior & Sanson, 1978), the outcome for rural children was better than that for city children, regardless of their level of intellectual functioning. Such findings do imply that less demanding, more relaxed, tolerant, and non-stigmatising environments may be extremely helpful at least in some cases.

A's entire life has been lived in the shelter of his family; it has been predictable, safe, relatively undemanding, and totally accepting of his interests and activities. This might be described as 'milieu' treatment, but it can hardly be described as a prescribed or constructed therapy. A happened to grow up in what was, for him, a very therapeutic environment, where the excellent management skills of his parents were almost certainly critical. His work life, marriage and fatherhood have provided recent growth experiences which have given him strength and confidence. There may be an element of fragility about his maturity, and he undoubtedly needs ongoing support to compensate for his cognitive shortcomings, but within his current environment he is functioning extremely well.

His recovery seems to have progressed in two stages — one rather brief, the other lengthy and gradual. The first stage was described above (Gajzago & Prior, 1974) and involved firm, consistent intervention by his mother with some help from a travelling teacher, and support from family, psychologists and a sympathetic and knowledgeable physician. The second stage involved his school and employment history as described above, in which small progressive steps towards competence and confidence led to an accumulating ability to cope successfully. This remarkable recovery seems to have occurred without the intrusive, continuous and rigorous behavioural approaches claimed by Lovaas (1987) to be required for such a positive outcome. It might also be suggested that A received a relatively light 'dose' of autism and with optimal rearing circumstances was able to overcome the most debilitating aspects of the disorder. One can only speculate on the possible outcome for A, had he grown up in a city environment, under multiple social and educational pressures and with a less accepting community around him. Even his relatively high level of intellectual functioning may not have produced such a benign outcome in this case. A himself expresses extreme anxiety about going to the city and seemed only able to cope through the 'mothering' of his wife, on the rare occasions where such a trip was unavoidable.

An inevitable question in rare cases such as that of A is whether the diagnosis in early childhood was in error. The history as described above, which was not retrospective but collected during the early and later life of the child, suggests that, by any current diagnostic criteria, A would have received the same diagnosis as he did at that time. Moreover he is certainly not the only case to make a good adjustment, as the literature in this field records. However, unlike some other recorded cases (see, for example, Bemporad, 1979; Happe, 1991), A is extremely inarticulate about his early history. He seems to have scarcely any memory at all of his early life and certainly no insight into anything other than his scholastic difficulties.

The prognosis for the majority of autistic people is very poor. Most require ongoing support, shelter, supervision and sometimes even basic custodial care. Relatively few are employable, and few can communicate with the world around them except in the most restricted and stereotyped way. 'Integration' into a normal environment as was characteristic of A's history, of itself does not normalise autistic children (Howlin & Rutter, 1987). Since the policy of 'normalisation' or integration into regular school and community life is a recent development in Australia, it remains to be seen how many children who progress through the normal school system with adequate support socially and educationally will show an improved outcome. It is well known that those cases who develop competent language skills and whose intelligence is in the normal range have the best prognosis, but such individuals number less than one-quarter of the population diagnosed as autistic. It is also known that the most beneficial treatment for autistic children is a highly structured, predictable, organised regime which teaches academic and social skills in a very focused and systematic way.

There are no pharmacological treatments of value for autism except perhaps in providing symptomatic relief for excessive anxiety, or aggression in the short term. There is no 'psychotherapy' which is useful, and no scientific support for the vast number of idiosyncratic methods of treatment which are occasionally publicised in dramatic and colourful ways, especially in the popular media. In most cases autism is a lifelong disorder requiring lifelong care.

A number of themes have been identified in this account of the development of A from a severely autistic child to a well-functioning and happy adult. First, his autism was extremely well 'managed' by determined parents within a context of strong family support, and a non-judgemental, non-critical community. A salient example of this point might be the fact that he is described as 'quiet' rather than 'withdrawn' with its connotations of pathology. Second, four younger siblings continuously stimulated and supported A's cognitive and social development. Third, despite school failure, A felt accepted by his peers and was perceived as a person with his own set of talents. Fourth, his adult work life and his marital and parenting skills have gradually developed and strengthened, building his confidence and self-esteem.

Residual signs of the disorder remain, however. These are his anxiety, his apprehension about new experiences, his lack of planning and judgement and his poor level of academic skills. Such descriptors however might reasonably be applied to a large section of the population. A's history appears to reinforce theories of the centrality of the cognitive deficits in the autistic disorder. It also provides support for the value of consistent, intrusive education and management strategies with young autistic children as the best tools we have at the moment for treating this very severe disorder.

Acknowledgements
I wish to acknowledge the contributions of Christine Gajzago and Wendy Hoffmann in the study of this case.

Mark R. Dadds and Martine B. Powell
Albert Einstein College of Medicine, New York City Monash University

3 Obsessive compulsive disorder

Every day, the same drama unfolded. Upon being picked up at school, Peta, 8 years old, and her mother would make the short walk from the school gate to the car. Peta would become more and more anxious, peppering her mother with questions about whether her books, pencils, pens and even her teacher would be safe during her absence. Peta was terrified that the world of her school classroom would somehow disappear during the night and that on her return the next day, she would find everything gone. Despite her mother's protestations and attempts to calm her, Peta would become increasingly anxious and upset until, extremely agitated and in tears, she would run back to the classroom to check if her desk, work materials and teacher were still there. On bad days, the returns to check on her things could last for an hour or more.

Similar problems were emerging in the home as well. Peta had begun checking the daily garbage to make sure that none of her possessions were being thrown out. If her parents tried to stop this checking, which sometimes was repeated over and over as if terrified she had missed something, she would become hysterical and act aggressively toward her parents. Similarly, Peta was developing a habit of checking on her parents, especially her mother, to make sure that she was 'still there'; that she had not disappeared or left home.

Clearly, Peta had little faith that her world would remain intact. She felt compelled to check on the important things in her life, lest her anxiety that they disappear overwhelm her. However, her checking offered only a temporary relief and the anxiety would return quickly, compelling her to check and check again, never fully satisfied that she had not missed something.

Peta's problem is a clear example of obsessive compulsive disorder, a relatively rare disorder in which the sufferer becomes trapped in a world of anxiety and repetitive behaviour. Obsessed with an anxiety-provoking thought, the sufferer compulsively engages in repetitive, ritualised behaviour in an unsuccessful attempt to cope with the anxiety. In this example, Peta's obsessive thoughts concerned the possibility that various aspects of her life would suddenly disappear. These frequent, intrusive thoughts caused her considerable anxiety; anxiety that she had no understanding of or skills for dealing with. Consequently, she would compulsively check the environment in vain attempts to relieve her worry.

No-one can say exactly what causes this disorder. However, a range of psychological and biological ideas and procedures has emerged from research and clinical experience with this disorder that allows us to engage in useful speculation about the nature and causes of the problem. Further, a number of treatments have been developed that, if not offering a full cure, often produce substantial symptom relief. In this chapter, we will review the research and clinical literature on the epidemiology, diagnosis, aetiology and treatment of this disorder, especially as it applies to children. We will examine how this literature can help us understand the case of Peta. Finally, by carefully examining Peta's case, we will attempt to make more sense of this unusual yet highly interesting problem.

The clinical picture

Obsessive Compulsive Disorder (OCD) is a rare anxiety disorder identified and defined by the presence of recurrent obsessions (thoughts, impulses, images) and compulsions that are repetitive, intentional and performed as a response to the obsessive thought (American Psychiatric Association, 1987). That is, the compulsions are a way of reducing the discomfort produced by the obsessive thought(s). However, these compulsions also produce anxiety (the individual realises behaviours are irrational or obsessional, but is unable to resist them) which feeds back into the obsessional cognitions, creating the obsessive-compulsive cycle (Sims, 1988). The obsessional thoughts usually have themes of contamination, fear of harming others, religious denial, and doubt (Riddle et al., 1990) and are involuntary phenomena which overwhelm the person. Avoidance is also an important element of this disorder. The person develops complex procedures designed to avoid situations which are associated with the anxiety and which have often become triggers for the obsessional thoughts (Kaplan & Sadock, 1988).

Unlike many other forms of psychopathology, OCD in children appears in a virtually identical form to that in adults (Rapoport, 1986). Further, while research on treatment for this disorder has predominantly dealt with adult patients it has been suggested that, due to the similarity between manifestations of OCD in children, adolescents and adults, treatment programs that are often successful with adults may be equally effective in treating child and adolescent cases (Allsopp & Verduyn, 1989; Hodgeman, 1983; Rapoport, 1989). Rapoport (1989), however, does mention several practical considerations which differentiate adult from childhood OCD, factors which may have major implications for the design and implementation of treatment programs:

1. Familial involvement in the child's disorder — the child's problem may be functionally related to particular family structures and interaction patterns and, thus, the family may need to change as well as the child.
2. The child may not be seeking help — the referral usually comes from the parents rather than from the person with the disorder.

3. If parents are involved in running the treatment program, issues of individuation and autonomy, common to adolescent development, may confound the therapeutic intervention.

As with all psychiatric disorders, the behavioural and emotional problems must be severe enough to interfere with day-to-day functioning before a psychiatric diagnosis is considered. This is important because many of the signs of psychological disturbance are present, albeit to a lesser extent, in people who are not considered to be disturbed. Thus, many people experience 'obsessive' thoughts and 'compulsive' behaviour but are reasonably happy and cope well with life. In fact, many religions teach such behaviour, for example, making the sign of the cross after experiencing an unpleasant thought. Throughout history, rituals, repetitive practices and ceremonies have been used as a way of warding off impending danger and disaster. The clear parallels between OCD and various religious practices led Sigmund Freud to speculate that the development of an effective understanding of OCD will necessitate a comprehensive understanding of the nature of religious experience and practice. Despite the fact that many people, including children, can show obsessive thinking and consequential compulsive behaviour, in its clinical form, OCD is a very serious problem that can be long lasting, problematic to treat and extremely distressing to the sufferer and his or her family and friends.

A number of disorders have many features in common with OCD. In order for a diagnosis of OCD to be made, the *Diagnostic and Statistical Manual of Mental Disorders,* third edition, revised (DSM-III-R) (American Psychiatric Association, 1987) requires that the diagnostician exclude the possibility that the obsessions or compulsions are due to another disorder. Ritualised behaviour can also be observed in neurologic disorders (Burd et al., 1988; Caine et al., 1988; Kaplan & Sadock, 1988), as well as in psychiatric disorders such as eating disorders (Rothenberg, 1990; Erdreich, 1988), developmental disability (Swedo et al., 1989) and schizophrenia (Kaplan & Sadock, 1988; Rapoport, 1989). Although these other disorders all may have obsessive and/or compulsive symptomology, they are not diagnosed OCD. Other disorders associated with OCD such as depression (Riddle et al., 1990; Swedo et al., 1989) and other anxiety disorders (Rapoport, 1989) do not exclude a diagnosis of OCD, rather they result in dual diagnosis.

Adams (1985) has pointed to the importance of distinguishing between common obsessional and ritualised behaviour and OCD in children. That is, many children display ritualised behaviour as a part of normal play, but it is usually temporary and does not cause distress or interfere with everyday life.

Incidence and prevalence

OCD is a relatively rare condition (Kaplan & Sadock, 1988). The incidence of OCD within psychiatric populations has been reported as between 0.1 per cent and 5 per cent, and as about 0.05 per cent in the general population (Beech & Vaughan, 1978). Figures for childhood/adolescent OCD are similar to the adult figures, with Judd (1965) reporting an incidence of 1 per cent in child psychiatric in-patients and Hollingsworth et al. (1980) reporting a figure of 0.2 per cent across all child clinical populations. In the general population, close to 0.3 per cent of children and adolescents can be expected to suffer from OCD (Flament et al., 1985; Rutter et al., 1975).

The age of onset is typically young. In one study of 1293 adolescent psychiatric patients, Honjo et al. (1989) reported on a subgroup of OCD with the earliest age of onset being 3 years and the average age of onset being 11.3 years. Likewise, Last and Strauss (1989) reported on a group of 20 adolescent OCD cases with a mean age of onset of 12.7 years. Even in a study of adult OCD, Rasmussen and Tsuang (1986) found age of onset to occur with peaks at 12–14 years and 20–22 years. In this study, it was also noted that men had a younger mean age of onset (15.5 years) than women (22.9 years). This finding has been replicated in studies of adolescent OCD, where the number of male sufferers has also been found to be greater than the number of female sufferers, sometimes by as much as two males for every female (Last & Strauss, 1989; Rapoport, 1989; Swedo et al., 1989). Personality traits have long been thought to be related to the risk of developing OCD. However, obsessional traits are commonly found in patients with other disorders and much research has found no clear relationship between personality factors and OCD in adolescents (Rapoport, 1989).

Like other psychiatric disorders, research suggests that the onset of OCD is related to the presence of environmental precipitants in the person's life that may serve to trigger the illness (Khanna, Kaliaperumal & Channabasavanna, 1986). Examples of such precipitants are sexual assault, poor peer relationships and social isolation, birth of a child, loss of a job and death of a family member (Allsopp & Verduyn, 1990; Murphy et al., 1988). Research into the long-term outcome of OCD has found that the illness, once established, is chronic. Through its course there may be many remissions; however, very few patients ever end up symptom-free (Flament et al., 1990; Rapoport, 1989; Kaplan & Sadock, 1988).

Theories of aetiology

Theories of the nature and causes of OCD have existed since the turn of this century (for example, Janet, 1903) and the first half of the twentieth century was dominated by psychoanalytic models. According to psychoanalytic theory, OCD arises as a result of an upsurge in unconscious impulses that are unacceptable to the conscious awareness of the sufferer. This upsurge is caused by some precipitating event in the individual's life, which contains elements of earlier childhood conflicts (Kulish, 1988). The emergence of OCD symptoms is the result of personality regressing to an earlier phase of psychological development (Kaplan & Sadock, 1988). Thus, the obsessive compulsive cycle, in particular compulsive rituals, are seen as defensive strategies designed to avoid experiencing unwanted unconscious conflicts and drives.

Psychoanalytic theories are rightly criticised by many researchers for being based on vague, unobservable concepts. Thus, their validity is largely untestable and little evidence exists to support the efficacy of the psychoanalytic approach to treatment of OCD. Notwithstanding this, it is generally acknowledged that issues of underlying anxiety, aggression, control and sexuality, all central to psychoanalytic theory, invariably arise during psychotherapy with OCD patients (Jenike, 1983).

Support for the involvement of biological factors in OCD comes from:

1. studies showing a genetic component in OCD (Rutter et al., 1990)
2. some evidence for brain cerebral dysfunction in OCD patients (Flor-Henry et al., 1979)
3. the beneficial effects of brain surgery for a subpopulation of OCD sufferers (Elkins, Rapoport & Lipsky, 1980)
4. the successful use of medication with many OCD patients (Rapoport, 1986).

Despite this collection of evidence, researchers have not been able to identify any definitive biological process that is uniquely associated with OCD. Perhaps the most promising line of research to date suggests an imbalance in neurotransmitters (the chemicals which permit nerve cells to communicate) which can be corrected by drugs (Hanna, McCracken & Cantwell, 1991).

The second half of the twentieth century has witnessed the widespread growth of learning models of mental illness, including OCD (Rachman & Hodgson, 1980). The underlying assumptions of this approach are that behaviour is learned through experience with the environment, that the specifics of this learning are different for different people, and that the best way to understand psychopathology is to break it down into a set of observable behaviours that can be systematically measured and analysed in relation to their environmental context. In the last few decades, learning theorists have increasingly incorporated cognitive as well as environmental factors into their models of psychopathology (Rachman, 1991). That is, the patient's way of processing information about the environment is increasingly coming under experimental and clinical scrutiny.

The most common learning mechanisms implicated in the development and maintenance of OCD are:

1. *Classical conditioning*. Various stimuli that have been paired with a traumatic experience can take on the qualities of the trauma themselves. For example, stimuli associated with illness (such as medical staff, bandages, coughs, skin eruptions) may come to elicit severe anxiety reactions because they have previously been associated with the illness or death of a loved one.
2. *Avoidance and escape*. People typically dislike stimuli that provoke anxiety, and many people with anxiety problems spend a good deal of energy ensuring that such stimuli are avoided. Unfortunately, avoidance strategies usually trap the sufferer in a vicious circle that escalates the fear. By avoiding certain stimuli, the sufferer never experiences these stimuli in the absence of trauma. Thus, the original conditioning experience in which the sufferer learned that these stimuli accompany trauma, is never overriden by new learning. Further, escape behaviour is, in itself, reinforcing. That is, escape or successful avoidance of a feared stimulus results in a decrease in anxiety. Such a shift from a negative to a more positive affective state is a powerful reinforcer that strengthens the behaviour that produced the change. Thus, avoidance grows and grows, trapping the sufferer in an increasingly restricted life dominated by fear. For the sufferer of OCD, one of the most common forms of avoidance and escape is the compulsive ritualising, which is designed to avoid the anxiety elicited by intrusive thoughts and external fear stimuli.

3. *Social reinforcement.* People are social beings and the responses made to us by other people, especially our friends, family and loved ones, greatly influence our behaviour. It would be highly speculative to argue that reinforcement from others plays any significant role in the genesis or maintenance of OCD. However, the role of social context is especially important when considering the behaviour of children and adolescents. That is, children are greatly influenced by the responses of parents, teachers and peers and a number of case studies have indicated that parental reinforcement can alter the course of OCD in children (Fine, 1973; Francis, 1988; Queiroz et al., 1981).

   Social reinforcement can play a major role in the maintenance of childhood behavioural and emotional problems. Once a particular behaviour appears, the attention it brings from parents, teachers and peers is often enough to ensure the problem persists. Further, unintentional reinforcement of a problem behaviour is often accompanied by a decrease in reinforcement at times when the child is not engaging in the problem behaviour. That is, the existence of the problem behaviour often ensures that the remainder of the child's behaviour gets less attention from others.
4. *Modelling.* Children learn much about the world by copying the behaviour of others, especially parents. Exposure to others suffering OCD would be expected to increase the likelihood of OCD symptoms in a vulnerable child.
5. *Cognitive style.* There is recent evidence that OCD sufferers may interpret environmental cues in a way that perpetuates their compulsive behaviour. Sher, Mann and Frost (1984), for example, recently demonstrated that compulsive checkers appear to suffer a trait-like inability to gauge the accuracy of their checking performance. Even though the checkers were able to accurately recall whether certain words were missing or not from a list of words, these sufferers rated their own performance as extremely poor. That is, they had little confidence that their checking had produced any reliable information about the presence or absence of a stimulus. It is unclear whether such cognitive phenomena are basic to the disorder or are symptoms of another underlying pathological process. However, they do alert us to the need to consider processing styles when working with these patients.

In summary, according to a general learning model of OCD, obsessions produce anxiety, while compulsions represent certain actions which the person learns to reduce the anxiety attached to the obsessional thoughts. These compulsive acts are reinforced by the relief from anxiety they provide. The compulsions, through a process of reinforcement, eventually become learned behaviours which can sometimes generalise and become relatively independent of the thoughts which initially generated them.

It is clear that this conceptualisation of OCD provides several useful hypotheses concerning the treatment of the genesis of the disorder. However, it fails to explain why common themes (such as dirt and contamination) exist in the obsessional thoughts. That is, the learning model of OCD only explains the maintenance and the generalisation of obsessions and compulsions. It does not explain what started the cycle off in the first place.

Approaches to treatment

Psychotherapy

Into this category fall many different clinical approaches that employ the patient-therapist relationship to explore the psychological conflicts of the patient. In adults, psychotherapies rely on open communication between patient and therapist; in children, exploration is often achieved through play. The research literature generally does not view any psychotherapeutic interventions as effective treatments for OCD, especially when it occurs in children. Despite this, these methods remain popular with clinicians from many professions. Psychoanalytic approaches to OCD attempt to track the unconscious conflicts underlying the obsessions back to their earliest childhood origins. Inadequate defences are exposed and replaced by more adequate ones as the client gains insight into his or her behaviour (Kaplan & Sadock, 1988). However, there is little evidence to support the effectiveness of this approach to treatment. The research in fact suggests that psychoanalysis is very poor in treating the compulsive behaviours (for example, hand washing associated with the disorder (Rapoport, 1989)).

Family therapy may be indicated when family conflict results from the child's disorder, or where family conflict may be a contributor to the onset or maintenance of the disorder. A number of family therapists have pointed to family conflict as a major factor in childhood OCD, claiming that the child's obsessive and compulsive behaviours are a symptom of a disturbed family system (Forster & Holthausen, 1979; Fine, 1973; Madanes, 1980). However, a lot of the initial enthusiasm about this approach has disappeared as evaluations have made it increasingly clear that the family lacks the power to alter OCD (Adams, 1985).

Pharmacotherapy

Until the rise in popularity of the cognitive-behavioural therapy (CBT) approach, drugs were the main form of intervention used to treat OCD and it is still extremely popular, either as a treatment on its own, or as a co-treatment with CBT. Research suggests that Clomipramine, an anti-depressant, is the most effective pharmacological agent used to treat OCD (Flament et al., 1985; Kaplan & Sadock, 1988; Lipsedge & Prothero, 1987; Leonard et al., 1989; Rapoport, 1986, 1989). The effects of Clomipramine may not be seen for as long as two months (patients are usually maintained on the largest tolerable dose), and it is most effective when specific compulsions are present. Another anti-depressant, Fluoxetine, has also been shown, more recently, to be effective in the treatment of OCD (Liebowitz et al., 1990; Rapoport, 1989).

Medications, however, cannot be used indiscriminately and without side effects. Many patients report nausea, lethargy, tremors, addiction and a lowering of self-esteem based on a perception that one is 'sick' and unable to cope with problems without the use of drugs. Further, the effects of medication for OCD are temporary; the symptoms usually return as soon as the medication is withdrawn.

Cognitive Behavioural Therapy (CBT)

This is currently the psychological treatment of choice for OCD. Because the behavioural approach emphasises individual differences in the causes of behaviour disorders, interventions for OCD can consist of a number of different therapeutic procedures. However, the most effective treatment appears to be that which systematically exposes the patient to the feared stimuli while preventing him or her from ritualising, teaches effective strategies for managing anxiety, and modifies the patient's tendency to always detect threat in the environment while under-estimating his or her ability to deal with it.

Prolonged exposure. Prolonged exposure involves exposure to external stimuli and thoughts that evoke high levels of anxiety, until the patient can face the stimuli without avoidance and without overwhelming levels of anxiety.

Imaginal exposure. When in vivo exposure is practically impossible or when the feared catastrophes of a situation are a major component of the patient's fear, exposure takes place in the patient's imagination.

Response prevention. During exposure, the patient refrains or is prevented from escaping or using compulsive rituals as a means of reducing anxiety. Thus, the patient rehearses alternative, more constructive, methods of reducing the anxiety such as positive self talk, deep breathing exercises and muscle relaxation. Exposure therapy in combination with response prevention has become the treatment of choice for OCD over the last decade (Beech & Vaughan, 1978).

Implementing an exposure/response prevention program consists of a number of stages:

1. Therapist and patient together generate a list of feared (anxiety-inducing) situations, objects and thoughts, and these are arranged in a hierarchy from lowest to highest anxiety ratings.
2. Treatment begins with a chosen item from the hierarchy (agreed upon by patient and therapist) being enacted while the patient, using newly taught coping skills and therapist support, stays in the situation and experiences the anxiety until it declines. Response prevention is incorporated here, with the patient not being allowed to escape from the situation or initiate any 'anxiety-reducing' compulsive rituals (cognitive or behavioural).
3. Exposure to a given item on the hierarchy continues until the anxiety ratings drop below an agreed level (indicating minimal anxiety).
4. The exposure process, using the same item, is repeated until the item evokes no more than minimal anxiety at any time.
5. Once this is achieved, treatment shifts to the next level up on the hierarchy and the whole exposure process begins again.
6. The exposure program is terminated when the most feared item has been confronted and shown to engender only minimal anxiety, usually after between ten and twenty sessions.

Homework, in the form of 'self exposure' or 'parent as therapist' exposure, is an essential component of these programs. Practice outside the sessions is vital to maintain the gains achieved in the sessions, as well as to foster generalisation of treatment effects to the patient's outside world. Due to the chronic nature of OCD, regularly scheduled follow-up sessions are usually recommended to consolidate treatment gains.

Controlled follow-up studies have demonstrated the efficacy of the exposure/response prevention treatment methodology, revealing that treatment effects may be maintained 12-15 months after program completion (Foa et al., 1983; Rapoport, 1989). The evidence is less clear with OCD in children. However, a small number of group studies and a larger number of case reports have supported the efficacy of exposure and response prevention with this population (Bolton, Collins & Steinberg, 1983; Bolton & Turner, 1984; Desmarais & Lallee, 1988; Fine, 1973; cf., Apter, Bernhout & Lyano, 1984).

Cognitive restructuring and thought stopping

Identifying, challenging and replacing obsessional thought patterns with more adaptive, rational ones is known as cognitive restructuring. Creamer (1987) refers to four levels of cognitive intervention which can be employed in parallel with exposure/response prevention.

1. The first stage is to attack the patient's 'fear of fear' or 'fear of the discomfort of fear'. A cognitive intervention is used to dispute such beliefs as 'I must not experience any discomfort', and to encourage patients to believe that while it is unpleasant to experience anxiety, it is not 'awful', and they can tolerate it if they choose.
2. The second level is to teach patients coping 'self statements' (Meichenbaum & Genest, 1980). This is recommended to aid patients in times when they are experiencing high levels of anxiety and find it difficult to employ cognitive disputation techniques.
3. The use of motivational self statements is recommended, as it is important to encourage patients to remember why they are deliberately putting themselves into unpleasant situations.
4. The last stage for cognitive intervention is when a patient later relapses, failing to prevent the ritualistic (or avoidant) response and indulging in compulsive behaviour. When this happens patients may often express feelings of guilt and worthlessness. It is important here to help them dispute this 'fear of failure'. Replacing the irrational thoughts with more rational ones (for example, giving themselves permission to make mistakes, not having to be perfect) will allow patients to persevere and complete the program.

Social skills training and maintenance

In social skills training, the therapist and the patient identify and rehearse positive behaviour patterns to help the patient reintegrate back into his or her social world. As compulsive behaviours are given up during the therapeutic process, a lack of appropriate social skills may become apparent in many children and adolescents. Therefore, when working with this population, the treatment program adopted must include provision for social skills training, to allow the patients to reintegrate with their peers more easily (Rapoport, 1989). Research by Welkowitz, Bond and Anderson (1989) demonstrated improved treatment outcome with 20 adolescent OCD cases when social skills training was built into the program.

Case study

Peta, an 8-year-old girl, lived with her parents Liza (32 years) and David (42 years). Two older step-siblings from her father's side of the family had recently left home. These included an older brother, Thomas (aged 19), and an older sister, Megan (aged 20 years). The parents were of Anglo-Irish working class origins and the father currently worked as a bus driver. The mother was engaged in home duties and worked part-time as an assistant in a cafeteria. Extended family living in the same city included a maternal grandmother, whom Peta had regular contact with, and a maternal uncle of Peta's, who was hospitalised in a psychiatric facility.

Both maternal and paternal sides of the family had a clear history of psychopathology. The uncle's hospitalisation was a result of chronic schizophrenia and the maternal grandmother had a history of depression and compulsive checking behaviour. The maternal grandfather, deceased at the time of the referral, had a history of alcohol abuse and according to Liza, physically and sexually abused her throughout her childhood. David reported that his father also abused alcohol and was rarely living in the family home due to a strong predilection for aimless wandering. During his times in the home, he was violent toward his wife and the children. David's mother also appeared to be disturbed, although it was difficult to discern the exact nature of the problem from David's descriptions ('she had a screw loose', and so on). It appeared that she was verbally and physically abusive of David, greatly favouring David's older sister. David's son by his first marriage and Peta's stepbrother, Thomas, had a history of severe conduct and learning problems that had resulted in school failure and dismissal, and repeated trouble with the police.

David and Liza reported that their marriage had been unstable and that at times in the past, David had been physically violent. However, both were able to speak openly about their past and future and expressed optimism that the improvements their relationship had seen in the last year or so would continue to grow. David presented as a generally happy and talkative fellow with no frank psychopathology or distress. He had a history of osteoarthritis and heart disease, the latter having required a period of hospitalisation approximately four years prior to referral. Peta was frightened by her father's heart problems, aware of the possibility that they could lead to further hospitalisation and even death.

Liza presented as mildly anxious with a history of recurrent unhappiness. She had poor self-esteem and this was constantly reinforced by the power structure of the family in which David made the decisions and afforded her little respect. Over the last eight years she had almost totally immersed herself in the care and upbringing of Peta as a way of undoing the painful memories of her own childhood, and to prove to herself that she could achieve something worthwhile.

Peta presented as a slender, pretty and intelligent 8-year-old girl. She spoke happily and confidently to the therapist, and appeared quite comfortable about disclosing the details of her fears and anxieties. At times, however, she would become visibly anxious while discussing her family, wringing and clasping her hands, frowning and shuffling about. The main problems she reported were:

1. Her need to go back and check the school classroom while leaving school for the day. She said she was scared that her things might be taken away or thrown out.

2. Her fear that her mother or father might not return from work one day.
3. Her fear that some of the things in her bedroom may be (accidentally) thrown out with the garbage.

In all of the above situations, Peta reported that she would find herself worrying that the target objects (school books, parents, personal belongings) were missing or being thrown out. These worrysome thoughts would increase in frequency and intensity producing uncomfortable increases in physical sensations of anxiety. Her only relief was to check on the target objects, this producing a temporary decrease in anxiety which would have to be repeated over and over to maintain anxiety at comfortable levels.

Her parents related almost identical concerns. Liza and David both agreed that their daughter's checking behaviour was the main problem. However, they were also concerned that Peta was becoming increasingly irritable, non-compliant and aggressive with her mother. During daily activities such as getting dressed for school, arguments between Peta and her mother were becoming increasingly frequent and many would culminate with Peta having a temper tantrum and repeatedly accusing her mother of not loving her. The father reported no such problems between Peta and himself.

Other details that the parents reported about Peta included the following: she was generally well adjusted at school and had a number of friends there and in the home neighbourhood; several times over the prior month, Peta had reported hearing a mature female voice quietly calling 'Peta, come here', when no one had called as such. Since an early age, Peta had had an imaginary friend who she would play with and talk to, even in front of other people. Peta was fully aware that this friend existed in her imagination only.

Her parents had vastly different interpretations of Peta's problems. For David, it was simply a matter of lack of discipline from his wife. He felt that Peta was becoming more and more out of control because his wife was unable to discipline her effectively. To Liza, the problem was far more ominous. Aware that both her family and her husband's family had a history of mental illness, she was scared that Peta was showing the first signs of schizophrenia. In particular, Liza said that Peta sometimes reminded her of her brother who had chronic schizophrenia. Thus, Liza was the main force behind the referral of Peta for assessment and treatment.

Peta was an unplanned but, nevertheless, wanted child and the birth was complicated by foetal and maternal distress with subsequent caesarian delivery. Apart from some mild asthma, Peta developed into a healthy and happy baby. During middle childhood, in the few years prior to referral, however, Peta suffered a number of losses. First, her older brother and sister both moved out of the family home and interstate. Peta was quite upset about this as she was very close to both. Next, her grandfather died, another close intimate of Peta's. Her parents reported that Peta's grandmother began teasing Peta about the possibility that others in the family could die soon as well. For example, it was reported that the grandmother would constantly remind Peta of her father's heart condition and that her mother could die any night while working late at the cafeteria. The grandmother appears to have been quite relentless in this attempt to upset Peta.

Next, Peta had to separate from her grade three teacher to whom she was extremely attached. At the time of separation and transition into grade four, the teacher had become ill, virtually disappearing from Peta's life. The parents reported that Peta would cry at night about not seeing this teacher, expressing constant fears that the teacher was either dead or dying. Soon after, Peta's mother then returned to work as a cafeteria assistant in a job that demanded working late at night. Peta found this stressful and would follow her mother out to the car, visibly distressed and asking her not to go. Over these two years, Peta had also suffered the loss of three pet cats. All were killed in traffic accidents outside the family home.

According to her parents, the first sign that anything was wrong came shortly after the death of the first two cats and her grandfather. Peta became more anxious than usual, fearful of her parents leaving her, expressing fear that she or her parents might die and intermittently accusing her parents of not loving her. Soon afterwards, the separation from her grade three teacher occurred, another cat died and her mother returned to work. Against this backdrop of loss in Peta's life, there appears to be a particular event that triggered off the actual checking behaviour. Her performance of daily chores was suffering and, in particular, she was refusing to clean up her room. One weekend her father, frustrated at the state of her room and tired of the constant battles to get her to clean it up, took matters into his own hands. In the space of an hour he had removed everything from her room that he did not consider necessary. Peta had become hysterical during the cleaning but she was unable to stop him. The parents reported that her checking of the garbage began the next day and the checking of her school possessions began the next week.

These problems had persisted at a reasonably stable level since that time with the exception of some recent improvement due to the parents seeking help from a clinical psychologist in private practice. The psychologist had recommended a reward system focusing on checking after school and this had led to some improvements (checking had reduced from an estimated mean of five down to two or three checks per afternoon). However, the parents had found the cost of this practitioner to be beyond their means and had asked their physician to refer them to a less costly clinic.

As a general measure of Peta's functioning, we asked both parents to complete the Revised Problem Behaviour Checklist (a list of problems — the parents are asked to tick each that applies) (Quay & Petersen, 1983). The overall levels of disturbed behaviour were not in the 'clinical' range, however, scores on items measuring anxiety were elevated, confirming the interview data that Peta was experiencing distressing levels of anxiety. There was no evidence that Peta was suffering any signs of depression according to parental report or depression tests (Petti, 1978; Kovacs & Beck, 1977). Although the mother reported a history of sad moods, her score on the Beck Index of Depression (Beck et al., 1961) indicated she was not currently depressed. Both parents scored in the normal range on a test of marriage adjustment (Spanier, 1976) indicating no major marital problems. However, scores on the Parent Problems Checklist (Dadds & Powell, 1991) indicated that David and Liza had considerable problems acting as a team in their parenting duties, and that fights would often occur over the best way to handle Peta.

Diagnosis and conceptualisation

Using DSM-III-R criteria, Peta has obsessive compulsive disorder with both obsessions and compulsions being present.

Treatment

It is important to consider Peta's overall adjustment in relation to the degree of stress she had experienced in the last two years. First, it is clear that the obsessive compulsive behaviour was not severely debilitating; she was still coping well at school, she had good peer relations and she showed no other emotional or behavioural problems apart from the OCD. Second, when one considers the nature of the stress Peta had experienced, the form of the OCD seems understandable. That is, the obsessions and compulsions were, to a large extent, realistic in that they represented her attempts to find stability and consistency in an unpredictable environment.

Peta's problems appear to be a clear result of genetic vulnerability mixed with environmental stress. Both sides of her family heritage have a history of schizophrenia, substance abuse and general conflict. Her mother's side also may have a history of OCD. Given this history, it is important to consider that Peta's current problem may be a precursor to more serious psychiatric problems in the future. On a more positive note, there are a number of factors present that are typically protective against the development of psychopathology. These include Peta's high level of intelligence (as evidenced by her behaviour in carrying out the treatment, her verbal skills and reports from her teachers), her good social skills and social adjustment, and her parents' attempts to rectify and improve both their own marriage and their daughter's problems.

In terms of the specific nature of Peta's obsessive thoughts and compulsions, we felt that a social learning conceptualisation offered the most parsimonious explanation and clearest directions for treatment. Such an explanation, while retaining an interest in the origins and development of a particular behaviour, focuses more on discovering the interpersonal and intrapersonal processes that are currently maintaining the problem. These factors may be very different from the factors that were associated with the onset of the disorder. For example, a therapist might consider that the loss of significant others was the original reason that Peta began obsessing and ritualising. Logically then, that therapist might prescribe a treatment that focuses on helping Peta to grieve appropriately and, thus, resolve her feelings about the losses. The social learning therapist may agree that the losses were associated with the onset of the disorder and that 'grief work' may be useful. However, there is no reason to hold that the loss continues to be the reason that the OC behaviour continues. On the contrary, it is likely that the problem behaviour, once established, is now being maintained by very different factors. We hypothesised that a number of social learning and cognitive factors were maintaining the problem.

For Peta, thoughts of important objects and people had taken on aversive qualities, that is, they produced unpleasant arousal. Upon thinking such a thought, she would experience increasing muscle tension, shortness of breath, a sick feeling in the stomach and thoughts of loss and separation and general feelings that some impending disaster was just around the corner. Having no other way of relieving these feelings, she would attempt to reassure herself that the content of the thought was not true. That is, no loss had occurred. This would temporarily reduce the anxiety until the thought would occur again.

Thus, thoughts of her school books, her possessions and her parents going to work had become conditioned stimuli, capable of producing severe arousal (conditioned response) because of their associations with various unconditioned stimuli (death, separation from loved ones, family violence). Engaging in ritualisation could temporarily reduce her arousal level; thus, ritualisation was being negatively reinforced by the reduction in anxiety it produced. A behaviour that is reinforced is more likely to occur next time the person is in a similar situation. Further, ritualisation has another insidious effect on obsessive thoughts; it prevents the conditioned aversiveness of the thoughts from undergoing extinction. That is, the thoughts are never not paired with arousal. The rituals remove both the obsessive thoughts and the arousal and the first is never experienced without the second.

In parallel with these conditioned effects, the anxious person increasingly allocates attentional resources to the detection of threat in the environment. That is, the sufferer becomes highly vigilant for any sign of threat and, thus, he or she may detect more threat cues in the environment and interpret ambiguous cues as threatening. For Peta, any signal of separation or removal thus became a potentially threatening cue (conditioned stimulus) for anxiety.

It is also important to consider the social context of the above factors. Interpersonally, we can also see a number of processes that were helping to maintain the problem. Inadvertently, her parents were reinforcing the problem. When another person displays unusual, inappropriate or aberrant behaviour, their 'normal' behaviour becomes less salient. Peta's parents were worried about her checking behaviour and were constantly on the lookout for it. When it would occur, they would immediately attend to her and employ various strategies in an attempt to stop her. These would range from chastising her to cuddling and comforting her. When she was not ritualising, her parents would either not notice her or would deliberately leave her alone in the hope of not upsetting the temporary cessation of rituals. For example, when leaving for work Liza would notice that Peta was calm and thus would try to sneak out without her noticing. Of course this would increase the likelihood of Peta becoming upset.

Thus, Peta's anxiety and ritualisation was being positively reinforced by her parents providing her with an increase in attention contingent upon the display of these behaviours. Conversely, non-ritualising and engaging in neutral behaviours was on an extinction schedule, being ignored by her parents.

Finally, it is quite possible that some of Peta's behaviour may have been learned, and may be being maintained, by direct observation of other family members. In particular, it is possible that she was directly copying some of her grandmother's checking behaviours as a way of coping with anxiety.

The conceptualisation of Peta's problem emphasised three components: conditioning/cognitive processes, reinforcement contingencies provided by her parents and broader imitation and stress coming from the extended family. Thus, the treatment we proposed to the parents was 'multiphasic', having various components that targeted each of the above putative causal factors in sequence.

1. *Conditioning/cognitive processes.* The aim of this component was to 'de-condition' the various stimuli that had taken on the potential to cause distress. We wanted Peta to be able to think about and experience such things as leaving school, her mother going to work, the garbage being thrown out and so on, without her ritualising and without her experiencing distress. To achieve this, we used a simple exposure and response prevention procedure. In preparation, Peta was trained to let her body relax and engage in a pre-planned self-talk script as a way of controlling her anxiety and not ritualising. Peta invented the script which, set in the form of a short poem, focused on feeling strong and confident.

   First, we rehearsed the use of these coping skills during our clinic sessions. The therapist would ask Peta to deliberately think of a 'yukky' thought (the hypothesised conditioned stimuli) about losing something important. As Peta's anxiety would start to rise, the therapist would then instruct her to engage in the coping procedure until the anxiety abated. Peta learned how to do this quite quickly and effectively so, next, she was instructed to use the procedure whenever she felt her anxiety climbing and the need to check.

   As with many anxious people, Peta was allocating a lot of her attention to the possibility of threat cues in the environment. To help her counter this, she was instructed to notice and list down 'happy, positive and friendly' things that she could notice at various times that were high risk for her becoming anxious. For example, during the walk from the school to her mother's car, Peta was increasingly able to attend to the presence of some friends, her mother's reassuring company and that she was soon going to be able to play with her toys at home, rather than focus on the possibility of her books being removed.
2. *Parental contingency training.* While Peta was being trained to implement the coping strategy, her parents were taught basic skills of reinforcement and extinction. This included training them to provide effective praise contingent upon Peta not checking, and to effectively ignore (not reinforce) checking behaviour. Because Peta was also showing evidence of increasing aggression to her mother and because her parents would often use verbal and physical threats and punishment in their interactions with Peta, the parents were also instructed to use praise and effective ignoring in their general interactions with Peta.

   To accomplish these training goals, we provided the parents with written materials, the therapist modelled the use of the procedures and then the parents rehearsed them while the therapist provided feedback. The details of these training procedures can be found in Sanders and Dadds (1982, 1992). This continued until the parents could demonstrate an effective praise comment and ignore repetitive complaining while the therapist acted as Peta.
3. *Modelling/general stress effects.* There was evidence that Peta's grandmother was suffering some form of OCD that included checking behaviour. Further, it appeared that she was not above teasing Peta about death and loss by repeatedly pointing out, for example, that her parents could die at any time. This behaviour obviously constitutes severe emotional abuse of a vulnerable child. Unfortunately, the grandmother refused to be seen by the therapist even though the approach made to her emphasised that her help and expertise was needed to help Peta. Thus, there appeared no alternative but to advise the parents to restrict the

grandmother's access to Peta to structured visits when another responsible adult was present.

Finally, there remained the issue of the general family conflict and how Peta would cope with any future loss. Sensitive to the fact that we had advised the parents to deliberately ignore checking behaviour, we were concerned that Peta was left with no method for discussing and solving emotional problems with her intimates. Thus, the parents were advised to regularly take time (approximately twice a week) to sit with Peta at bedtime and encourage her to talk openly and, if possible, find solutions to her fears and problems. The parents were briefly trained to actively listen and encourage exploration and problem solving rather than be directive with Peta.

The treatment plan specifies the content of therapy. Just as important is the process by which a therapeutic plan is implemented, especially when treatment involves the cooperation of multiple parties such as therapists, children, parents, teachers and others. The method used with Peta's case has been comprehensively described by Sanders and Dadds (1992) and Dadds (1989). This approach emphasises the team aspects of the intervention; the parents and child(ren) are afforded equal status with the therapist and all information and psychological knowledge is shared equally among the group. Similarly, parents are expected to openly share all information they have that may be relevant. Assessment information and the treatment plan is discussed, formulated and openly agreed upon as a team before any action is taken.

In this case, we agreed to begin treatment by training Peta in the coping strategy and the parents in the contingency management skills as the first treatment component. Thus, the weekly sessions were divided into 30 minutes spent with Peta, 30 minutes then with the parents, followed by 15 minutes with everyone together in order to review how everything was going.

A major hallmark of the scientist-practitioner approach to clinical psychology (Barlow, Hayes & Nelson, 1984) is the objective assessment of treatment outcome. In this case, measures of checking behaviour were to be the main criteria for determining treatment effectiveness. The target behaviours were defined as follows:

1. School checking: Peta returns or attempts to return to classroom after leaving the building after school is dismissed. The number of times was to be recorded.
2. Garbage checking: Peta either checks through or attempts to check through the garbage or makes a comment to her parents about the possibility of one or more of her possessions being in the garbage. Because this behaviour was sometimes happening many times each day, we decided to only score 'yes' (the behaviour occurred that day) or 'no' (the behaviour did not occur that day).
3. Checking on parents: Peta moves into vicinity of parents, in the home, with no other purpose than to check on their presence, or she expresses concern that one or more of them may leave or die. This was scored 'yes' or 'no' for each day.
4. Overall happiness: At the end of each day, an estimate of how happy Peta had been that day (mean level) was to be recorded using a five-point scale — 1 = extremely unhappy to 5 = extremely happy.

The above measures were completed by both Peta and her mother using specially designed daily score sheets.

Treatment outcome

Figure 3.1 (see page 50) shows the effects of treatment on measures of checking and general happiness according to Peta and her mother respectively. It is clear from the similarity of the two figures that Peta and Liza agreed moderately well on the frequency of checking and on Peta's general level of happiness. The only obvious exception to this is the frequency of school checking for which Peta reported higher frequencies due to some checking occurring prior to her mother arriving at the school.

At baseline, Peta was returning to the classroom to check on her school possessions at an average of twice per afternoon. There is a decreasing trend through the baseline period, indicating that school checking was improving prior to the formal intervention beginning. This could be due to a number of factors, but the most likely explanations are that the treatment suggestions made by the previous therapist were having an effect, or the general effects of coming into therapy were motivating Peta to change her behaviour.

Checking of the garbage was occurring on average one in every three days at baseline and it can be seen from figure 3.1 that mother and daughter agreed 100 per cent on these occurrences. While the frequency across days is quite low, these episodes were reportedly quite severe, with Peta actually climbing into the garbage bin while crying and fighting off her parents' attempts to restrain her. At baseline, most recorded episodes of checking on parents involved seeking out the mother and expressing concern that she would leave or die. From figure 3.1, these occurred approximately one in every three days.

During the first phase of intervention, checking on the garbage reduced to zero and stayed at that level. School checking and checking on parents both showed minor improvements over baseline frequencies, however, they stabilised without ever reducing to zero rate. It was decided then that a more intensive intervention was required and the therapist set about discussing different strategies with Peta and her parents. Everyone agreed that Peta was trying really hard and had made substantial improvements. However, at times she would be distracted or temporarily lose motivation and become engrossed in the obsessive thought. Thus, we decided that a more intensive reward program would help to increase the salience of the program.

In the next phase of treatment, a contingency management program was established using a 'differential reinforcement of zero rates (DR0)' system. By this strategy, the periods in which the problem behaviour is likely to occur are divided up into a number of short intervals. Whenever the child abstains from engaging in the problem behaviour for the length of the interval, the pre-determined reward is given. This occurs for each interval and rewards are accrued or can build up hierarchically. For the problem of checking on parents, the times at which Peta was at home was divided into a series of one-hour intervals. Each hour without checking was rewarded with a happy face being placed on a publicly displayed poster, a small amount of money, a hug and verbal praise. Happy faces could be saved up and, at Peta's discretion, could be traded in on a range of other rewards that had been agreed upon during the design stage of this system.

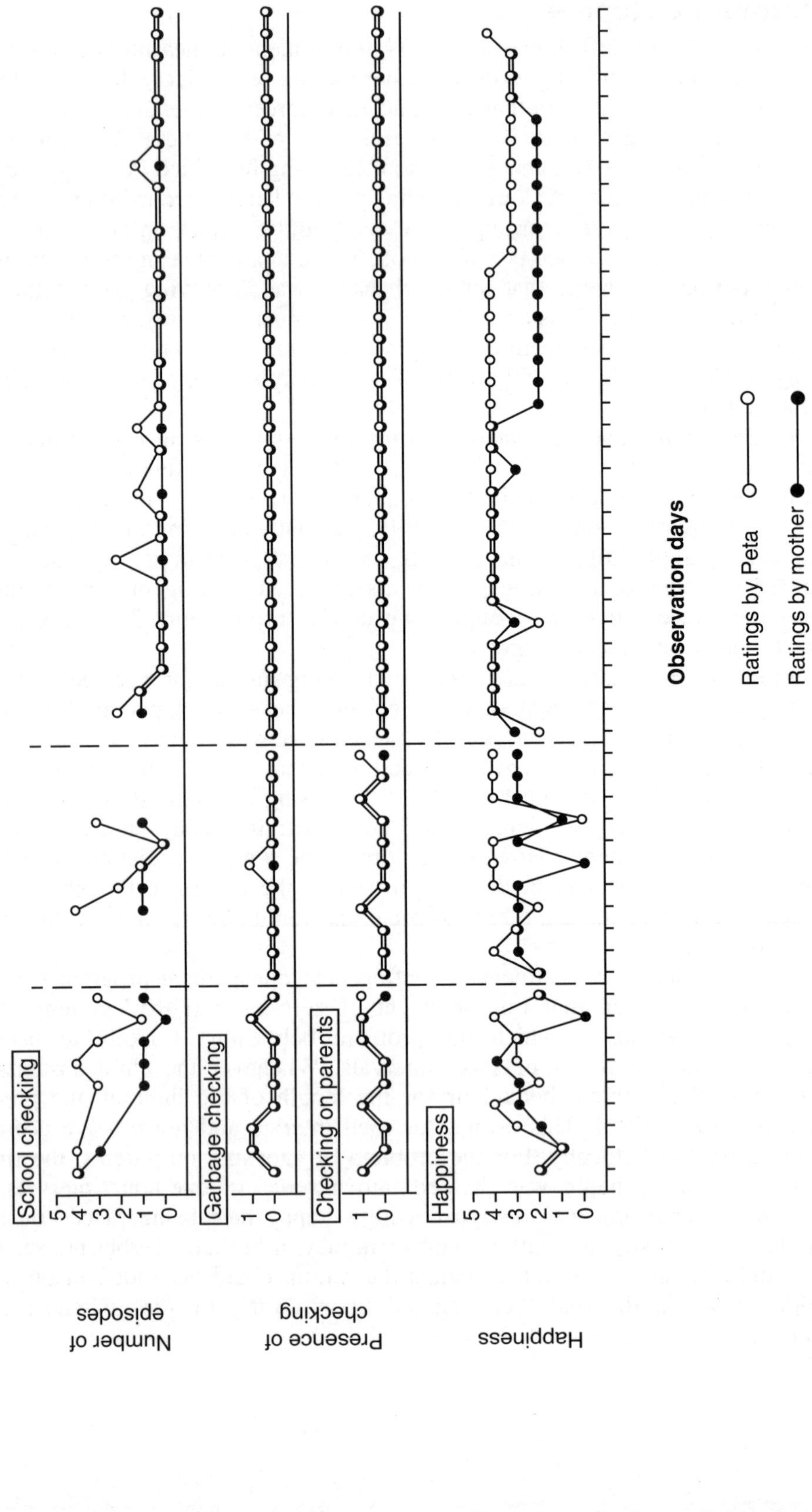

Figure 3.1: Ratings on four measures for Baseline, Treatment 1 and Treatment 2

For school checking, the 10 minutes that it typically took to get from the classroom to inside her mother's car was divided into five two-minute intervals. Each interval in which attempts to return to the classroom or expressions of anxiety about her possessions were absent was rewarded with a happy face in a system similar to the above. Peta was able to work toward a range of rewards that had been agreed upon, including a family day trip to a swimming centre and a new desk. Figure 3.1 shows that the implementation of this system was associated with a reduction to zero in checking of her school possessions and her parents.

Clinical experience has shown that it is usually much more difficult to phase out such a contingency management system than it is to start it. The child may resent having the rewards stopped and thus it is very important that the system be phased out gradually so that the changes in the child's behaviour continue, supported by new systems of cognition and environmental contingencies rather than by the temporary and artificial rewards of the therapeutic system. Thus, fading of the system began after day six, with the length of the intervals, the type of rewards and the amount of independent self-monitoring of Peta's behaviour all varying over the next few weeks. Peta was actively involved in the design of this phase and she fully comprehended the need for her to be able to avoid checking without artificial prompts. From figure 3.1 it can be seen that her checking behaviour remained at zero until the system was completely phased out in the final stage of therapy.

Figure 3.1 also shows daily happiness ratings made by both Peta and her mother. It is clear that treatment was associated with a small but consistent improvement in Peta's overall mood state. In particular, the second phase of treatment was associated with the extreme troughs of unhappiness that occurred intermittently during baseline and treatment phase 1.

In all case studies and evaluations of therapy it is important to follow up clients to assess the longer term effects of interventions. This was especially true in Peta's case because of the chronic nature of OCD and the elevated risk for psychopathology that existed in her family. Unfortunately, we were not able to build a maintenance program into the treatment because the family moved to another state a few weeks after treatment ended. Thus, the follow-up assessment was limited to some telephone calls. The parents indicated that Peta had shown no signs of checking or ritualisation up until 5 months after the end of treatment, and that her general adjustment was good. However, we have no independent evidence to corroborate this conclusion.

Discussion

Many people, including children, can experience obsessive thoughts and the need to ritualise behaviour at some time in their lives. Despite how common these phenomena are, obsessive compulsive disorder is clearly one of the most bizarre and complex forms of human emotional distress. In contrast to most psychiatric disorders, it is very rare and appears in a similar form in children and adults. Despite the significant improvements in treatment that have come with the development of cognitive-behavioural methods and anti-depressant medication, the nature and causes of this disorder continue to baffle clinicians and researchers.

In this chapter, a cognitive-behavioural conceptualisation and treatment of an 8-year-old child with OCD was described. We saw how the cognitive behavioural approach was useful in formulating a plan that is practical and easily understandable to children, parents and clinicians alike. This approach allows the clinician to assess the idiosyncracies of each particular case and then design a treatment program which incorporates these idiosyncracies, while also being based on laws of learning that apply to all organisms. For example, while the type of attention that a child's compulsive behaviour will attract from parents and siblings will differ from family to family, that attention and its effects on the child will still follow the general laws of reinforcement. We also saw how the social learning approach alerted the therapist to influences of the broader family context through general stress and modelling/imitation processes. Of course the approach taken in this case is not without limitations. For severe cases of OCD, more intensive and structured interventions may be needed. For example, where the patient or his/her family are less compliant with therapeutic instructions or the rituals are so severe that the patient cannot resist them, medication or hospitalisation may be required in the short term. As with most psychosocial therapies, social learning theorists have only recently begun to appreciate the many levels of causal factors that can interact to determine and maintain a psychological problem. Complex psychosocial problems may involve interactions between factors ranging from a biological disposition in the patient, to interactional patterns in the immediate family, to cultural norms and attitudes about behaviour and experience (Dadds, 1987). It is difficult to conceptualise and integrate such diverse factors within a social learning model, or almost any other psychosocial approach to mental illness.

While the social learning approach is increasingly paying attention to the role of thinking processes in the origins and maintenance of psychological disorders, the theory and technology for altering cognitive processes is still in an early stage of development. For OCD, the main thrust of therapeutic success usually comes from altering the rituals and then targeting the obsessional thinking. Patients who are predominantly obsessional and do not have marked rituals are notoriously difficult to treat with behavioural and most other therapeutic methods. Enormous energy is currently being invested into the study of cognitive processes in OCD and other psychological disorders (Williams et al., 1989). Hopefully the next few decades will witness a further improvement in our knowledge of how to conceptualise and treat these problems.

Stephen W. Touyz and Peter Beumont
Westmead Hospital and University of Sydney

4 Overcoming anorexia nervosa

It is apt to commence this chapter which deals with both the complexities and struggle to overcome anorexia nervosa with a quotation from the seminal text by Bruch (1973) entitled *Eating Disorders, Obesity, Anorexia Nervosa and the Person Within* (page 3):

> There is no human society that deals rationally with food in its environment, that eats according to the availability, edibility, and nutritional value alone. Food is endowed with complex issues and elaborate ideologies, religious beliefs and prestige systems. It is these aspects that give the eating habits and food traditions their special cultural and national character, and to the food habits of one's background and family, the emotional connotation of warmth and home.

This quotation vividly illustrates the complex interrelationship between food and human behaviour and it indicates some of the contextual difficulties inherent in the treatment of patients with anorexia nervosa.

Anorexia nervosa is a complex, multi-dimensional disorder characterised by the relentless pursuit of thinness. It was recognised about 100 years ago, but there are earlier descriptions in the literature of patients who appear to have suffered from the condition, although they were not diagnosed as such. One of the earliest descriptions of the illness was that of an 18-year-old girl treated by Richard Morton in 1684 whom he diagnosed as having 'nervous consumption' (quoted in Bruch, 1973, page 212).

> In the month of July she fell into a total suppression of her monthly courses from a multitude of cares and passions of her mind, but without any symptom of the green-sickness following upon it. From which time her appetite began to abate, and her digestion to be bad; her flesh also began to be flaccid and loose and her looks pale she was wont by her studying at night, and continual pouring upon books, to expose herself both day and night to the injuries of the air. I do not remember that I did ever in all my practice see one, that was conversant with the living so much wasted with the greatest degree of consumption (like a skeleton only clad with skin) yet there was no fever, but on the contrary a coldness of the whole body ... only her appetite was diminished, and her digestion uneasy, with fainting fits, which did frequently return upon her.

Morton's patient refused the medications offered to her and died a few months later following a fainting fit.

The illness usually occurs in adolescent girls and young women, hence its German name Puberstatsmagersucht. Less frequently it occurs in pre-pubertal children and rarely in young males. The percentage of anorexic males varies between 4 and 6 per cent of the total.

The behaviours which are most commonly used to bring about excessive thinness include food refusal, dieting (avoiding carbohydrates and fats), strenuous exercising, self-induced vomiting and surreptitious disposal of food. Patients with the illness have been observed to have peculiar eating patterns in that they often nibble at food all day long, cut foods such as cheese into many tiny pieces which they eat one at a time and refuse to eat in front of relatives and friends. Abnormal eating and the consequent emaciation lead to disturbances of physiological function and hence to physical symptoms such as amenorrhoea (the cessation of menstruation) and unsightly hair.

The illness is relatively common in the western world, particularly in the more affluent sections of the community. There is indirect evidence that the incidence of anorexia nervosa has been increasing over the past decade. A study in Britain found that one out of every two-hundred 12-year-old girls, who were attending boarding school, were likely to develop the illness. In Australia, a significant number of young girls with anorexia nervosa are admitted each year to acute psychiatric or general hospital units, and many more are either treated at home or avoid treatment altogether. Anorexia nervosa is an uncommon illness in less affluent communities.

The term anorexia nervosa is a misnomer as patients with the illness rarely lose their appetites until they reach an extreme stage of emaciation. Although the patients deny being preoccupied with food, they may be observed collecting recipes, preparing the family meal which they refuse to eat and, in extreme cases, mothers of anorexia patients are banished from the kitchen by their daughters.

Although it may appear that the diagnosis of anorexia nervosa is a relatively easy one to make, it can often be quite difficult as many patients with anorexia nervosa are not motivated to engage in treatment and tend to deny their symptoms. It is, therefore, important that one obtain additional information from close relatives or friends.

Although the term anorexia nervosa is sometimes used to refer to all patients in whom weight loss is associated with psychiatric disturbance, it should really be restricted to those in whom there is a primary disturbance in the eating process. The *Diagnostic and Statistical Manual of Mental Disorders*, third edition, revised (DSM-III-R) (American Psychiatric Association, 1987) lists the following criteria for making the diagnosis:

A. Refusal to maintain a body weight over a minimal normal weight for age and height, for example, weight loss leading to maintenance of body weight 15 per cent below that expected, or failure to make expected weight gain during period of growth, leading to body weight 15 per cent below that expected.
B. Intense fear of gaining weight or becoming fat, even though underweight.

C. Disturbance in the way in which one's body weight, size or shape is experienced, for example, the person claims to 'feel fat' even when emaciated, believes that one area of the body is 'too fat' even when obviously underweight.
D. In females, absence of at least three consecutive menstrual cycles when otherwise expected to occur (primary or secondary amenorrhoea). (A woman is considered to have amenorrhoea if her periods occur only following hormone administration, e.g., estrogen).

Psychiatric illnesses such as schizophrenia, depression and anxiety states or even brain lesions may occasionally lead to emaciation. But their presentation and optimal treatment are quite different from true anorexia nervosa. For example, depressed patients complain of a loss of appetite, are not preoccupied with the caloric content of their food and do not have a weight phobia. Likewise, schizophrenic patients may have delusions concerning foods (for example, someone is trying to poison them) but they are rarely concerned about the caloric content.

Like most psychiatric diagnoses, anorexia nervosa is a syndrome (a recurring group of associated symptoms) diagnosis, and it has a specific clinical presentation. The patient's main problem is perhaps best thought of as one of control. Just as an alcoholic is unable to regulate the use of alcohol, so an anorexia nervosa patient appears unable to control eating, dieting and related behaviour.

In anorexia nervosa there is a clear relationship between psychological trauma, disordered behaviour and consequent physiological symptoms. For this reason, it is a good example of one of several types of psychosomatic disorders (disorders with both psychological and physiological signs) that are of special importance to general medicine.

There is evidence to suggest that there are two types of patients who present with classical symptoms of anorexia nervosa. The first are obsessional, intense, introverted individuals who commence dieting apparently inappropriately, when under psychological stress. They become preoccupied with dieting and emaciate themselves to the extent that they develop malnutrition. Their illness has some resemblance to an obsessional state. That is, they behave similarly to people who cannot get an 'idea' out of their head, even when that idea has clearly been shown to have no basis in reality. Patients belonging to the second group tend to be more extroverted, have less denial of their illness and are more motivated to seek treatment. They also tend to be more anxious and depressed and have more somatic complaints. Most of the patients have always had a problem with their weight. Their desire to reduce their weight is reasonable at first, but when they are unable to maintain a normal weight by dieting, they are soon frustrated by their failure and become unreasonable in their attitudes. They come to depend on methods of weight reduction such as self-induced vomiting and laxative abuse which may cause serious physical illness, even death. Patients in this category have a poor prognosis in that they tend to have had the illness for a longer duration than those who simply abstain from eating. They also tend to have more hospitalisations, poorer social adjustment and a higher incidence of attempted suicide. Despite their personality differences, both groups deserve the diagnosis of anorexia nervosa because of the presence of symptoms such as an aversion to regaining a normal weight and a denial of the severity of their emaciation.

Psychological aspects of anorexia nervosa

Quest for thinness

The deliberate pursuit of thinness is the essential psychopathological feature of anorexia nervosa. Some patients do not admit that they have this morbid preoccupation, but even in these instances there is usually ample evidence to suggest that patients are concealing their true feelings in an attempt to avoid appropriate treatment.

Obsessionality

The patient's preoccupation with body weight, with food and with the desire to become thin is probably more closely related to an obsessional thought than to any other form of mental phenomenon. The patient realises that these attitudes and behaviour are morbid, but is unable to escape this preoccupation with food and thinness. It is relevant that many anorexia nervosa patients have marked obsessional traits in their pre-morbid personality. They are often perfectionistic, conscientious, hard-working and somewhat competitive people whose anorexic symptoms are related to other behaviour aimed at rigidly controlling themselves and their environment.

Interpersonal relationships

Many anorexia nervosa patients are shy, reserved girls. They have withdrawn, and have become isolated, from their peers. Furthermore, they are sexually inexperienced, even in comparison to other girls of their age. The illness often appears to be precipitated by some sexual challenge, such as the physical change of puberty, the first experience of heavy petting or intercourse or an impending marriage.

Patients' relationships with their families, and particularly their mothers, is often disturbed. Many complain that their lives are controlled by their parents, and that they feel quite helpless and unable to do anything for themselves. Their mothers, on the other hand, appear domineering and over-directive. It is difficult to be sure, of course, that these behaviors were actually present before the onset of the illness and are not themselves the result of the anorexia. Any mother must find it extremely distressing to have an anorexic child, and may respond by trying to force her to eat. Indeed a feature of anorexia nervosa is the extent to which the family gets involved in the patient's illness.

Somatic aspects

Weight control

Many patients are significantly overweight before the onset of their anorexic behaviour, and become obese again on recovery from their illness. They appear to have a basic disturbance of the mechanisms that control body weight. The similarities that are alleged to exist between anorexia nervosa patients and obese people may be due to the existence of this group.

Methods used to induce weight loss

The usual methods of inducing weight loss are food refusal and dieting, that is, the avoidance of carbohydrates and other fattening foods. As the diet is low in calories but relatively high in proteins and vitamins, resembling the typical 'health diets' of women's magazines, the malnutrition which results is very different from that found in the victims of famine. Some patients adopt more drastic measures to induce weight loss, including self-induced vomiting, the ingestion of massive quantities of purgatives, and the abuse of liquid-reducing medications. These methods may lead to even further physical complications.

A characteristic feature of the anorexia nervosa patient is the preservation of a high level of physical activity despite severe emaciation. Strenuous exercising and overactivity are themselves used by many patients to increase their rate of weight loss.

Amenorrhoea

A disturbance of menstrual function is invariably found in anorexia nervosa. It usually starts early in the illness, before there has been significant weight loss, and persists for some months after weight has been regained. The mechanism underlying the menstrual disturbance remains unclear. Emaciation reduces the level of hormones circulating in the body. Levels of these hormones are probably influenced by body weight, and they are restored to normal once the patient regains weight. The cyclical release of hormones, which is associated with ovulation and hence the menstrual cycle, does not return immediately. At this stage, the amenorrhoea of anorexia nervosa resembles the post-pill amenorrhoea found in some women after stopping a contraceptive pill.

Many anorexia nervosa patients first come to their doctors complaining of secondary amenorrhoea. Failure to recognise the syndrome and its basic psychiatric nature still leads to the needless investigation of anorexia nervosa patients in the quest for non-existent hormonal pathology, even in the best teaching hospitals!

The following case history describes the intense struggle over several years of an adolescent girl to overcome her anorexia nervosa. It raises many complex issues such as factors pertaining to the aetiology of the disorder, management (including the vexed issue of involuntary hospitalisation) and the role of the family in both aetiology and treatment. Controversial issues such as forced 'tube' feeding and the use of strict operant conditioning programs are discussed. Furthermore, the dilemmas that so many of us confront when dealing with the oppositional patient who flatly refuses treatment are also addressed. Our society seems more willing to tolerate those persons who cause serious bodily harm to themselves through excessive drinking or smoking than those who insist on starving themselves. In the latter case, ethical considerations are often brought to the fore. The story of Sally B embraces many of these issues which will be dealt with in the discussion.

Case study

Sally B, a 17-year-old unemployed young woman, was referred to us by a psychiatrist in private practice. She attended the interview accompanied by her mother who had consulted the same psychiatrist a month before on her own behalf because she was having difficulty coping with both Sally and her older sister Jenny, aged 20. Both girls had left home but Sally had since returned. Sally had had a 13-week admission to a psychiatric clinic earlier in the year where she was diagnosed as having anorexia nervosa. In late January, she had become ill with a viral infection and was unable to keep food down and it was at this time that she decided to diet. In her own words:

> *... everytime I ate something, I brought it straight back up. So I didn't eat much at all. Perhaps a couple of pieces of dried toast and flat lemonade got me through a day. It was one of those days that I thought, well, if I can live on two pieces of toast a day, surely I could live on one. So it was the next day that I tried it. I succeeded and I felt really wonderful ... But I had fallen into a trap. This was no ordinary little trap but a huge shaft, a pit of darkness. My innocence and naive nature at this stage did not let me know or see how deep the hole was. The trouble was that I was a curious 16-year-old and this shaft had intrigued me. I chose to explore.*
>
> *My mystery illness seemed to end shortly after. I was ready to once again tackle school. So off I trotted. I still wasn't eating anything. Just drinking lemon juice every now and then throughout the day. My all-juice diet lasted well. My parents were perhaps a bit bewildered by my behaviour but I can't remember if anything in particular was ever said. I think after the first few days the hunger pains stopped as well as that terrible nauseating feeling you experience when you haven't eaten. No one could understand as to how someone that ate as much as I did, could suddenly stop and eat nothing. In fact I was quite surprised at my endurance but overall it was gaining me a lot of recognition.*
>
> *Girls at school started to notice I wasn't eating. My parents noticed and so did my sister. I'm not sure how they felt and what their first reactions were. They probably thought that I was going through a 'dieting stage' like most teenage girls. But little did they know inside me a seed had been planted and it was growing very rapidly. This seed was an unusual one. It did not thrive on water, sunlight and nutrition but exactly the opposite. It thrived on being deprived. It was an evil seed. I managed to get through two weeks quite easily. Perhaps the only thing I felt different was an excessive tiredness. Of course if I had no food in me, I wasn't going to be the usual active girl that I had previously been.*
>
> *I remember getting huge 'highs' when someone used to ask me how long it had been since I had eaten. I would get the biggest buzz out of informing them how many days it had been. The more the better. In my third week, things started to drastically change, the week before I had lost energy and I could no longer even manage to get up the stairs at school. It was then that people began to recognise that the so-called diet phase had got out of hand and the so-called seed had well and truly started to blossom.*
>
> *My tremendous game was coming to a halt though. Unfortunately, people noticed I was losing weight quite rapidly and no one but me liked it. However, by this stage I had no intention of giving in. I did not starve myself stupid just for the fun of it. Mum and Dad decided at this stage that it was well and truly time that we sought medical advice. We went to our local doctor who gave me a thorough physical examination and weighed me. During my three-week fasting*

period, I had lost a whole 10 kgs. 'Wow' was probably my first reaction. I must say though that I was quite proud of myself. I wanted to lose more. Dr X had different ideas. She referred me back to a psychiatrist we had previously seen for behavioural problems at the psychiatric clinic. He was the first person to diagnose me with having anorexia nervosa. He suggested that I stay at the clinic and simply put on the weight that I had lost. My anorexia did not like getting this thumb on its head but instead of decreasing its power, it rebelled. It was angry. It wanted no food, no weight and definitely no-one telling it what to do. It was determined to get this doctor back and it fought. It fought in my body.

My stay at the clinic was awful. Being 16 years old, I hadn't really stayed away from home that much except on the odd occasions like a sleepover at a girlfriend's house. So I was very lonely. I also hated the dark and the bigness of the place. My room accommodated ten people, yet I was the only one. In fact I was the only anorexic in the whole place. I think right from the word go I had no intention of putting on any weight. My anorexic friend, though, seemed to have that all under control. I didn't even have to try. I could just lie back and take it easy while he did all the work.

After about a week or so and not gaining weight, the nursing staff started to crack down on me. I couldn't handle this for some time as I was kind of on a line of choosing to beat my best friend in my head or lying back to die. I loved anorexia: I didn't want it hurt in any way but then one day I had an amazing idea. Just perhaps I could get a balance between the anorexia and the nursing staff. If I ate, I could please them (not that the anorexia liked it) but later I could make myself sick and he would be in heaven. Now, don't you think that was a good idea? At least this way, both people could be happy. As for me though — the real me — I was feeling pretty drained and sapped. This whole business was exhausting me but at least I was still in control.

My stay at the clinic was a long one. As for my weight gain, it had gone up a whole 3 kg in my 13-week stay! My anorexia really had a hold on me at this stage and I considered hospitalisation to be nothing but a good waste of time and money. I discharged myself. I was 47 kg and that was just too much for my liking, so when I left I had all intentions of losing more. Probably, now more so as a type of revenge. My anorexia was tired of being bossed around for three months. He didn't like it at all. Therefore the fight became worse. His poisonous flowers bloom and grow stronger everyday. In his favour ... death!

At the clinic, Sally was placed on a strict operant program which required strict bed rest and no visitors, music or books (near total isolation). She was reported to have rebelled against the program and failed to gain much weight. Sally complained that the registrar who was insisting she eat more was in fact underweight herself. Her doctor's discharge summary indicated that progress had been slow and was adversely influenced by significant difficulties within the family. Hospital staff were not able to involve the family in Sally's therapy. Sally gained weight extremely slowly and caused much disruption on the ward. Eventually, she coerced her parents into taking her home against medical advice. It was felt that she remained a troubled girl who was in need of ongoing help. But they still felt there was little to offer while she remained so resistant to treatment. They were happy to take her back if her attitude towards treatment improved. Picking up Sally's words again:

Well now I was out I was once again free to do as I chose. I could exercise when I wanted, I could see my parents (whom I so much wanted by my side) and I didn't have to eat. I decided that I didn't want to sit around (on my so-called fat buttocks) all day but to get a job and do something practical and worthwhile.

I ended up with a job as a computer secretary. God only knows how, but I did. At first, like anything new, it was a novelty but the longer I was there the worse it became.

My family was not happy with me. They were just worried about my bizarre eating habits. I was treated in a funny way. People tended to have no patience with me so they ignored me. This was not what the real Sally liked; as for the anorexia, it became angrier. Another shoot grew off my tree. The real Sally didn't know what to do anymore. Everything was now just a straight-out fight between anorexia and its enemy. For example, Mum was trying to fight it and my friends. It seemed that everyone hated it but me. How could people hurt my friend. They were saying wicked things. They wanted to kill it. I kept my head low — I had nothing to offer the world anymore. Everything I ever had or could do was absorbed. My talents, my personality, everything. It was now gone. Sally had died. Anorexia was there to fill her place.

Although anorexia had taken everything off me, I wasn't cross or angry with it, for it was my friend. I was prepared to do anything to let this strong, controlled, thing stand in my place.

It was during this that there was a lot of turmoil at home. My sister had a new boyfriend and decided to leave home. I decided that if my sister was to leave home, I had to do so as well. So off I trotted. I went to a friend's house. I stayed there for two weeks. It was fun, however, deep inside I knew I didn't belong there but rather home with my family where it would be better now.

My eating throughout this time was satisfactory from what I remember. But as for the emotional side of me, I had been slaughtered. I think at this time I, Sally, was giving anorexia the big boot, yet little did I know, I was going to one day fall again and the anorexia was going to be even angrier with me. I just felt like dying.

It was during my two-week stay with my friend that I lost my job. I didn't really mind too much as I was getting pretty frustrated working in an office with four computer heads! After I lost my job I decided that my 'little run away' game would have to end. I called my Dad who fetched and took me home.

Because of my recent 'no position' stance in society, I had a hell of a lot of spare time. I hated being left by myself, trying to find something to do but as time progressed realised that I could spend even more time with my so-much-loved new hobby, dieting.

I had to eat but each day I would write myself out a new menu plan which consisted of things such as yoghurt, fruit, rice and vegetables. If I considered that I had eaten too much (which I always felt) I would make myself sick. Now looking back on it, I, the real Sally, didn't consider that I had eaten too much, but my anorexia had and it was now starting to take its revenge.

I hated being alive now. I didn't have any sort of life anymore. Sure I wanted it but that so-called seed that was first planted in me was now a fully matured tree. This tree was now bigger than I could ever be and I could not kill it. Its branches spread far and wide. It spread to my arms, my legs, both inside and out.

I think that this growth probably continued for about 3-4 months before things really got out of hand once more. Mum and Dad and the doctors could see and knew that I should be back in hospital again but weren't too sure as to where I should go.

Sally was referred to us for an opinion regarding her management in June 1988.

Sally impressed as an underweight 17-year-old young woman who was most articulate in her presentation of her past history. She had been dieting for six months and had been taken to a nearby general hospital by her mother one morning after she induced vomiting after drinking a glass of orange juice and black coffee. She was discharged after a day and referred to the psychiatric clinic where she remained for 13 weeks. She had not eaten adequately since discharge and was receiving no follow-up treatment. Sally was inducing vomiting up to six times a day, and after leaving hospital took 100 laxatives over a three-day period. She was exercising compulsively, 150 sit-ups each night as well as an hour of running or walking each day. ('I hated my job because I was sitting behind a desk all day and couldn't exercise.') She weighed 45.1 kg. (She was 167 cm tall.) When asked why she wanted treatment now, Sally replied, 'I am fed up with it. I want to get better, I don't want to drop dead'. Prior to coming to the clinic, she had broken up with her boyfriend with whom she had been going out for two months. Sally had been attending year 12 at a local public high school prior to her hospitalisation. She enjoyed high school but felt she didn't mix nearly as well as in primary school.

Her mother was very forthcoming and produced the following history. She had been married for over 20 years to her husband who worked as a security officer. He loved his job, which included shift work on weekends. Their marriage was good and they were financially secure living in their own home which Sally's mother had inherited from Sally's maternal grandmother, the same house Sally's mother had grown up in. Sally's parents enjoyed playing golf together which they did when Sally's father was not at work.

Because Sally's mother was unable to have children, the couple had adopted two girls, Sally when she was 10 days old. Sally's sister, Jenny, was now studying to be a technician (aged 19 years) and had a boyfriend whom she had met two–three years previously.

A neighbour had told Mrs B that Sally wanted to know her real mother but feared that she would be rejected, so took her resentment out on her mother. Sally's biological mother was a single woman aged 19 years who had previously given birth to a daughter when she was 16 years old. This child was also given up for adoption. Sally has said:

I came into the world in 1971. I apparently was or created complications for my mother who was just 19 herself at the time. Right from the word go, I gave this poor young woman discontent and pain. On 27 February, I gave a false alarm, my mother went into false labour (what an eager beaver I must have been to get out, into the big, vast, new world). My mother then returned home, back to the country and returned at the end of March. She went into labour this time. I was for real, no false alarms. I punched and fought for15 hours and 12 minutes and then arrived at 10.09 in the morning. (I have always been a day person so my timing was nice.) Although there were some complications with my birth, I came out a healthy baby girl. My crying rated well, my life was about to commence.

Unfortunately, my mother being so young could not physically, mentally or economically afford me. She returned to the country after five days. As for me, well, I was to stay behind and another young couple were to receive me, love me as their own and raise me. Who was to know where, what or whom I would go to?

As a child, Sally would fly into a temper but come out of it quickly. She was a bubbly child who took interest in all around her. Sally was a very excitable child and was often naughty. She had never been tidy and her room was always in a mess. She followed her sister around like a puppy dog but Jenny wouldn't include Sally at all in any of the activities she was involved in. Jenny was jealous of Sally and Sally was jealous of Jenny. If Jenny thought that Sally had anything better than her, she would take it and replace it with an item of lesser value. Sally started pre-school twice weekly and loved it. She was a real little leader. Jenny was the naughty one at pre-school, refusing to sleep. Sally did well academically at primary school (except for mathematics) and her mother described her as a real little actress.

Mrs B became aware of Sally's visual difficulties when she was 7 years old. She had experienced visual difficulties during a mathematics examination. Sally was referred to an ophthalmologist and was diagnosed as having Stargadts Disease (a disease of the retina). Her parents were told that she would be blind by the time she left high school. They were advised not to tell Sally because she was too young. They would take her out a great deal to enable her to see as much as she could before she became blind. Her parents told her what was likely to happen to her vision when she was in year 7 at school. At this time her behaviour became erratic, she would have terrible temper tantrums and would become physically violent. She would damage the home, smash furniture and strip wallpaper from the walls. Sally would kick her parents and slapped her mother across the face on at least one occasion. She would slam doors until they came off their hinges. Mrs B stated that she dealt with it in everyway she could. 'I hit her, ignored her and loved her but none of these methods succeeded.' Mrs B and her husband consulted a psychiatrist who felt Sally was acting out because of her eyesight (Sally now couldn't see at night) and would grow out of it. Sally accused her mother of starting arguments. Mrs B secretly taped her tantrums and her verbal abuse. Sally would throw glasses of jam against the wall as well as bottles of cosmetics, making a terrible mess. On one occasion while her mother was vacuuming up pieces of wallpaper Sally had stripped off the wall, Sally kept switching the power supply on and off. Mrs B became angry and hit Sally with the nozzle of the vacuum cleaner. The next day she received a visit from a Youth and Community Services (YACS) officer who allegedly warned her that if she physically abused Sally again over a two-year period, they would remove Sally from their home. Sally had gone to school the next day complaining of a sore hand saying her mother had broken it. The school had contacted YACS and sent her for X-rays which turned out to be normal. Sally then derided her mother, trying to provoke her into hitting her.

With some trepidation, we decided to admit Sally to hospital. Her physical examination was essentially normal. She complained of weakness, palpitations and other symptoms. She had no periods. Sally had a history of exercise-induced asthma and had been prescribed medication. Her heart function was normal.

She was admitted to our unit weighing 45.1 kg. Shortly after admission, the nursing staff described her eating behaviour in the following way: 'She ate poorly at dinner — only had small quantity of salad. Ate her meals with difficulty — she doesn't let food touch her lips. At one point I thought that she was going to cry when her dessert was given to her. She picks at her food, leaves meat and sweet foods on her plate. She says she wants to get better but not to put on weight. She also worries that if she starts to eat normally, we will consider her cured and send her home'.

Sally felt that her sister was a major contributor towards her problems. She idealised her sister and felt rejected by her. It was decided that she needed intensive family therapy and we referred the family to a psychiatrist who specialised in family therapy whom they could see while Sally was in hospital and after discharge. Sally was found to have lesions under both eyes from crying and rubbing her face. It was felt that Sally was not clinically depressed but rather was becoming increasingly frustrated and distressed at the thought of resuming normal eating behaviour. After more than four weeks in hospital, Sally had lost rather than gained weight and was being prescribed 3300 calories per day by the dietitian. She was, however, not taking her full diet. For example, she was rolling her scones into little balls and then only eating a quarter. Her behaviour was becoming increasingly rebellious and disruptive and she began to miss meals. She told staff that she wanted to lose weight to 39 kg as it would be a great achievement and she would only start to eat again once she reached that weight.

Since Sally was so oppositional to the program, she was discharged from hospital to see the family psychiatrist with her family as an outpatient and her family doctor if her physical condition deteriorated. The family psychiatrist described the family dynamics as follows:

> ... it would appear to me that the family dynamics are that the daughters are both at war with their adoptive parents. Jenny's battleground is over her boyfriend and this has been attentioned for some years. She left home in June 1988 for her own unit but her parents are most critical that she continues to see him. The chronic conflict over the boyfriend has involved Sally, initially as the meat in the sandwich, and more recently as a supporter of her sister.
>
> The war with Sally is, of course, over her eating. Apart from being a struggle for independence, the anorexia has provided a mechanism whereby Sally feels that she gets the attention that was previously totally centred on Jenny. In view of the intensity of the parental war with Sally, she needed to find a fairly striking avenue and anorexia fits.

A week following discharge, Sally pleaded to be readmitted. While at home, she refused food, lost weight, destroyed the house and abused her parents who could no longer cope with her acting out behaviour and food refusal. Sally was readmitted to hospital under the clear understanding that: (i) she would gain weight each week; (ii) would not disrupt the ward; (iii) would continue to see the psychiatrist for individual and family therapy; (iv) would see her ophthalmologist for a definitive opinion regarding her eye problems. Sally agreed to these conditions.

Sally weighed 40.8 kg on admission, having left hospital a week before at 42.9 kg so she had, in fact, lost a further 2.1 kg while at home. Whilst at home, she only managed half a piece of fruit for the first two days and thereafter only drank three cups of black coffee and very diluted cordial each day.

She insisted that she now wanted to get better but expressed her anxiety regarding gaining weight too quickly. Sally insisted that her parents paid little attention to her before she became ill and complained that '... they will ignore me again when I am well'. She accused her parents of being preoccupied with her sister's problems to her detriment.

By the fourth day in hospital, Sally had become uncooperative, was eating poorly and was abusive towards her mother. It was made quite clear to her that if her behaviour didn't improve, she would be discharged. A day later, she insisted on discharging herself from hospital. She was asked to see her general practitioner on a regular basis as she was eating little and was also restricting her fluid intake. She was also encouraged to continue her sessions with the family psychiatrist. Sally described the events leading up to her discharge as follows:

> *Anorexia had taken over, not only parts of me, but again the whole of me — mind, body and soul. This time it was out to kill … All the fighting I had done had been pointless, a non-progressive waste of time. All I wanted to do was to go home. I wanted to curl up into a ball, go to sleep and never wake up. I kept wishing that this existence I had acquired was not real, just merely a dream. I prayed for my mother to wake me up and tell me to hurry along or I would be late for school. But unfortunately times were now a lot rougher and no-one, not anyone, was prepared to let me go.*

Sally returned home under the care of her distressed parents. She described her trip home:

> *My mother was in tears; I was feeling pleased that I no longer had people trying to help me … When we arrived home, Mum decided it was time for me to have a drink. Yes, I was indeed very thirsty but anorexia did not want any fluid, either, now. I think it was a fear of drowning, so Sally didn't have any. I remember Mum measuring out water in measuring cups. I finally gave in and had 25 ml. I cried and it hurt me but I did it for my parents. That night I cried myself to sleep.*

Sally refused to eat or drink at home and by the third day felt acutely ill.

> *I was trembling, weak, tired and dizzy and I smelt it. The smell was that of something decaying but now I look back at it, it was not just something, it was me. My body had just about had it. I was literally on death's door.*

Sally was taken to a large general hospital where she was promptly admitted especially since there was some uncertainty as to whether Sally had taken an overdose of medication. She was transferred from casualty to the in-patient psychiatric facility where her disruptive behaviour continued. She threatened to take an overdose of her asthma medication and was eventually involuntarily transferred to a psychiatric institution where she could be forcibly treated. She only stayed for a week because the transfer order was revoked. Despite having hardly drunk or eaten, her metabolism remained relatively normal. She returned to the psychiatric in-patient facility, where her physical condition deteriorated rather rapidly. Her behaviour became increasingly disruptive, her blood tests suggested that she was going into renal failure and she was transferred to a medical ward for forced feeding and intravenous feeding. She was judged to be suicidal and unable to care for herself and was sent back to the psychiatric institution where she was previously treated after she had attempted to run away from hospital.

A strict operant conditioning program was introduced after attempts at a more lenient program failed. She was given high protein feed, through a tube while manacled to her bed; if she ate a small meal as well, she would be rewarded with a 30-minute television privilege. Sally slowly gained weight from 35 kg to 41 kg, when tube feeding was ceased. At her lowest weight of 35 kg, she was extremely emaciated. When she was discharged from the psychiatric institution after a five-week stay, she had gained weight but was still quite severely malnourished. It is worth noting that when Sally was admitted to hospital, another anorexia nervosa patient had already been admitted weighing only 30 kg, which made even Sally look 'fat'.

A further development occurred while Sally was in hospital. There was legal argument as to whether anorexia nervosa came under the Mental Health Act and whether patients with such a disorder could be treated against their will. It appears that this is only permissible if the patient's physical health is imperiled or they are actively suicidal or a danger to others. Sally's parents felt they were unable to care for their daughter at home and supported the hospital's endeavours to have her made an involuntary patient for up to one month. This medico-legal issue will be addressed later.

While in hospital Sally was initially prescribed a major tranquilliser. Her dosage was increased when her behaviour became increasingly violent, resulting on one occasion in her smashing windows in the hospital.

Although operant conditioning programs are relatively easy to develop and implement, this is not usually the case with patients with anorexia nervosa. The in-patient staff experienced significant difficulty in Sally's case. It was predictable but surprising to all, the amount of 'splitting' that occurred between all levels and types of staff that had to deal with her case. From the experience of drawing up appropriate behavioural programs, they learnt much about how precise and inclusive they had to be and also, how they had to be straightforwardly adhered to by all members of the staff. An enormous amount of ill-feeling and tension was caused.

Sally was discharged from the psychiatric institution with the clear understanding that she would seek further treatment at our Anorexia and Nervosa Clinic. She later decided that she didn't feel ready for further in-patient treatment and chose instead to see the family psychiatrist for both individual and family therapy sessions with her parents and sister.

Sally sought readmission about 18 months later. Her relationship with her parents had improved significantly but she still wasn't getting on well with her sister. She felt that the sessions with the family psychiatrist were going well and wished to pursue these while in hospital. She was attempting to complete her Higher

School Certificate at Technical College. At the time of this admission, she weighed only 34.5 kg.

Her physical examination revealed an emaciated young woman who was finding it difficult to breathe and had lost some of her hair. Her pulse rate was slow, at 40 beats per minute, and she had blue extremities, indicating poor circulation. Her heart sounds were fine and her chest was clear. Sally's heart tests were normal but several of her blood tests were outside normal limits.

Sally admitted to taking up to 30 laxatives per day over the preceding year and had induced vomiting on three or four occasions. She would walk for hours per day and do stretching exercises while in the shower as well.

Her eating behaviour was most problematic. She had been fasting during the day and at 2.00 p.m. would drink a can of diet coke. At 10.00 p.m. at night she would drink another can of low joule soda. Around this time, she would prepare a plate of All Bran and water, microwave it for four minutes and then freeze it for three hours. She would let it thaw until 3.00 a.m. Sally avoided all food except All Bran and 100 g of carob on some days. She limited her caloric intake to 250 calories per day. She had kept to this schedule religiously over the preceding month and exclaimed that 'If I did break this ritual, I would feel like a failure, as if the whole world had come to an end'. Once in hospital, her problematic eating behaviour became quite evident, scoring highly on a psychological test designed to measure eating disturbance (Wilson et al., 1989). She scored highly on the following items: (i) picking at food; (ii) food disposal; (iii) distaste for food; (iv) slow eating; (v) ritualistic eating; (vi) preference for low-energy foods.

Sally once again failed to make any progress and after a week in hospital had gained no weight. She became increasingly ambivalent about staying on but was strongly encouraged to do so by her mother.

She had been placed on our lenient, flexible operant conditioning program (Touyz et al., 1984; Touyz, Beumont & Dunn, 1987) which required her to gain 1.5 kg per week in order to avoid being restricted to the confines of the unit and making her ineligible to go on ward outings to interesting places. The failure to gain the weight would also have precluded her from going out for drives with her family or visiting local shopping centres. Sally pleaded for a special dispensation. She wanted immediate rewards for very small weight movements. One of the most important rules when working with such patients is tolerance and flexibility, but remaining firm with one's conviction that weight gain is an integral component of the recovery process and cannot be compromised. We acceded to her request and the following interim program was developed, for example:

34.7 kg by Thursday (one hour out with mother)
34.9 kg by Saturday (two hours out with mother)
35.2 kg by Tuesday (one hour out with mother).
Plus, if she gained 1 kg over the week, she could go out to a movie with her mother.

Despite Sally's assertion that she really wanted to get better and the introduction of a special incentive program at her own request, she gained only 1 kg over a five-week period. We were concerned about her lack of progress but were impressed with her general good behaviour in the unit. We decided to persevere despite reservations from some members of the treatment team. Our patience and flexibility were well rewarded. During her seventh week in hospital, Sally gained 1.6 kg and then proceeded to gain weight at a very acceptable rate reaching her minimum weight of 54 kg after 117 days in hospital. She ended up gaining 19.5 kg and averaged over 1 kg per week.

At the time she reached her minimum weight, she decided to work part-time in a nursing home but, much to her distress, found the work too demanding. She decided to become an enrolled nurse but was unable to gain acceptance into such a program. Sally maintained her weight for five weeks before being discharged from our unit. However, since reaching her minimum weight, her adolescent behaviour had re-emerged with gusto, and she was causing her parents significant concern over returning home in the late hours of the morning at weekends and drinking to excess. These issues became the centre of discussion in her family therapy sessions.

Discussion

This case history encompasses many pertinent issues regarding the aetiology, diagnosis and treatment of patients with anorexia nervosa. It could be assumed that since there has been such widespread interest and proliferation of research on the topic, that there is now a general consensus with regard to treatment and that no patient should go uncured as suggested by Venables in his review of the topic more than 60 years ago. Venables (1930) went on to say (page 213) that:

> Every patient with anorexia nervosa can be persuaded to eat normally. The condition is hysterical and no patient should remain uncured … the doctor should sit down with the patient and fight for every mouthful of food, which may take an hour or two per meal. The doctor must never lose his temper. With each successive meal, eating becomes easier, and the patient may eat alone in about a week. The patient must be given a full diet from the first. One must cure the anorexia before one starts on the psychology of the patient's symptoms.

Venables indicated that he was never in favour of prolonged or deep analysis; the immediate cause was seldom hard to find. He believed a few frank discussions, coupled with any necessary adjustments in circumstances, should be all that was necessary to prevent future relapse. Venables recommended that patients should be kept in bed and special nurses were needed. He further added that '... the patient should never be treated at home and the parents should be excluded'.

From his description, it appears that Venables regarded anorexia nervosa as a relatively minor illness from which all patients recover. Sally B's struggle to overcome her anorexia nervosa reminds one that it is a much more serious disorder than previously believed, often with marked morbidity and a not insignificant mortality rate. Despite Sally's admissions to hospital, individual and family therapy and nutritional counselling, she is yet to completely recover from her illness. The degree of suffering and distress invoked within the family is often not appreciated. Sally's parents were placed in an awful predicament. Did they support their daughter in a legal challenge to be discharged from an involuntary admission to a psychiatric institution or ask the magistrate to keep her in hospital so that she could receive treatment which she refused to accept previously? A difficult dilemma for any parent. In Sally's case, her parents felt that they were unable to cope with her at home and acknowledged her urgent need for treatment. It should be pointed out at this stage that most patients fortunately can be persuaded to eat or drink again although this often requires much patience and effort, especially on the part of the nursing staff who spend a great deal of time with such patients. A question worth asking is, if a unit specialised in treating such patients is unable to succeed, what chance has an institution with little or no experience in doing so? Every effort should be made in trying to engage the patients in accepting treatment even if this involves feeding the patient by hand initially. Patients with anorexia nervosa resent being force-fed and this does little to establish a meaningful therapeutic alliance with the patient (Garner, 1985). Russell (1973) argued that tube feeding 'should be quickly dismissed as a crude method of forcing food into the patient and is no longer justified because of enlightened nursing methods' (page 47). Anderson, Morse and Santmyer (1985) have not needed to implement tube feeding in any of their more than 170 patients, whereas Strober and Yager (1985) have used it in less than 5 per cent of their cases. There are significant dangers associated with tube feeding patients with anorexia nervosa.

1. It represents a direct intrusion into the gastrointestinal tract of someone who is already preoccupied and misguided about bodily functions.
2. It may be perceived as an assault or act of hostility which the patient attributes to her worthlessness.
3. It may be done with minimal patient cooperation and as such leads to increased mistrust.
4. The physiological side-effects are not insignificant.
5. It is almost always unnecessary (from Garner, 1985, page 709).

It seems preferable to transfer a patient to a medical unit if he or she fails to respond to conventional treatment, with the opportunity of returning to the anorexia nervosa unit once normal eating has resumed. This minimises the hostile conflict between patient and therapist when tube feeding has to be enforced. Sally described her experiences of being force-fed as follows:

I didn't know what it was going to involve. I hated pain ... I was afraid, so scared. The tube looked so hard and so long. I began to cry ... this hideous piece of plastic tubing was being forced down my left nostril ... I was screaming ... my head thrashed wildly on the bed whilst my body squirmed or moved like a wounded fish out of water.

I cried ... Nothing can or will ever remove the memory of that tube.

However, this tube was going to save my life ... But I decided that I didn't want this tube inside of me nor the fluid flowing into me through the tube. The most sensible thing in my eyes to do was to pull it out. But I didn't want any pain.

I gently pulled the tube protruding from my nose and it was sore. I was so afraid and scared of what I could do to myself and also scared of what the staff would do to me ...

I lifted my feeble arms and fingers. I placed the tube between my thumb and forefinger and gently yanked it. Something moved inside me. I could now feel the tube inside my stomach. My mind ran amuck. I was so confused. Out came the tube, one hell of a long tube. I hadn't realised how long it actually was. (I later found out that it was 3 feet long).

Sally even learned how to regurgitate her nasogastric feeds.

I taught myself how to vomit through the tube … I learnt that by holding my breath and blowing out through my nose, I could regurgitate any fluid that had been passed down through the tube into my stomach.

Tube feeding is an invasive procedure with not inconsiderable risks and for these reasons every effort should be made to encourage the patient to recommence eating. Time and effort expended will have been well worthwhile if recourse to tube feeding is avoided. However, as in the case of Sally, this was necessary as a lifesaving procedure, however unpalatable it may have been.

Sally responded well to our lenient flexible behavioural program gaining nearly 20 kg in two weeks. There are several advantages in using a lenient, flexible behavioural program when re-feeding patients with anorexia nervosa:

- the program is seen as acceptable by the majority of patients
- the patients require less nursing time
- the program is more economical and allows staff to engage in individual and group psychotherapy.

Patients such as Sally, who need to gain a substantial amount of weight, often complain of discomfort and a distended abdomen. Supervised anaerobic exercise with the specific aim of toning muscles appears to be effective in reducing the degree of body shape disparagement which so often results in this situation. Similarly, patients who have lost weight because of an inability to control the amount of exercise they do may also be helped by learning how to moderate their behaviour on a controlled exercise program.

There is no general consensus as to what constitutes an optimal weight for patients with anorexia nervosa, although most clinicians probably use a low average weight for height and sex as a general guideline. This is one of the most emotive issues confronting clinicians and its resolution often requires both the wisdom of Solomon and the patience of Job. Fortunately, there are some guidelines to use when coming to a decision:

- it is preferable to specify the minimum target weight at the onset of treatment rather than later during the course of an admission
- the weight should be one that the patient can maintain without continued dieting
- there should be a range of approximately 2 kg rather than a specific set weight.

Quetelet's body mass index is a useful means of determining target weights (Beumont, Al-Alami & Touyz, 1988). It is derived from the following formula:

$$\frac{\text{weight (kg)}}{\text{height}^2\text{(m)}}$$

For those patients aged 17 years or older, a body mass index of 20 should be used as a guide to minimum weight. For those aged between 15 and 16 years, a body mass index of 18.5 appears to be appropriate. However, for patients aged 14 years and under it is best to consult standardised data. Sally was aged 17 years with a height of 167 cm. A body mass index of 20 was derived by squaring her height in metres (1.67 m × 1.67 m) and multiplying it by 20, that is, 2.79 × 20 = 55.80. There will always be exceptions to any rule, and there is much to be said for using a pragmatic approach.

Finally, it is preferable to weigh patients no more than three times a week, in their pyjamas and before breakfast. Once they have reached their target weight they should be 'range' weighed. The scale should be set at the lowest acceptable weight and then at a weight 2 or 3 kg higher. This enables the clinician to document whether an individual is maintaining his or her weight within an acceptable range without focusing upon a specific figure, hence avoiding reinforcement of the patient's preoccupation with weight as such.

Sally received individual group and family therapy. All family members living in the patient's home are called to attend an initial family therapy session just before or shortly after admission. At this interview an assessment of family interactional patterns is made and a decision regarding ongoing family therapy is taken. Not all families require regular therapy and a deliberate decision should be made for each family as to the number of sessions required and the family members who will be asked to attend. For example, if the parents of the index patient have marked marital difficulties, the family therapist may choose to work with the parents alone for a number of sessions before including the patient and siblings. The objectives of family intervention are as follows:

- to enable family members to understand the illness and the goals of treatment
- to bring about a readjustment of family interactional patterns where appropriate
- to encourage participation in post-discharge planning activities.

In Sally's case, there was no question that family therapy was indicated. Family therapy sessions usually included all members of the family but at times Sally's parents were seen on their own.

Individual psychotherapy is an integral part of treatment but is only effective when combined with an overall plan of management.

Undoubtedly, many patients need dynamically oriented psychotherapy to deal with the emotional and relationship problems that underlie the anorexic illness. The general goals are:

- to increase the patient's self-esteem
- to increase the feeling of power and control which the patient can then express in a healthy way
- to resolve underlying conflicts.

Therapy should also allow the patient to become more mature, enabling him or her to establish rewarding relationships with family and friends. It may also be helpful to explore career options so that the patient can eventually become financially as well as emotionally independent and self-reliant.

How does one engage the patient in meaningful psychotherapy when he or she wishes to be free of any adult influence? As a rule, psychotherapy ought to be initiated with the clear understanding that psychological change requires months, if not years, to attain. It also involves self-observation and self-reflection: the discovery of the unknown. In anorexia nervosa, a willing, self-observant patient desirous of change does not exist as a result of the regressed isolation into self-sufficiency; instead, an obstinately resistant patient must be engaged. Furthermore, psychotherapy requires sincerity and trust, virtues which are often distorted in these patients (Casper, 1987).

Thus, there are innumerable obstacles to overcome in successfully engaging the anorexic patient in psychotherapy and, unfortunately, there are no simple answers. However, it is imperative that the psychotherapist be well versed in all aspects of the disorder and accept that psychotherapy with such patients requires not only tact and patience but time as well. Casper (1987) has articulated this rather well: 'Any treatment intervention is experienced by the anorexia nervosa patient as an overpowering attack and coercion, and she defends herself in every way possible, not infrequently by cheating and manipulating her environment. Thus, in anorexia nervosa, more than in any other psychiatric disorder, the soil for psychotherapy needs to be prepared'.

Some authors have advocated the use of cognitive procedures based upon the 'assumption that maladaptive feelings and behaviours are mediated by distorted or maladaptive thinking and that the primary aim of clinical intervention is to alter these cognitive processes' (Garner & Bemis, 1985).

The fundamental goals of cognitive behaviour therapy are:

- to heighten patients' awareness of their thought processes and to encourage them to monitor their own thoughts.
- to enable the patient to recognise the connection between certain dysfunctional thoughts and maladaptive behaviours and emotions.
- for the therapist and patient to evaluate the validity of particular beliefs; the implications of certain attitudes and beliefs should be followed to their logical conclusions.
- to enable the patient to learn to gradually substitute more realistic and appropriate interpretations for his or her dysfunctional thoughts and maladaptive behaviours.

The ultimate challenge for the therapist is to modify the underlying assumptions which give rise to the specific dysfunctional beliefs. One of the advantages of the cognitive behavioural approach is that it is not necessarily incompatible with other approaches to treatment. The course of therapy will vary depending on the orientation of the therapist and the circumstances of the patient.

Conclusion

Anorexia nervosa is a potentially serious illness which may lead to prolonged psychosocial dysfunction, physical morbidity and a significant mortality. It is important that it is recognised early and treated appropriately. Although there is no definitive treatment accepted by all clinicians, there is a general consensus among most psychiatrists and psychologists who are experienced in the area (Vandereycken, 1987).

In the short term, many patients relapse, but with continued care the majority recover fully and lead happy and useful lives.

Sally B has had a long struggle to overcome her illness. She has maintained her weight for a year, left home and found employment in a restaurant as a waitress. She has also recently developed a heterosexual relationship and has a good social life. It is too early to say whether she has recovered from her illness but the case of Sally B clearly illustrates what a potentially serious illness anorexia nervosa can be.

Acknowledgement

We would like to thank Sally B for permission to quote from her own story of the struggle to overcome her illness.

Susan H. Spence
University of Sydney

5 Sexual dysfunction

Human sexual behaviour involves a fascinating interplay between emotion, cognition and physiology. To complicate matters further, each of these aspects is influenced by a multiplicity of biological and psychosocial factors. Although the complex nature of sexual behaviour is acknowledged, sexuality may be subject to applied behaviour analysis in the same way as any other form of human behaviour. The assessment and treatment of sexual problems is therefore within the range of abilities of any clinical psychologist who is trained in cognitive-behavioural assessment and therapy and who has a satisfactory understanding of the determinants of sexual behaviour. One of the aims of this chapter is to illustrate the complex interaction between cognitive factors and the more overt aspects of sexual behaviour. A major role of the therapist is to integrate cognitive therapy methods with those approaches to the treatment of sexual dysfunction which focus primarily on overt responding. Similarly, the interplay between a couple's sexual relationship and their general relationship is emphasised, making a case for the integration of marital and sexual therapy methods.

Phases of sexual responding

Sexual behaviour has traditionally been described as a sequence of interacting stages. Various models of sexual responding have been proposed (Jehu, 1979; Masters & Johnson, 1970), but for the present purposes sexual behaviour will be simplified to include four major stages: desire, arousal, orgasm and resolution. Traditionally, sexual behaviour has been described primarily in terms of physiology. For assessment and therapy purposes, however, it is important to examine the emotional, cognitive, physiological and overt behavioural aspects of sexual responding. Each of these components plays a varying role at different stages of sexual behaviour. For example, sexual desire refers to the cognitive and affective components of the appetitive aspects of sexual behaviour. As such, desire refers to thoughts or fantasies about sex or 'urges' to engage in sexual activity, which typically, although not necessarily, trigger sexual arousal and may lead to behaviours designed to elicit sexual activity. In many respects the desire phase can be seen as a drive state in which a 'need' or 'urge' is created to engage in sexual behaviour. Desire may be triggered by a range of stimuli. These may be external cues, such as the sight of a partner or a certain perfume, or they may be internal or cognitive events such as a thought or image about a particular stimulus which in turn triggers off thoughts, fantasies or subjective feelings of sexual desire.

Although the current trend is to emphasise the distinction between sexual arousal and desire, in practice it is extremely difficult to make such a differentiation. Typically, sexual desire is conceptualised in terms of cognitive events, with sexual arousal being seen as a network of physiological responses which may or may not be accompanied by overt sexual behaviours. Stage models of sexual responding tend to oversimplify the picture, in that sexual behaviour does not necessarily involve a progression of events from cognitive desire to physiological arousal. Desire does not suddenly end when sexual arousal begins. Indeed, both may occur simultaneously and independently.

From a physiological perspective, the aim of sexual arousal is to produce changes within the body that will enable intercourse and conception to take place. Sexual arousal therefore brings about the changes required for erection of the penis, lubrication of the vagina and preparation for the orgasmic response. In the male, the excitement or arousal phase involves a combination of penile arterial dilation (widening of the arteries supplying blood to the penis), increased arterial blood flow, active relaxation of the smooth muscles of the tissue of the copora cavernosa (a sponge-like tissue in the penis) and constriction of outflow of blood from the penis (Williams, 1987). These processes result in an engorgement of blood which causes the penis to become erect and the foreskin to retract. Additional responses include tightening of the scrotal sac, raising of the testicles within the scrotum, nipple erection and general bodily reactions such as increased muscle tension, blood pressure, heart rate and respiration rate.

Similar blood vessel changes occur in the female, causing vaginal lubrication, vaginal lengthening, and formation of what is known as the orgasmic 'platform' around the base of the vagina. Engorgement of the clitoral area typically results in the raising of the clitoris towards the mons veneris and the labia may become darker in colour as the result of increased blood flow. General body responses during this phase mirror those found in the male.

A complex network of physiological changes and accompanying subjective feelings are also involved in the orgasm stage of sexual responding. In the male, two separate components can be identified during orgasm (ejaculation), namely emission and expulsion. Emission involves contractions of the vas deferens (which carry sperm), seminal vesicles and ejaculating ducts as semen is placed at the entrance to the urethra. Simultaneously, the internal sphincter of the urethra contracts which prevents ejaculation backwards into the bladder. The result is the formation of a pressure chamber which prepares for expulsion of the ejaculate. At this point most males report a feeling which is usually described as 'ejaculatory inevitability'. Expulsion then involves a series of rhythmic contractions of the penile urethra and muscles at the base of the penis, propelling the ejaculate through the penis. The orgasm phase in women involves rhythmic contractions of the muscles around the base of the vagina and pelvic floor, preceded by a retraction of the clitoris under the clitoral hood. It remains unclear whether orgasm produced through clitoral stimulation is identical to that produced by vaginal stimulation. Evidence suggests that the physiological responses of orgasm are the same for the two forms of stimulation, but many women report differences in the subjective feelings that accompany clitoral versus vaginally triggered orgasm (Rosen & Beck, 1988).

The final stage of sexual responding that follows orgasm is termed the resolution phase. In the male, this involves a 'refractory' period during which the penis becomes flaccid and the physiological responses of sexual arousal do not occur in response to further stimulation. The length of this period varies according to the individual and the age of the man involved. In women, the physiological responses of sexual arousal gradually subside, but the period of insensitivity to further stimulation is typically much shorter.

Types of sexual dysfunction

Sexual difficulties may occur at any one or all of the stages of sexual responding outlined above. The case to be described here concerns a woman who presented at a university psychology clinic complaining of an inability to attain orgasm under any circumstances. Because of space limitations, the following discussion will focus primarily on female sexual disorders. Many of the points made, however, are equally relevant to cases of male sexual dysfunction.

The categorisation of sexual problems according to the stages of the sexual response are reflected in the *Diagnostic and Statistical Manual of Mental Disorders,* third edition, revised, (DSM-III-R) (American Psychiatric Association, 1987). The DSM-III-R criteria for a diagnosis of a psychosexual dysfunction require that the problem cannot be attributed entirely to organic factors, a mental disorder such as a major depression, or to inadequate sexual stimulation. Sexual dysfunctions are categorised into disorders of sexual desire, arousal, orgasm and sexual pain. Diagnosis also requires the specification of the degree to which a sexual problem can be categorised as psychogenic or biogenic, lifelong or acquired and generalised or situational.

The following section outlines the types of psychosexual disorders which are relevant to the presenting case and provides the definitions of relevant terms used within the DSM-III-R.

Hypoactive sexual desire disorder

Hypoactive sexual desire is defined by DSM-III-R as 'persistently or recurrently deficient or absent sexual fantasies and desire for sexual activity. The judgement of deficiency or absence is made by the clinician, taking into account factors that affect sexual functioning, such as age, sex and the context of the person's life' (American Psychiatric Association, DSM-III-R, 1987, page 293). The overt behavioural characteristics of this problem may vary considerably, with responses ranging from active avoidance of sex, to participation in sexual activities upon partner initiation despite a lack of desire. The emotional features also vary and may or may not include negative feelings about sexual activity, such as disgust, anxiety or guilt. In cases where negative emotional reactions are severe, extreme aversion or avoidance of sexual contacts may occur and a diagnosis of sexual aversion disorder may be given (see below). The lack of desire may be limited to a particular partner or type of sexual activity, or it may be a more global problem. Factors such as a mismatch in desire between partners or unrealistic expectations need to be considered during the assessment process. The consequences of low sexual desire for subsequent stages of the sexual response also varies. In many cases, the lack of desire leads to a low frequency of sexual interaction, with the result that arousal and orgasm are rarely experienced. Other clients may engage in sexual activity despite the lack of desire and may or may not experience subsequent sexual arousal and orgasm.

Nathan (1986) suggests that low sexual desire is relatively common, with prevalence rates varying according to the sample studied and the question being asked. Only a small proportion of married men and women report never having any desire for sex at all (1–3 per cent), whereas the figure is much higher for unmarried heterosexual women (15–20 per cent). If questions are phrased so as to ask whether lack of interest in sex constitutes a problem, both men (16 per cent) and women (35 per cent) report a greater incidence of low sexual desire (Nathan, 1986). Lack of sexual interest appears to be extremely common among sex therapy referrals, with around 50–70 per cent of couples reporting a lack of sexual desire to be a problem (Freidman et al., 1982; Schover & Lo Piccolo,1982), albeit not necessarily the primary reason for seeking help.

Sexual aversion disorder

Sexual aversion disorder is defined by the DSM-III-R as 'persistent or recurrent extreme aversion to, and avoidance of, all or almost all, genital sexual contact with a sexual partner' (American Psychiatric Association, DSM-III-R, 1987, page 293). It appears from the limited information available in the DSM-III-R manual, that this category includes those cases of low sexual desire which are accompanied by extremely negative affective and cognitive reactions, leading to marked avoidance behaviours.

Aversion to and avoidance of some forms of sexual activity, such as oral-genital contact, is relatively common and would not be labelled as dysfunctional. A sexual aversion disorder is only said to exist when the aversion and avoidance responses are sufficiently generalised so as to exclude all forms of genital sexual contact with a partner. The relatively recent recognition of sexual aversion disorder as a category of sexual dysfunction means that minimal information is available concerning its incidence and aetiology.

Female sexual arousal disorder

Female sexual arousal disorder may be defined as '(1) persistent or recurrent partial or complete failure to attain or maintain the lubrication-swelling response of sexual excitement until completion of the sexual activity or, (2) persistent or recurrent lack of a subjective sense of sexual excitement and pleasure in a female during sexual activity' (American Psychiatric Association, DSM-III-R, 1987, page 294). A distinction is made, therefore, between the physiological and subjective components of arousal, given that these aspects are not always in agreement. Some women may experience the physiological responses of arousal and yet not report any pleasurable feelings or arousing thoughts. Others may experience the cognitive aspects of arousal and yet fail to lubricate or exhibit other physiological aspects of the sexual arousal response. The degree to which desire and orgasm are also affected is variable. Some women may attain orgasm (for example through the use of a vibrator) without the experience of sexual arousal, whereas, for others, problems of desire and orgasm accompany lack of sexual arousal.

Data concerning the incidence of sexual arousal disorders in women is lacking and the few studies available have typically failed to make a distinction between lack of desire and lack of arousal.

Inhibited female orgasm

Inhibited female orgasm may be defined as 'persistent or recurrent delay in, or absence of, orgasm in a female following a normal sexual excitement phase during sexual activity that the clinician judges to be adequate in focus, intensity and duration' (American Psychiatric Association, DSM-III-R,1987, page 294). Previous terms used in the literature include 'female orgasmic dysfunction' and 'anorgasmia'. As with other psychosexual disorders, anorgasmia may be situational or global and may also be lifelong or have developed after a period of orgasmic ability in the situation(s) of concern. The most common situation in which orgasm does not occur is intercourse, with estimates suggesting that around 70–80 per cent of women are unable to experience orgasm during coitus if they rely purely on vaginal stimulation by the penis (Kaplan, 1983). The majority of women appear to require some form of direct clitoral stimulation in order to reach orgasm during intercourse. This raises the question of whether lack of orgasm during coitus, in the absence of additional stimulation, should be classified as a sexual dysfunction. Perhaps it may be necessary for some women to accept that orgasm by penile thrusting alone is an unrealistic goal. Failure to experience orgasm through any form of stimulation, including self-pleasuring, is much less common, with estimates ranging from 5–15 per cent (Nathan, 1986). Female orgasmic dysfunction is a frequent cause of referral for therapy. Hawton (1985) reported that 19 per cent of his female referrals concerned orgasmic dysfunction whereas Masters and Johnson (1970) found that 56 per cent of female sexual dysfunction referrals concerned primary orgasmic dysfunction (lifelong — in all situations) with another 44 per cent reporting problems of situational anorgasmia.

Biological causes of sexual dysfunction

Before discussing the psychosocial factors that are implicated in the aetiology of psychosexual dysfunctions, it is important to note the enormous range of organic factors that may produce sexual disorders. A thorough medical assessment is generally recommended before the onset of psychological intervention, to exclude the possibility of organic aetiology. Questions relating to possible organic causes should be asked during the psychological assessment as a further check for biological aetiology. Diseases, illnesses and injuries which interfere with the hormonal, vascular or neural systems involved in sexual responding, may lead to sexual dysfunction. Sexual difficulties may also occur not through the direct physical effects of a disease or illness, but as the result of anxiety, fatigue, fear of further injury or just from general feelings of ill health. Some illnesses may also cause disfigurement of the body, producing self-consciousness about one's physical attractiveness (Anderson & Wolf, 1986).

A wide range of chemical substances may interfere with sexual functioning, the exact nature of which will depend on the biological action of the drug involved. Any drug which affects the neural, endocrine or vascular systems involved in sexual functioning may impair sexual responding. Particular attention must therefore be paid during assessment to any substance use by the client whether it be prescribed medication, illicit drugs or alcohol. The age of the client is another factor that should be considered in sexual dysfunction cases. Although changes in sexual responding take place with age, sexual dysfunction is not part of the normal ageing process. The majority of people are capable of sexual activity, sexual desire, arousal and orgasm throughout their lives. Nevertheless, subtle changes in sexual responding typically occur which may be misinterpreted as an indication of sexual dysfunction and produce performance anxiety in the older person if not understood. Menopause warrants a separate mention in that this process may produce specific difficulties for some women, particularly if lubrication is affected.

A detailed discussion of the major biological causes of sexual dysfunction is beyond the scope of the present chapter and readers are referred to more extensive reviews such as Kaplan (1974), Jehu (1979) and Spence (1991).

Psychosocial causes of sexual dysfunction

Psychosocial factors may be responsible directly for the development and maintenance of sexual difficulties or may be superimposed upon organic causes. Psychosocial determinants involve environmental factors (the physical environment, family influences and partner behaviour) and factors relating to the individual (sexual knowledge, attitudes and beliefs).

The physical environment, family relationships and life events

A variety of external environmental factors may influence sexual responding. Lack of opportunity for sexual interactions, lack of privacy, or a cold, uncomfortable setting are typical examples of events which may be associated with an unsatisfactory sexual relationship. Similarly, family relationships impinge upon the couple's sexual interactions. Negative life events, such as loss of employment, death of a family member, excessive work demands, unwanted pregnancies, abortion, sexual abuse or childbirth may also trigger sexual difficulties. It is generally not the event itself, but the person's appraisal of the event and subsequent emotional reaction to it, which results in sexual dysfunction.

Partner behaviour

Partners obviously play a crucial role as the source of both antecedents and consequences of sexual behaviour. For those cases presenting for therapy which involve a partnership, the problem is, therefore, typically viewed as a problem of the couple, rather than of any one individual. A partner's skills in providing sexual stimulation and in communicating effectively play an essential role in the development of a sexual problem. Similarly, the partner's reaction to the occurrence of a sexual difficulty is an important factor in determining whether such problems are likely to recur. Reactions may vary considerably, ranging from calm reassurance to overt criticism and obviously the impact varies accordingly.

Quality of the general relationship

Marital and sexual difficulties are closely associated (Zimmer, 1987). Hence, it is essential that general relationship difficulties are explored during assessment and therapy if a successful outcome is to be achieved. For many couples, negative emotions associated with marital distress are likely to interfere with sexual desire and arousal. Similarly, sexual difficulties may produce tensions and conflicts within non-sexual aspects of the relationship. Hence, the direction of influence between sexual and marital problems tends to be two-way, requiring that both aspects be considered during intervention.

Sexual knowledge, sexual skills and communication skills

Knowledge of sexual anatomy and sexual techniques is important in enabling individuals to provide their partner and themselves with appropriate sexual stimulation (Derogatis & Meyer, 1979). It is insufficient, however, to be knowledgeable about sexual matters and techniques at a cognitive level if this knowledge cannot be put into practice. This requires a combination of sexual performance skills and communication skills. Each person needs to be able to stimulate their partner appropriately and to achieve positions during sex from which they can obtain the greatest amount of arousal and pleasure themselves. Communication skills are also required to deal with situations such as initiating sexual interactions, giving feedback to the partner, requesting certain activities and turning down requests for sex, all in a manner that produces a positive outcome.

Attitudes, beliefs and thoughts

Thoughts, attitudes and beliefs about various aspects of sexuality may have a considerable influence over the type of sexual activities people engage in and their response in terms of desire, arousal and orgasm. Irrational or maladaptive thoughts and attitudes about events or situations may result in inappropriate or unsatisfactory responding in all areas of behaviour, including sexual responding. People hold beliefs and attitudes relating to a wide range of subjects concerning the acceptability of particular sexual activities, sex roles and the role of orgasm, spontaneity, passion, physical affection and mutual orgasm in a sexual relationship. A range of irrational or maladaptive attitudes and beliefs concerning such topics has been identified in relation to sexual dysfunction (Baker & De Silva, 1988; Sanders & Cairns, 1987; Zilbergeld, 1978). Maladaptive attitudes, beliefs and thoughts are not only proposed to play an important role in the development of sexual problems but they are also suggested to play an important role in the continuation of sexual difficulties. For example, Masters and Johnson (1970) placed considerable emphasis on thoughts of fear of failure, focusing on one's performance rather than on pleasure ('spectatoring'), and anticipation of pain or hurt. A detailed outline of the role of maladaptive attitudes and thoughts in the determination of sexual problems is provided by Spence (1991).

It is clearly important to explore patients' specific thoughts during different stages of sexual encounters and those beliefs and attitudes which tend to govern their behaviour. This may pinpoint maladaptive beliefs which are impairing sexual responsiveness and which may become the focus of a cognitive therapy component during intervention.

Emotional reactions

A wide range of emotions such as anger, guilt, disgust, fear or shame may interfere with sexual functioning if they are experienced during sexual interactions. Hence, emotional reactions before, during and after sexual activities should be considered during assessment and therapy. The couple's emotions and thoughts with regard to each other during sex should be given particular attention. It may also be possible to identify fear, anxiety, guilt or anger reactions about sexual activity or the non-sexual aspects of life which are inhibiting sexual responding.

Sexual preference

Individuals vary in their preference for a particular type of sexual partner or sexual activity. Assessment should therefore explore this area by examining the content of sexual fantasies, targets of sexual desire and arousal and content of any erotic material used. For some individuals, erotic preferences may not be for traditional hetero- or homosexual activities but may be for some type of anomalous stimuli such as voyeuristic, sado-masochistic or transvestite situations (Freund & Blanchard, 1981).

Fantasy ability and use of erotic material

There is considerable empirical evidence to demonstrate the effectiveness of erotic stimuli such as pictures, literature and videotapes in creating sexual arousal (Gillan, 1977). Couples vary, however, in their attitudes towards and use of erotic material. Similarly, individuals vary in their use of fantasy, in the form of visual imagery or verbal rehearsal, in producing sexual arousal (Heiman, Lo Piccolo & Lo Piccolo, 1976). The use of fantasy and erotic materials should therefore be considered during assessment, as it may be feasible to use these aspects as components of intervention, if sexual arousal levels are lacking.

Ability to focus on sexual sensations

It is possible that some individuals lack the ability to attend to and interpret correctly the sensations associated with sexual stimulation and arousal. Distractibility may occur if a person is preoccupied with other thoughts relating to anxiety or non-sexual events. It is also possible that arousal cues may be misinterpreted as an aversive feeling rather than pleasurable, or may be interpreted as a sign of anxiety rather than sexual arousal.

Mental and physical health

Various forms of psychopathology are associated with sexual dysfunction, in particular problems associated with anxiety and depression. Physical ill-health and fatigue may also be triggers for the development of sexual difficulties, hence these factors should be examined and dealt with prior to the onset of intervention for any sexual problem. There is an extensive literature relating to the role of anxiety and depression in the development of sexual disorders (for example, Barlow, 1986; Schreiner-Engel & Schiavi, 1986) but detailed discussion of this area is beyond the scope of the present chapter.

In summary, there is an enormous range of organic and psychosocial factors which can influence sexual responding and which may impair sexual responding. Careful examination of these factors and integration of the obtained information permits the assessor to identify those variables which were initially responsible for the onset of the problem and those that are currently maintaining its occurrence. This information provides the basis for designing an individually-tailored intervention program.

The assessment process

As with the assessment of any form of behavioural problem, the major sources of information include the cognitive-behavioural interview, personal history, self-report questionnaires, reports from significant others (in this case the partner) and self-monitoring information. A detailed description of the content of the cognitive-behavioural interview for psychosexual difficulties is provided by Wilson, Spence and Kavanagh (1989) and Spence (1991). Detailed guidelines for sexual history taking are also outlined by Hawton (1985), Lobitz and Lobitz (1978) and Lo Piccolo and Heiman (1978).

Many practical issues should be considered in designing the interview. The assessor must decide whether to include both partners in assessment and therapy, how to deal with issues of confidentiality and how to develop an interviewing style that makes clients feel comfortable and willing to divulge accurate, personal information. Ideally, both members of the partnership should be included in assessment and therapy, but there are some instances when this is not feasible or desirable. The present case study provides an example of a client who did not wish her partner to be involved at the onset of intervention and did not want him to be aware of her attendance at the clinic. Although this situation may not be ideal, it is relatively common and the client's wishes should be respected. In many instances, significant benefits may be produced through therapy without the attendance of both partners. Indeed Ersner-Hershfield and Kopel (1979) found minimal difference in outcome in the treatment of female anorgasmia whether or not the partner was involved in therapy sessions.

The cognitive-behavioural interview

The interview can be divided into two main sections: (a) identification and specification of the presenting problem; and (b) identification of determinants of the problem. The first step in the assessment interview is to determine the exact nature of the problem and why the client is seeking help. In specifying the presenting problem, the assessor needs to identify exactly what the client does overtly, how he or she responds physiologically and what thoughts and emotions are experienced in the cognitive domain. It can therefore be determined whether the client's sexual response differs in any way from normal and whether a problem can be said to exist. In some instances the referral is a reflection of unrealistic expectations on the part of the client(s) which would be best dealt with by giving them appropriate information and reassurance. If a genuine dysfunction is evident, this first phase of the assessment permits identification of the exact stage of the sexual response at which the problem occurs, whether it be before sexual interaction begins (avoidance of sex, or lack of desire to engage in sexual activity), in the arousal stage or the orgasm phase. In addition, the components of the sexual problem, in terms of observable behaviours and physiological and cognitive responses, may be identified.

The second part of the interview aims to identify the historical and current determinants of the problem. The content of the interview therefore examines the many organic and psychosocial factors that are possible causes of sexual dysfunction and which may be manipulated during therapy to produce behaviour change. The interview should therefore examine health-related determinants and drug and alcohol use, in addition to the psychosocial factors outlined above.

Self-report assessment measures

A wide range of questionnaire measures are available to assist in the assessment of sexual dysfunction. Some of these are extensive and cover many aspects of sexual functioning. Others focus on specific areas, such as sexual arousal or sexual anxiety. Only those methods used in the present case will be described here.

The Bentler Scale (Bentler, 1967, 1968) is a measure of current sexual activity and assesses the frequency of occurrence of 21 heterosexual behaviours. It does not, however, assess whether the activities were satisfactory for those involved nor whether any sexual problems occurred. The Sexual Arousal Inventory (Hoon, Hoon & Wincze, 1976) is frequently used to assess sexual arousal in women. This involves a list of 28 sexual activities for which clients must rate the degree to which arousal is affected adversely or positively. A measure of marital satisfaction, the Dyadic Adjustment Scale (Spanier, 1976), was also used in the present case. This 32-item scale incorporates scales of consensus, satisfaction, cohesion and affectional (emotional) expression and a total score.

Case study

Assessment information

Personal information

Miriam referred herself to the University of Sydney's Badham Clinic complaining of a lifelong inability to experience orgasm under any circumstances. At the time of referral, Miriam was 28 years old. She was a physically attractive woman, always well dressed and neatly groomed. She had been married to 30-year-old Michael for the past 3.5 years and they had no children. Both partners were employed full-time in stable, clerical jobs in a government department and had left school at 18 years of age. They were buying their own home in the suburbs and did not have any financial worries. According to Miriam, they were not particularly ambitious and were content with their lifestyle. The couple did not plan to have children for several years and were using pessaries as a form of contraception. Attempts to use other forms of contraception had not proved to be satisfactory and fears of pregnancy did not appear to be an issue.

Miriam had lived in Sydney all her life and had a wide family and social network. She was the only child of parents who were both in their late 30s when she was born. She described her parents as having a good marital relationship but physical contact or expression of affection were minimal. Her parents were both devout Catholics and Miriam viewed them as conservative and inhibited, and yet supportive and kind. Personal and sexual issues were rarely, if ever, discussed. Miriam lived at home with her parents until she married Michael at the age of 25.

Miriam did not report any other problem areas in her life and did not exhibit any symptoms of anxiety disorder or depression. She appeared to be relatively happy and contented with other aspects of her life. Her interpersonal skills were good and she was able to communicate with the therapist in an open and skilled manner. Miriam did not report any medical conditions or drug usage and there was no history of excessive alcohol use. An examination by her medical practitioner failed to identify any biological causes for her lack of orgasm. It was, therefore, considered that a psychogenic aetiology was most likely.

Sexual history

Miriam reported a relatively uneventful sexual history. As a teenager, she had experienced several non-sexual romances and did not recall any sexual activity being involved. No incidents of sexual abuse, sexual violence or previous pregnancies were reported. Her education about sexual matters was acquired from girlfriends, novels and magazines. The local Catholic school that she attended did not provide any form of sex education. Until she was in her early twenties and read a magazine article on female sexuality, Miriam was unaware of what an orgasm was or that a woman could have one. She had never attempted to masturbate until this point and her attempts produced little pleasure and no orgasm. Feelings of guilt and general disappointment were experienced and Miriam did not attempt to masturbate again. Her first sexual experiences occurred with her husband prior to their marriage and these were reported to be enjoyable but did not lead to orgasm on her part. According to Miriam, both she and Michael did not have much idea about sexual techniques. Although she felt sexually aroused, there was minimal foreplay and Michael typically ejaculated very quickly in the early stages of their sexual relationship. With time, Michael's ability to control his ejaculation improved but Miriam reported that she began to find sexual activity unrewarding and distressing. Although the couple attempted to discuss Miriam's lack of orgasm and tried to use additional forms of sexual stimulation, such as oral sex, this was not successful in producing orgasm. Furthermore, Miriam reported feeling anxious and guilty about varying their sexual repertoire. The couple then sought treatment from a person described as a 'sex counsellor' who had prescribed the use of a vibrator. Therapy had not been successful and had resulted in conflict within the marital relationship. Miriam reported feeling a failure and humiliated. She was insistent that she did not wish her partner to be involved in the present treatment, nor for him to be aware of her attendance at the clinic.

In recent months, a set pattern of sexual activity had developed. Miriam and Michael engaged in sexual intercourse approximately once per week, generally on Saturday evenings. Careful questioning by the therapist revealed that sexual activity typically involved about 10 minutes of foreplay which was limited to touching of each others' genitals. This led on to 5–10 minutes of sexual intercourse which always involved the face-to-face position. Miriam did become lubricated, indicating that the physiological component of arousal was not problematic. She did not, however, experience strong subjective sensations of sexual arousal. Foreplay and intercourse was described as being moderately arousing, and left Miriam feeling disappointed and frustrated. She frequently avoided opportunities for sexual intercourse and stated that she felt 'obliged' to engage in sexual activities once per week in order to be fair to Michael.

Current sexual functioning

At the time of referral, Miriam reported being extremely dissatisfied with her sexual relationship. Miriam completed a modification of the Bentler Scale designed to assess sexual anxiety. This measure assessed degree of anxiety concerning a range of sexual activities, being rated from 1 (extremely anxious) to 5 (not at all anxious). Miriam's responses on this scale indicated considerable feelings of anxiety about foreplay and oral sex but not in relation to basic sexual intercourse. Further questioning revealed a dislike of touching semen, although ejaculation within the vagina did not produce negative feelings. Miriam reported many anxious thoughts relating to her ability to become aroused and reach orgasm during stimulation by her partner. These thoughts typically reflected concerns about her ability to reach orgasm and anticipation of failure ('What's wrong with me, there must be some reason why nothing happens?') or anticipating the likely thoughts of her partner ('He thinks I am useless in bed. I bet he wishes he had married someone else').

Miriam's responses to the Sexual Arousal Inventory (SAI) suggested a problem in the area of sexual arousal, with most sexual activities being rated as only slightly or moderately arousing. Her score on this measure (see table 5.1 on page 92) was more than one standard deviation below the mean score of 80.9 (s.d. = 22.7) reported by Hoon, Hoon and Wincze (1976) for a sample of women in the USA. It must be acknowledged that cultural and sample differences in response to the SAI are possible, which should be borne in mind in interpreting this result. When questioned further about arousal to clitoral stimulation by her partner, Miriam reported adequate lubrication. Her subjective feelings of arousal, however, were reported to be limited and were frequently inhibited by a range of negative, anxious thoughts as outlined above. Interfering and distracting thoughts were also reported which related to non-sexual topics, such as events that had occurred at work.

Miriam did not admit to engaging in sexual fantasies or to the use of erotic materials. When asked about her attitude towards such activities, Miriam stated that she considered them to be acceptable activities for other people to engage in, but 'did not feel right' about using sexual fantasies or erotic materials herself.

Quality of the marital relationship

The information provided from the interview and the Dyadic Adjustment Scale (DAS) indicated that Miriam was dissatisfied with her marriage. Spanier (1976) reported a mean total score of 114.8 (s.d. = 17.8) for the DAS with their sample of married couples. The main problem areas identified concerned differences in personal goals, lack of time spent together, lack of common interests and leisure activities, lack of expression of affection and being too tired for sex. Religion was also a source of dispute, Miriam being a practising Catholic and Michael, her husband, being agnostic. Further questioning revealed that both partners tended to work long hours and Michael played squash two to three evenings per week. Miriam tended to stay home on her own on these evenings or would visit friends or family. The couple rarely went out together to social events. Miriam reported that she found Michael physically attractive and she wanted very much for their relationship to succeed.

Case formulation

Miriam clearly met the criteria for DSM-III-R inhibited female orgasm which was a lifelong, global problem. She perceived her marital relationship as slightly unsatisfactory, with the major areas of dissatisfaction relating to the lack of shared quality time and positive experiences. This was a reflection of the minimal time that the couple spent together engaging in enjoyable activities and shared interests. Her emotional feelings towards Michael were essentially positive and she found him sexually attractive. Although she did not report any problems of sexual desire and lubrication occurred during sexual activity, it was noted that Miriam did not experience strong subjective feelings of arousal.

It was hypothesised that the level of cognitive and physical stimulation that Miriam was receiving was not sufficient to trigger orgasm as a result of either (a) insufficient intensity and duration of appropriate physical stimulation, (b) interfering cognitions relating to performance, (c) inadequate focusing of attention on sensations as the result of distracting cognitions, or (d) feelings of guilt and mild anxiety concerning sexual activities. Further, it was proposed that transfer of orgasm to coital situations and improvement in the couple's sexual relationship generally would be unlikely to occur unless the aspects of marital dissatisfaction were dealt with.

The treatment of inhibited female orgasm

The treatment of inhibited female orgasm has typically involved a masturbatory training approach (Heiman, Lo Piccolo & Lo Piccolo, 1976; Barbach, 1980). Such programs are based on the suggestion that orgasm in women is most likely to be experienced during self-stimulation and that the intense stimulation provided by a vibrator is the method most likely to produce orgasm. Furthermore, Barbach (1980) suggests that it is easier for a woman to establish orgasmic skills on her own to begin with and, once she is confident of being able to experience orgasm on her own, therapy may begin to generalise orgasmic skills to activities with the partner. The aim is then to teach the partner the skills necessary to trigger orgasm and to gradually generalise orgasm to intercourse situations.

The components of therapy are typically based upon the methods of systematic desensitisation (graded exposure to a hierarchy of anxiety-provoking situations while in a relaxed state), education regarding sexual anatomy and sexual responding, physical skill development and attitude change. The treatment of female orgasmic dysfunction generally begins with a discussion about attitudes related to sexual activities, sexuality and sexual responding. Information is provided about the female body, with home-based tasks including relaxation exercises, body viewing and touching of non-genital areas of the body, to determine what forms of touch are pleasurable. A ban is usually placed on attempts to achieve orgasm at this point in order to produce a non-demanding situation in which performance anxiety will be minimised. A series of exercises to tense and relax relevant muscles commonly known as Kegal exercises may also be used to increase awareness of sensations in the vaginal area. Information regarding anatomy and physiology is then provided, which involve the use of pictures of genitalia to enable the woman to identify the various parts and to demonstrate the wide variation in appearance. Education is provided about sexual responding and frequently-held misconceptions are discussed.

Therapy then moves on to discussion of myths, attitudes and methods about masturbation. Some therapists (for example, Barbach, 1980) use films to illustrate methods of masturbation and also as a form of desensitisation. The inclusion of film material does not appear to be crucial to the effectiveness of therapy (Spence, 1985). Methods of self-stimulation are then practised at home, although the aim at this point is not to progress to orgasm. Attempts are then made to increase attention to pleasurable feelings and to encourage the use of fantasies. Women are also asked to read erotic literature at home, prior to or during self-pleasuring, as a means of enhancing sexual arousal. The duration of sensual touching (self-stimulation) is gradually increased and clients are asked to experiment with different movements and positions to identify the most arousing forms of stimulation. Some therapists introduce the use of a vibrator at this point, given that a vibrator is suggested to be the most likely means of producing orgasm for women. For most clients, orgasm is experienced for the first time during this phase of therapy. With other women, it may be necessary to deal with various factors which may be inhibiting orgasm, such as fear of losing control, performance anxiety or negative cognitions about self-stimulation.

When orgasm has been experienced regularly through self-stimulation, intervention aims to generalise the occurrence of orgasm to situations which gradually become closer to intercourse. At first, the woman is asked to carry out her self-pleasuring exercises in front of her partner. This is designed to demonstrate the type of touch and stimulation that is needed to produce orgasm and also to teach the woman to feel relaxed and comfortable about having an orgasm in the presence of her partner. Many couples find this aspect of therapy difficult to accept and its inclusion may not always be appropriate.

The introduction of the partner into therapy usually commences with non-genital pleasuring exercises as outlined by Masters and Johnson (1970), followed by genital pleasuring tasks. These exercises aim to increase communication skills in relation to sexual matters and to provide a desensitisation experience to physical and sexual contact. Intervention may then move on to prolonged genital pleasuring in an attempt to produce orgasm from partner stimulation. Alternatively, the woman may be instructed to practise self-pleasuring during intercourse. The couple are advised to select a position in which the clitoral area is easily accessible. Once orgasm can be reached in this situation, clitoral self-stimulation is stopped just before the point of orgasm, allowing orgasm to be triggered by vaginal stimulation from thrusting. The aim is then to gradually stop the clitoral stimulation earlier in the sequence, until orgasm may be triggered by the movements of intercourse, following less direct clitoral stimulation. In practice, only a minority of couples appear to reach this stage of orgasmic ability and the majority are required to rely upon direct clitoral stimulation from the partner, from self-pleasuring or from the use of a vibrator (Spence, 1985).

Although there have been many attempts to evaluate the effectiveness of treatments for inhibited female orgasm, it is difficult to draw firm conclusions regarding outcome given the variation in the criteria to determine success. Some studies have used subjective ratings of satisfaction with the sexual relationship to define successful outcome whereas others have used various measures of orgasmic ability. These have ranged from the single occurrence of orgasm (the woman is then technically no longer anorgasmic), to the ability to achieve orgasm by any means (including use of a vibrator), or to the ability to achieve orgasm during coitus with penile thrusting alone. Some authors such as Wakefield (1987) have suggested that the generally accepted definition of successful orgasm held by most of the adult population would refer to orgasm which is triggered through penile thrusting alone and not to orgasm that occurs during intercourse that is triggered by simultaneous use of a vibrator. Views such as this have led other authors (for example, Wilcox & Hager, 1980) to point out that the vast majority of women require some form of clitoral stimulation in order to experience orgasm during intercourse and that to aim for orgasm through penile thrusting alone is frequently unrealistic.

Several studies have demonstrated that masturbatory training approaches can be successful in triggering orgasm for the first time in previously anorgasmic women. The degree to which orgasm is then experienced consistently, and is generalised to partner stimulation or intercourse, is variable. For example, McMullen and Rosen (1979) found that 24 of the 40 therapy clients who participated in a masturbatory training program experienced orgasm by post-treatment. However, only 13 out of the 40 women were able to attain orgasm during intercourse (by any means). Both approaches to treatment produced improvements in sexual attitudes, adjustment and responsiveness. This study illustrates the relative difficulty in generalising orgasm to intercourse situations, with the results being in keeping with those of Spence (1985) who found that only 5 out of 17 anorgasmic women successfully generalised orgasm to intercourse by the end of treatment or during the three-month follow-up period (using any additional means of stimulation).

Wakefield (1987) presented an extremely critical review of two early studies by Wallace and Barbach (1974) and Ersner-Hershfield and Kopel (1979) which claimed exceedingly impressive results in terms of the proportion of women achieving orgasm and being able to generalise this to intercourse. Wakefield pointed out that both of these studies included some women who were technically not anorgasmic in the sense of never having experienced orgasm. He also noted that both studies accepted orgasm by any means during partner-related activities as being successful generalisation. This could include self-stimulation with a vibrator while the partner is watching, which Wakefield suggested is not what the majority of the population would consider to be a successful outcome with the partner. Wakefield re-analysed the results of the Ersner-Hershfield study to exclude those women who were technically already orgasmic and to separate out different forms of sexual activity with the partner. This re-analysis showed that 14 out of 15 women experienced orgasm by some means following treatment. However, even by follow-up, only 3 out of 15 women were able to experience orgasm during partner-manual stimulation and no women were orgasmic during coitus, even if self- or partner-stimulation was used. It seems therefore, that generalisation of orgasmic skills to coitus is relatively difficult to achieve using traditional masturbatory training approaches.

The effectiveness of masturbatory training has been compared with a traditional Masters and Johnson approach and has been shown to be superior in producing orgasm (Riley & Riley, 1978). Similarly, masturbatory training has been found to be more effective than systematic desensitisation in the treatment of primary orgasmic dysfunction (Andersen, 1981).

Content of therapy

The therapy program used in the present case study involved an adaptation of the masturbatory training approach outlined above. This form of intervention was selected given the evidence that it is highly effective in producing the experience of orgasm during self-stimulation. It was recognised, however, that generalisation of orgasm to partner stimulation and intercourse may be more difficult to achieve using this method, or indeed any other method available. Thus, the initial goal of therapy was to generate orgasm during self-stimulation, with specific attempts being made to generalise orgasm to partner and intercourse situations in the later stages of the program. The therapy program selected had several aims. First, it was designed to increase sexual arousal levels through increased physical and cognitive stimulation. Increased physical stimulation was achieved through education regarding methods of self- and partner-stimulation and the use of a vibrator. Cognitive stimulation was increased through training in sexual fantasy skills and encouragement in the use of mild erotic literature. Attention-focusing skills were also taught in order to increase awareness of sexual sensations. Second, therapy dealt with those factors which were proposed to inhibit sexual arousal or to reduce the probability that orgasm would occur. 'Cognitive restructuring' methods were used to reduce maladaptive and interfering cognitions. Similarly, graduated exposure and relaxation methods were included in order to reduce anxiety and feelings of guilt regarding sexual responding. Finally, an important focus of therapy was to increase couple communication skills and enhance the marital relationship generally. This was considered important to increase affection toward the spouse, to reduce inhibiting negative thoughts about the partner and to develop the intimate communication skills necessary to enable the couple to learn to transfer orgasm to intercourse situations.

The first phase of therapy involved eight weekly sessions which Miriam attended on her own. In the initial session, Miriam was given a copy of Heiman, Lo Piccolo and Lo Piccolo (1976), *Becoming Orgasmic: A Sexual Growth Programme for Women*. It was necessary to adapt the program outlined in this text somewhat, given that Miriam was adamant that she did not want her partner involved in therapy. The first session discussed sexual responding, what is normal to expect and the myths of female sexual behaviour. It was stressed that lack of orgasm is relatively common, but that high expectations could be held for successful outcome from the program. The home readings covered sexual anatomy, exploring one's sexual history and looking at one's own genital areas in a mirror in order to identify the relevant parts. In addition to an educational purpose, these tasks also provide steps towards anxiety reduction relating to sight and touch of one's own genital areas. Subsequent sessions included relaxation training, practice of Kegal exercises as outlined above and gradual introduction of sensual touching (self-pleasuring). These exercises revealed that Miriam held a range of negative attitudes and beliefs regarding touching of her own genitals, their appearance and the acceptability of self-stimulation. Home-based self-monitoring was used to identify specific irrational or maladaptive thoughts which were suggested to inhibit sexual arousal to sensual touching. These thoughts were subject to discussion during the therapy sessions, with instructions to continue 'cognitive challenging' at home. For example, Miriam identified several negative thoughts such as 'I don't like looking at myself down there. It's just not natural to be doing this' and 'I shouldn't have to do this to myself in order to feel sexy. There is definitely something wrong with me'. Discussion of information relating to the frequency of self-stimulation among women and the statistics relating to the significant number of women who are unable to experience orgasm from partner stimulation only was helpful in challenging these maladaptive thoughts. The therapist avoided imposing her own values at this point, but gave Miriam an opportunity to evaluate the rationality of her thoughts and beliefs in the face of factual information about female sexual behaviour.

To enhance levels of sexual arousal, Miriam was trained in the use of fantasy skills and asked to read mild erotic short stories at home. She was also instructed to focus her attention on bodily sensations, initially while touching non-sexual body parts and later on the sensations produced by genital massage at home. The training of fantasy skills commenced with non-sexual imagery prior to instructions to practise sexual fantasy content at home. Within the therapy session, Miriam expressed some reluctance about engaging in sexual fantasy and reading the erotic stories as a homework exercise. The therapist explained that sexual fantasy and use of erotic materials is relatively common amongst women. Once reassured, Miriam was able to carry out her homework tasks successfully. During the homework assignments relating to touching of her genital areas, Miriam initially reported very few pleasurable sensations, even when she used a massage lotion. She did not find the feelings unpleasurable, but described them as 'nothing much', although she did experience vaginal lubrication. Reading the erotic stories was more successful in producing feelings of sexual arousal and Miriam reported feeling some pleasurable sensations when she combined genital massage with sexual fantasy or reading of the erotic literature.

Miriam was then asked to vary the type of physical stimulation used during genital massage in order to identify the most arousing methods. Once this stage was reached, by session four, Miriam was instructed to use a vibrator at home for a short period only, alternating with manual forms of clitoral stimulation. Interestingly, Miriam was not repelled by the vibrator and in some ways preferred its use to direct physical contact. She reported thinking that the use of a machine was more acceptable to her than actually touching herself and she was able to feel strong, pleasurable sensations when she used the vibrator after reading erotic stories.

The duration of vibrator stimulation was increased for the home-based assignment following session five. At this point, Miriam reported experiencing orgasm for the first time, using the vibrator. Over the next two weeks, Miriam reported achieving orgasm on several occasions with the vibrator, but not from self-manual stimulation. She still reported some negative thoughts about touching her own genitals but interestingly was accepting of vibrator or partner stimulation. At this point, Miriam agreed to inform her partner about her attendance at the clinic and to ask him to participate in her home-based assignments. Miriam continued to insist that she did not wish her husband to attend the clinic, despite suggestions from the therapist that his attendance would be helpful. Michael was enthusiastic and supportive when Miriam asked him to participate in home-based tasks, the first of which consisted of non-genital pleasuring. The therapist produced written guides which Miriam took home to Michael at the end of her therapy sessions and the couple was asked to provide a written summary of their homework experiences. Very briefly, each partner was instructed to take turns in the giving and receiving of sensual massage to non-genital areas. Based on the work of Masters and Johnson (1970) these exercises are designed to facilitate couple communication, to provide a desensitisation experience in a non-threatening and non-demanding situation and to provide an opportunity for each individual to learn about the types of stimulation preferred by their partner. Once these exercises had been completed, the couple progressed to genital pleasuring exercises. During these tasks, Miriam and Michael were asked to take turns in giving and receiving pleasure during touching of the genital areas. It was made clear that the aim was to concentrate on giving and experiencing pleasure and not to use the exercises as a preliminary to sexual intercourse. Miriam and Michael had no difficulty with these exercises, reporting them to be pleasurable and informative. During the genital massage tasks, Miriam reported pleasurable feelings of sexual arousal.

Given the evidence of dissatisfaction with non-sexual aspects of the marital relationship, home-based tasks were set which were designed to enhance the quality of the marriage. Initially, these tasks were very simple and included attempts to increase the amount of enjoyable time that the couple spent together, such as going out for a cheap meal, to a movie and for a walk in the Botanical Gardens. Michael agreed to participate in this approach and the tasks were reported to be pleasurable.

The Heiman, Lo Piccolo and Lo Piccolo (1976) program suggests that, once the woman is able to reach orgasm and the genital massage exercises have been completed with the partner, the woman should demonstrate to her partner how she produces orgasm. For Miriam, however, this suggestion was extremely anxiety provoking and aversive. It was therefore agreed that this aspect should be omitted and the genital pleasuring exercises should progress to include partner stimulation of longer duration and partner use of the vibrator. In response to this task, Miriam reported experiencing orgasm through partner-manual stimulation and during coitus with Michael using the vibrator. At this point, the therapist suggested that Miriam ask Michael if he would be willing to attend two therapy sessions at the clinic. Although considerable progress had been made with Miriam attending sessions on her own and involving Michael in the later home-based assignments, it seemed important that both partners should be involved in attempts to generalise orgasmic ability to include self- or partner-stimulation during intercourse. Miriam expressed a desire to be able to experience orgasm during intercourse without having to use the vibrator. In the first of these sessions, the therapist pointed out that it is relatively uncommon for women to be able to experience orgasm without some form of additional clitoral stimulation during intercourse and that Miriam was not in any way unusual. Hence, the goal of orgasm through vaginal stimulation alone was suggested to be a secondary goal, and therapy should not be regarded as a failure if this goal could not be reached. The aim of therapy at this stage was presented as an attempt for the couple to produce orgasm through partner- or self-manual stimulation during coitus.

Given that Miriam could reach orgasm through partner stimulation during the genital pleasuring exercises, a home-based program was drawn up which attempted to transfer the skill of orgasm to intercourse. It was suggested that the couple engage in partner stimulation, with penetration being attempted just prior to orgasm. The couple were then instructed to gradually bring penetration forward earlier in the sequence of partner stimulation. Unfortunately, this method was not successful in producing orgasm during intercourse and penetration appeared to inhibit the occurrence of orgasm, unless vibrator stimulation was used. Miriam was unable to identify specific interfering thoughts which could be proposed to inhibit orgasm, arousal levels during intercourse were reported to be high and partner stimulation was reported to be pleasurable and appropriate. Hence, it was unclear exactly why Miriam did not experience orgasm during coitus without the use of the vibrator. Miriam continued to feel discomfort at touching her own genitals and was reluctant to try this as a means of producing orgasm during intercourse. At this point, the couple decided to end therapy, feeling that they had made satisfactory progress and had developed a satisfactory sexual relationship. Although orgasm during intercourse without the use of vibrator stimulation of the clitoris remained an important longer term goal for the couple, they did not wish to attend further therapy sessions, feeling that they were now able to manage their own intervention.

Michael's attendance at the clinic in the latter two sessions provided an opportunity to conduct problem-solving, 'role-playing' exercises in which unresolved areas of conflict could be discussed. For example, an important area of dissatisfaction for Miriam was the amount of time that Michael spent at work, playing sport or socialising with friends in the evenings or at weekends, leaving her on her own. With only minor prompting about basic problem-solving and communication skills, the couple were able to express their feelings about this problem and to suggest possible solutions. A compromise was reached in which Miriam identified recreational activities that she could participate in on her own, the couple agreed to take turns to organise at least one joint social activity each week, while Michael agreed to limit his sporting or social evenings to two per week. Other problems relating to the distribution of home duties and decision making were dealt with in a similar way.

Outcome of therapy

Miriam completed all assessment measures before treatment, at the end of the eight sessions which she attended on her own and three months after Michael had attended the two therapy sessions with her.

Orgasmic activity

In the two-week period following the eight sessions in which Miriam was seen on her own, she reported having reached orgasm on three occasions. Two of these occasions involved stimulation with a vibrator, with one occasion resulting from partner stimulation. Furthermore, Miriam experienced orgasm on all three occasions of sexual intercourse, with Michael using the vibrator. Miriam reported being unable to experience orgasm through self-stimulation without a vibrator, although she had attempted to do so on several occasions.

By the three-month follow-up, which included two sessions attended jointly by the couple, Miriam reported being able to experience orgasm through self-stimulation without the vibrator and the couple were using the vibrator to produce orgasm during coitus. In the two weeks of monitoring at the three-month follow-up, Miriam reported engaging in intercourse with her husband five times, and experienced orgasm with a vibrator on four of these occasions. She was not able, however, to reach orgasm during intercourse with partner or by self-stimulation of the clitoris or through vaginal stimulation alone. Nevertheless, Miriam reported being much more satisfied with her sexual relationship.

Table 5.1: Response to assessment questionnaires at pre-treatment, post-treatment (8 sessions) and 3–month follow-up

	Pre-treatment	Post-treatment	3–month follow-up
Dyadic Adjustment Scale	81	108	110
Bentler Sexual Behaviour Inventory	37	58	74
Sexual Arousal Inventory	52	60	72
Sexual Anxiety Inventory	65	87	90

Overall sexual activity

Following individual treatment, Miriam reported an increase in the frequency and range of sexual interactions with her husband as indicated by interview data and the increased scores on the Bentler Sexual Activity Inventory. This effect was further enhanced at the three-month follow-up. A marked increase in overall rating of satisfaction with the sexual relationship was reported, from a rating of 2 on a 7–point scale (1 = dissatisfied to 7 = satisfied) at pre-treatment, to 4 at post-individual treatment, and 5 at the three-month follow-up.

Sexual anxiety and attitudes

Miriam reported a marked reduction in anxiety levels relating to sexual activities at the end of the individual treatment period, which was maintained at the three-month follow-up. Anxiety levels declined in relation to a wide range of other situations which had previously produced anxiety, such as kissing of nipples and partner stimulation of the clitoris. She continued, however, to report high levels of anxiety in relation to oral or manual stimulation of her partner if it resulted in ejaculation. It was clear, therefore, that her dislike of direct contact with semen remained. Miriam stated that she did not wish to change her views with regard to contact with semen and her attitudes were not considered to be crucial to the progress of therapy. Her wishes were therefore respected, and no attempt was made to challenge these views. Interestingly, Miriam found oral and manual stimulation of her partner acceptable and non-threatening as long as it did not result in ejaculation *outside* the vagina. Ejaculation within the vagina was not perceived as unpleasant or anxiety-provoking.

Although Miriam had clearly improved in terms of reductions in sexual anxiety and increased orgasmic ability, she continued to report some feelings of guilt relating to sexual activities and still disliked touching her own genitals.

Sexual arousal levels

By the end of individual therapy, Miriam's score on the Sexual Arousal Inventory had increased slightly, with a further increase occurring by the three-month follow-up (see table 5.1). Despite this increase, the majority of stimuli on the SAI were rated as only slightly or moderately arousing rather than very or extremely arousing. From a clinical perspective, therefore, this improvement was marginal. Even though Miriam reported being better able to focus her attention on sexual feelings and enjoyed sexual activities, she did not experience such events as highly arousing. The physiological responses of sexual arousal, such as lubrication, were reported to be satisfactory prior to intervention and remained so.

Quality of the marital relationship

The post-treatment and follow-up assessments showed a marked improvement in Miriam's overall rating of marital satisfaction. Interestingly, this improvement occurred during the individual therapy phase, prior to the joint sessions in which communication skills and problem-solving skills were taught. In particular, the couple were spending more time together, sharing responsibilities and decisions, quarrelled less often and communicated with each other more often. These benefits may reflect the increase in enjoyable time spent together or the sensate focus (sensual pleasuring) exercises, all of which were instigated by Miriam in sessions seven and eight. At the three-month follow-up, Miriam rated her marriage as extremely happy. Michael did not complete formal marital evaluation measures but reported that he perceived a considerable improvement in the quality of their relationship.

Summary

In summary, the outcome of therapy was successful in several respects. First, the quality of the couple's general relationship improved markedly from the perspectives of both partners. Overall satisfaction with the sexual relationship also improved and the frequency and range of sexual activities increased. The client reported a considerable decrease in anxiety concerning sexual activities and a reduction in the degree of guilt experienced in relation to sexual behaviour. In terms of orgasmic responding, the effectiveness of therapy is debatable, according to the criteria taken for success. Certainly, Miriam was able to experience orgasm in a range of situations, through partner- and self-manual stimulation and use of a vibrator. The couple were not able, however, to generalise this to intercourse situations except with the use of the vibrator. Whether this aspect of outcome can be classed as successful depends on whether one considers orgasm from penile thrusting alone to be a realistic goal for all women. Certain authors have suggested that a normal distribution of ease of attaining orgasm may exist for women, reflecting inherent constitutional factors, with some individuals unfortunately finding it much harder to experience orgasm than others, particularly through penile thrusting alone (for example, Derogatis et al., 1986). It would seem inappropriate to over-emphasise orgasm of this type as the primary target for intervention if this results in the clients' failure to attend to other pleasurable, positive outcomes that may have been achieved through therapy.

The therapy program used in the present study included a variety of components, each of which may have contributed to the relatively successful outcome. It is obviously not possible to determine which component was either necessary or sufficient to produce the changes observed. The approach taken was based on the outcome of the assessment process, with intervention being tailored to the needs of the client and subsequently her partner. This required the modification of existing package programs in order to take into account the specific characteristics of the case. For example, Miriam held strong beliefs about the unacceptability of certain sexual activities (for example, stimulating herself in front of her partner) which made it difficult to apply the standard approach outlined by Heiman, Lo Piccolo and Lo Piccolo (1976). Bearing in mind the comments of Brown and Sollod (1988), that therapy can frequently take place without requiring the modification of clients' attitudes towards specific sexual activities, it was decided to omit this aspect of the program. Similarly, the client's dislike of touching semen, either by hand or mouth, was not tackled given the client's reluctance to change in this area and the therapist's view that such beliefs were not preventing the client from attaining her therapy goal.

Although these attitudes were not tackled, considerable attention was paid to the cognitive restructuring of maladaptive thoughts and beliefs which were considered necessary to the progress of therapy. These maladaptive thoughts typically related to the client's concern over her ability to experience orgasm and her predictions of her partner's thoughts during sexual activity.

This case also illustrates the need for integration of interventions for both the sexual and non-sexual aspects of the couple's relationship. Again, it is not possible to separate out the relative contribution of the sexual and marital therapy components to the overall success of the program. It seems likely that the masturbatory training approach produced a specific effect upon the client's ability to experience orgasm in the first instance. Increasing the positive aspects of the couple's general relationship, however, is likely to play an important role in determining the satisfaction with the sexual relationship overall. Finally, the case demonstrates the feasibility of conducting sex therapy programs without requiring the attendance of both partners and yet illustrates the advantages that joint therapy can produce.

Murray J. Dyck
University of Central Queensland

6 Mood disorder

In considering a topic like depression — its description, causes and treatment — it is tempting to focus exclusively on all that has been learned about the disorder in recent years. Such a focus would, after all, not only help us to consolidate what we have learned, but also bolster our sense of professional self-efficacy, of having something worthwhile to offer the psychological marketplace. But if such a focus would be reassuring (and make my task of writing much easier), the result would also be highly misleading. Our understanding of depression is not so complete as we sometimes like to think.

The case that I have chosen to present is one that happens to illustrate several of the most pressing problems in contemporary depression research. It does so because it is typically untypical; if less 'messy' than some of the cases that clinicians meet on a regular basis, it is also not without its complications. In particular, this case highlights problems in how depression is diagnosed and how it is treated; these, in turn, may illustrate concerns about how depression is to be understood.

Before actually presenting the case, I provide brief reviews of several of the sub-literatures of depression. My aim in reviewing these literatures is not to be comprehensive or by any means exhaustive; rather, my aim is simply to underscore some of what remains unknown about depression.

The diagnosis of depression

The development of a consensual diagnosis: an overview

If asked to nominate an uncontroversial diagnostic category, many clinicians might nominate the *Diagnostic and Statistical Manual of Mental Disorders*, third edition, revised (DSM-III-R) diagnosis of Major Depression (American Psychiatric Association, 1987). It is certainly true that diagnosing depression is much less controversial than it was before the appearance of the first DSM-III. Those were the days when authors referred to the 'contemporary confusion' in the classification of depression (Kendell, 1976). Indeed, we can feel almost smug about just how far we have come since researchers were preoccupied with distinguishing between such quaint-sounding conditions as 'neurotic' and 'endogenous' depressions (Kiloh & Garside, 1963) or 'psychotic depressive' and 'involutional psychotic' reactions (Friedman et al., 1963).

From our present perspective, it is apparent that many of the old disputes concerning whether or not there are different subtypes of depression, and what the subtypes might be, were simply premature. Researchers had to first agree on whether a person was depressed before they could consider whether the depression was a response to life events (reactive/exogenous) or to things that were happening within the body (endogenous).

That agreement on a core concept of depression was possible was amply illustrated by studies showing that clinicians could agree on how severe a depression was even when they disagreed as to what type of depression it was (Beck et al., 1961). Further, despite substantial disagreement when deciding even between major diagnostic categories (Ward et al., 1962), clinicians could agree on the presence and severity of 'depression' within diagnostic categories such as schizophrenia that were ostensibly unrelated to depression (Beck et al., 1961). Thus, there was clear evidence for a unitary depression syndrome (a set of symptoms) that could be identified without regard to putative depression subtypes and other diagnostic entities.

That clinicians were able to agree on the severity of a depression suggests that they were using shared, if implicit, diagnostic criteria for the syndrome. The research that has since been devoted to improving the reliability and validity of the depression diagnosis can be regarded as an attempt to state explicitly those previously implicit criteria. What all of the innovative diagnostic systems proposed during the 1970s share with their offspring, the DSM-III-R criteria, is the aim of achieving the same consensus for defining the category of depression (among other diagnoses) that had already been achieved for defining the severity of depression.

How, then, is depression defined? The DSM-III-R makes use of Beck's early work on depression severity to define a depressed 'mood syndrome'. The first essential feature of a depressed mood syndrome is, obviously, either a depressed mood or a significantly decreased interest in life or the ability to enjoy life. In addition to one of these essential symptoms, a depressed mood syndrome may include significant weight loss or weight gain, disturbed sleep, restlessness or lethargy, loss of energy, feelings of worthlessness or guilt, difficulty in concentrating or in making decisions, and repeated thoughts of death or suicide. Five of these symptoms, always including either depressed mood or loss of interest, are required to define the depressed mood syndrome.

Once a depressed mood syndrome has been identified, the clinician determines whether criteria other than the presence of specific depression symptoms are also satisfied. For example, in addition to a person having a depressed mood syndrome, a diagnosis of Major Depressive Episode is made if (a) it cannot be shown that an organic or physical factor caused the problem, (b) the mood disturbance is not a normal grief reaction, (c) the person was not delusional or hallucinating during the times when mood symptoms were not prominent, and (d) the person did not already have schizophrenia or a similar disorder.

Current issues in the diagnosis of depression

Granted that the DSM-III-R diagnosis of Major Depression was intended to be consensual (and has been criticised for being consensual — Ban, 1987), does it then follow that the diagnostic problem is resolved? In a word, the answer is 'no' for at least two reasons. First, many of the issues that were suppressed two and three decades ago in the hope of achieving consensus about basic classifications are now resurfacing. And second, the appearance of consensus concerning the criteria for Major Depression was gained partly by an act of diplomacy. One historically important subtype, 'endogenous' depression, was artfully shifted from the Mood Disorders category to that of Organic Mental Syndromes and Disorders, where it appeared under the heading, Organic Mood Disorder, Depressed. The only reliable difference between an 'endogenous' depression and an 'organic' depression is that in an organic depression, the clinician is required to say what physical factor is believed to have caused the mood disturbance whereas in an endogenous depression, no specific physical factor is named.

Not all of the old diagnostic controversies are reappearing. Some traditional concepts of depression, such as 'neurotic' depression, are seemingly revived these days only so that they can be knocked down again (Klerman, 1985). Others, however, have proved remarkably resilient. For example, evidence for an 'endogenous' subtype within the major category of depression continues to accumulate from highly divergent kinds of studies (Andreasen et al., 1988; Duggan, Lee & Murray, 1991). But in addition to these old issues, the need to rethink the way in which depression is diagnosed is becoming more apparent for quite other reasons.

For example, recent articles suggest that the existing diagnostic consensus concerning major depression has never been as complete as is usually supposed (Farmer & McGuffin, 1989). In particular, the DSM-III-R diagnosis of Major Depression does not correspond with parallel diagnoses in other diagnostic systems (Philipp, Maier & Delmo, 1991a, 1991b). But one of the greatest challenges to the validity of the diagnosis of depression is the fact that the response to treatment of depressed people is unpredictable for individual cases. Perhaps some people don't respond to standard treatments for depression because their depressions are nonstandard? I shall return to the question of treatment-resistant depressions after briefly discussing organic depressions.

Organic mood disorders

The essential feature of an organic mood syndrome (in this case, depression) is 'a prominent and persistent depressed mood, resembling a Major Depressive Episode, that is due to a specific organic factor' (American Psychiatric Association, 1987, page 111). What is the difference between an organic and a major depression? The only difference is the presumption of a specific cause in the case of an organic depression. It is important to note that there are no symptoms specific to an organic mood disorder that would permit its reliable discrimination from major depression on empirical grounds; in other words, there is no observable difference between the two syndromes. Further, in almost all cases, the presumption of an aetiological role for some organic factor in the mood disorder is a matter for clinical judgement, an inevitable consequence of the absence of observable indicators of organic depressions.

The specification, in the DSM-III-R, of a class of causal factors necessary to make a given diagnosis is interesting because the DSM-III-R is usually touted as being atheoretical. However, the authors of the DSM-III-R argue that 'for some of the mental disorders, the aetiology or pathophysiologic processes are known,' and give the example of the 'Organic Mental Disorders' (American Psychiatric Association, 1987, page xxiii). Although it may well be the case that the aetiologies or causes of some organic mental disorders are known, it is an overstatement at best to suggest that the aetiology of depression is known.

Organic mood disorders are usually diagnosed when depression accompanies some identified medical illness, often one of the neurological disorders (Berrios & Samuel, 1987). And, indeed, depression is frequently associated with stroke (Parikh et al., 1988), Parkinson's Disease (Mayeux, 1990), Alzheimer's Disease (Burns, 1990), Multiple Sclerosis (Berrios & Quemada, 1990), tumour (Tanaghow, Lewis & Jones, 1989), and the neurological catch-all, 'old age' (Alexopoulos, 1989). The question that must be asked is whether an association between depression and some neurological disorders indicates a causal relationship between them, whether such a causal relationship is also to be inferred when depression is associated with other common or garden-variety physical disorders (Mai, 1989), and if the inference is not always to be made, on what grounds is it ever to be made? In other words, are we to make organic mood disorders an exception to the rule that correlation does not imply causation?

One reason why the diagnosis of organic mood disorder seems peculiar is that the DSM-III-R system is one which in any case 'permits the clinician to indicate any current physical disorder or condition that is potentially relevant to the understanding or management of the case. In some instances the condition may be aetiologically significant (for example, a neurologic disorder associated with Dementia)' (American Psychiatric Association, 1987, page 18). What this means is that the category of organic mood disorders is entirely redundant given the mood disorders category and judgements about presumed organic aetiology (Popkin, Tucker & Caine, 1989).

Clearly, the diagnosis of organic mood disorder serves no function other than to provide a form of official recognition to the idea of endogenous depression. Because it makes aetiological assumptions that are not borne out by evidence, it is a category that is inconsistent with the movement towards empirically-derived classifications, and should be discarded. This is not to suggest that organic depressions do not exist, only that there are no reliable means of distinguishing organic from non-organic depressions. Hence, there is no possibility that the category, as it stands, is valid. Indeed, the presence of the category of organic mood disorder is likely to impede the identification of a specific endogenous subtype by virtue of the fact that it confuses descriptive hypotheses with aetiological ones.

Unfortunately, there is small reason to hope that this diagnostic anomaly will soon be a thing of the past. Although among the possible changes to the diagnostic system canvassed in *DSM-IV Options Book: Work in Progress* (American Psychiatric Association, 1991) is the elimination of the Organic Mood Disorder category, its suggested replacement is a new category of Secondary Mood Disorder Due to a Non-psychiatric Medical Condition. Unless this new category refers to explicit methods for reliably identifying the disorder — other than correlation with a medical condition — nothing of substance will have been accomplished.

Treatment-resistant depression

If depression is a unitary syndrome, how is it that no treatment for depression is effective in more than about two-thirds of cases (Ban, 1987)? Although it has already been established that individual difference factors (for example, the presence of a personality disorder) reduce the effectiveness of all depression treatments (Shea et al., 1990), the usual inference is that because depression is sometimes resistant to treatment, the existence of at least two depression subtypes (treatment-responsive and treatment-resistant) is presupposed (Ban, 1987; Nierenberg & Amsterdam, 1990). Although the presupposition is not warranted at a time when we are uncertain about what makes any treatment of depression effective, it has had the salutary effect of stimulating research into those patient characteristics, including specific symptoms, that might differentially predict treatment outcome.

For the most part, the attempt to distinguish signs that predict treatment outcome has not been successful. For example, although certain hormone levels vary among diagnostic groups, systematic differences tend not to be related to outcome (Krasnov & Kohanenko, 1989). Although there are correlations between the amounts of various chemicals in the nervous system and treatment outcome (Petit & Dollfus, 1986), the correlations are likely the result of the drugs that are used to treat depression; anti-depressant drugs affect both the concentration of chemicals in the nervous system and a person's symptoms (Ban, 1987). In this respect, not much has changed in the quarter-century since researchers tried to identify the symptoms that would predict response to electroconvulsive therapy (Carney, Roth & Garside, 1965).

Cognitive theory and the diagnosis of depression

Apart from his work in developing an index of depression severity (Beck et al., 1961), one of Beck's most enduring contributions to depression research has been his focus on cognitive symptoms as a means of describing a depression syndrome and as a potential means of discriminating depression from other syndromes (Beck, 1963, 1964, 1987). Beck argues that depression is a thought disorder that is distinguishable from other disorders in terms of the characteristic thought form and content expressed by depressed people. Briefly, depressed people inevitably exhibit repetitive, unintended thoughts reflecting themes of loss and revealing negative views of the self, the world and the future. This kind of thinking is believed to typify all depressions; the extent to which a person demonstrates such thinking predicts the severity of other depression symptoms.

Cognitive symptoms have not been emphasised in the major diagnostic systems. In the DSM-III-R, cognitive symptoms of depression include only 'feelings of worthlessness or excessive or inappropriate guilt', 'diminished ability to think or concentrate', and 'recurrent thoughts of death' (American Psychiatric Association, 1987, page 222). Should cognitive symptoms be given greater emphasis?

Research evaluating cognitive descriptive hypotheses indicates that some cognitive characteristics of depression are by now so well established that they might be regarded as defining characteristics of depression. In particular, negative thinking about one's self and biases favouring 'mood-congruent recall' (a tendency to remember things that are consistent with one's mood, in this case, sad things when one is sad) and an extremely negative outlook are each basic to depression (see Haaga, Dyck & Ernst, 1991, for a review).

If certain cognitive symptoms are common to all depressions, it might appear to follow that cognitive theorists would oppose the notion of depression subtyping. But although negative cognitions as measured by such tests as the Automatic Thoughts Questionnaire (Hollon, Kendall & Lumry, 1986) are equivalent across unipolar and bipolar depression (Hollon, Kendall & Lumry, 1986), 'primary' and 'secondary' depression (Norman, Miller & Klee, 1983), 'endogenous' and 'nonendogenous' depression (Eaves & Rush, 1984), and 'melancholic' and 'nonmelancholic' depression (Norman, Miller & Keitner, 1987), cognitive theory supports the notion of subtyping.

There are two main reasons for maintaining a willingness to subtype depressions. The first reason is the belief that depression can result from different precipitating causes. Cognitive theory purports to explain non-endogenous depressions (Beck, 1987); thus, the possibility of eventually distinguishing among depressions on the basis of their distinct aetiologies is left open. Second, however, Beck (1983; Beck, Epstein & Harrison, 1983) has argued that at least two subtypes of major depression (a sociotropic or dependent depression and an autonomous or self-critical depression) can already be distinguished empirically, that is, in terms of systematic differences in depression symptoms. These differences, for which there is as yet scant evidence (Dyck & Stewart, 1991), are thought to be related to personality characteristics (Beck, Epstein & Harrison, 1983).

The treatment of depression

If there is one question that was decisively answered during the last decade, it is whether psychological therapies are effective in the treatment of depression: they are (Dobson, 1989; Elkin et al., 1989). In fact, it isn't entirely tongue-in-cheek for me to suggest that a more interesting question is: what treatment might not be effective for depression? For example, not only is pill-placebo plus clinical management an effective treatment (Elkin et al., 1989), Ban (1987) reminds us that the combination of a warm bath and moral treatment (exhortations to 'get on with life') was known to be an effective therapy for 70 per cent of depressed in-patients as early as 1813.

One answer to the question of which treatments are ineffective is easily provided. All treatments are ineffective in approximately one-third of cases; no treatment, pharmaceutical or psychological, has been found to be significantly more effective than the drug Imipramine was shown to be in the first major review of controlled studies (Klerman & Cole, 1965). As suggested above, this utterly consistent result has been one of the major reasons why some people have wondered whether those depressions that resist initial treatment might be essentially different from those that respond to initial treatment. This result has also prompted research concerned with evaluating therapies for treatment-resistant depression.

Biological treatments for treatment-resistant depression

If nothing else, biological approaches to treatment-resistant depression are noteworthy for their variety. The range of treatments on offer includes anaesthetic-induced electrocerebral silence (Langer et al., 1985), electroconvulsive therapy (Allen, 1984), periodic sleep deprivation (Dessauer, Goetze & Tolle, 1985), amphetamines (Linet, 1989) and a potpourri of drug combinations (Price, Charney & Heninger, 1987; Charney, Price & Heninger, 1986; Deicken, 1987). These treatments have not been evaluated in controlled trials and none appears especially promising. The two biological treatments that have received most attention have been lithium augmentation therapy (where the drug lithium is added to some other drug treatment) and thyroid hormone augmentation therapy (where thyroid hormone is added to another medicine).

Although strong claims for the effectiveness of lithium augmentation in the treatment of resistant depressions are regularly made (Chalmers & Cowen, 1990; Poirier & Benkelfat, 1986), the evidence to support these claims is remarkably weak. The problems with the evidence are several. First, the treatment itself is highly variable; the drug lithium (most commonly used as a treatment for mania, one expansive mood disorder that often accompanies depression) is as likely to be added to a 'standard' anti-depressant drug as to an 'experimental' one (Ontiveros, Fontaine & Elie, 1991; Pope, McElroy & Nixon, 1988), or even to a drug used for some other condition (Kramlinger & Post, 1989). In other words, lithium augmentation is anything but a specific treatment. Second, treatment histories tend to be remarkably complex and varied. For example, in reporting on the effectiveness of one lithium combination, Price, Charney and Heninger (1985) report that the patients had already received two weeks of treatment with a placebo (an inert substance) then four weeks of another drug. When lithium augmentation had failed, the patients were treated with still other drug combinations. Third, as may be typical of new treatments, there is a tendency to report only what works rather than what doesn't. But, in many cases, there are clear failures of recommended treatments that occur prior to the eventual 'success'. Finally, where there is an attempt to impose reasonable methodological controls on the study of lithium augmentation, the results show minimal effectiveness for the treatment, with complete symptom remission in only about 15 per cent of cases (Kantor et al., 1986).

When it comes to thyroid hormone augmentation therapy, there are two essential points to be made. First, in general, the evidence supporting the treatment is no better than is the case for lithium (Cooke, 1990; Extein & Gold, 1988; Hullett & Bidder, 1983). However, unlike lithium, there is a strong rationale for using thyroid hormone in some depressions.

The rationale for the use of thyroid hormone is that not only is there an established relationship between hypothyroidism and depression symptoms (Norman, Sartor & McIntyre, 1988), among depressed patients who do not respond to treatment, approximately one-third have been found to have a form of thyroid dysfunction (Gewirz et al., 1988; Targum et al., 1984). The patients responding to thyroid hormone augmentation are those with thyroid dysfunction (Gewirz et al., 1988; Targum et al., 1984).

Cognitive therapy for treatment-resistant depression

Research evaluating cognitive therapy as a treatment for drug-refractory depressions differs from that evaluating biological interventions in several respects. Besides being substantially fewer in number, cognitive therapy outcome studies are not based on single case reports, are much more standardised and controlled in their methods, and much more cautious in their interpretation of results.

Based on the four studies that I have been able to locate, cognitive therapy results in complete remission of symptoms in between 20 (Fennell & Teasdale, 1982) and 40 per cent of cases (Antonuccio et al., 1984; see also Harpin et al., 1982). Partial or complete remission was observed in at least 60 per cent of cases. When cognitive therapy was combined with standard pharmacotherapy, complete improvement was noted in 67 per cent of cases, and all cases showed at least partial remission of symptoms (Miller et al., 1985). These results, unimpressive though they be, suggest that cognitive therapy is as or more effective than any biological intervention in the treatment of drug-refractory depression.

Summary of depression treatments

There is abundant evidence that many treatment approaches are effective for most depressed people, but each of these approaches is unsuccessful in treating a significant minority of cases. These treatment failures, or refractory cases, also generally fail to respond to second and third treatment attempts. Research reports of specific therapies for these refractory cases are highly 'exploratory' in character; they lack the methodological controls necessary to draw sound inferences about the specific elements of a treatment that may have been responsible for the occasional success. It is therefore not possible to conclude that any treatment is consistently more effective than any other treatment for initially refractory cases.

Case study

Notwithstanding the fact that controlled clinical trials have indicated that cognitive therapy for depression (Beck et al., 1979) is an effective treatment (Dobson, 1989), there has been considerable reluctance among clinicians to prescribe cognitive therapy for depressions associated with organic pathology. Indeed, Beck et al. (1979) list 'organic brain syndromes' among the conditions for which cognitive therapy alone is not indicated. This was a peculiar position to adopt, for there has never been an adequate a priori reason to doubt its efficacy in such cases. Just as an association between medical illness and depression does not mean that the former is a cause of the latter, the simple presence of 'biological' pathology does not preclude the effectiveness of a 'psychological' therapy.

Fortunately, several researchers have ignored the advice of Beck et al. (1979) and evaluated the effectiveness of cognitive therapy in cases of depression that were associated with various forms of medical illness. Apart from case studies illustrating the potential applicability of cognitive therapy to a range of illness-related mood problems (Bates, Burns & Moorey, 1989; Lustman, Kulkarni & Amado, 1983), two controlled studies have also been reported. Davis et al. (1984) report the successful treatment of depressed epileptics, and Larcombe and Wilson (1984) report the successful treatment of depressed people suffering from multiple sclerosis, in both cases with short-term cognitive-behavioural therapy.

There is evidence that cognitive therapy is no less effective than biological treatments in cases of drug-resistant depression (Antonuccio et al., 1984), and evidence that cognitive therapy is effective in treating depressions associated with physical, and in particular neurological, illness (Davis et al., 1984). Might cognitive therapy also be effective in cases where depression associated with organic pathology does not respond to standard biological treatments?

A case history

Happily married and the doting father of six children, pleased with his position as purchasing coordinator for a large international industrial concern, well-ensconced in an upmarket suburb, John Boxton seemed to have everything. At least, he once seemed to have everything. Things had changed markedly by the time John first came to the university research clinic for a preliminary assessment. One of the problems the 55-year-old John faced was that he had been given his retrenchment notice. Why? The company had decided that the quality of John's work just wasn't what it had been before his neurosurgery.

History of the organic disorder

Approximately two and a half years before coming to our clinic, John had been experiencing symptoms that are usually associated with allergy. As part of a medical evaluation to determine whether his sinuses were inflamed, John underwent a series of head scans (known as computerised axial tomography or CT scan, for short). The scans revealed a tumour in the right lateral ventricle (a storage area for the cerebrospinal fluid or CSF, a liquid that bathes the entire central nervous system) that was blocking the foramen of Monro (a channel through which CSF passes) and causing early hydrocephalus (which literally means 'water brain,' in this case an enlarging of the ventricles due to the damming of the CSF). The tumour, subsequently diagnosed as benign, was removed. Surgical notes indicate that John's skull was opened and that it was necessary to split his corpus callosum, the main bundle of nerve fibres connecting the right and left halves of his brain, in order to reach the tumour. Post-operative brain scans indicated bleeding in the right frontal region of John's brain after surgery.

Following surgery, John was plagued by a series of medical complications. Not long after his discharge from hospital, he developed a severe bacterial infection of the skull, an infection which proved very resistant to treatment. Time after time the infection would be treated, only to return shortly after treatment was stopped; even a return to hospital for intravenous antibiotics ultimately proved futile. Finally, about 11 months after his operation, a decision was made to remove the area of John's skull that was carrying the bacteria. That seemed to do the trick: with the offending piece of bone gone, the infection was at last eliminated. It was then only necessary to replace the missing bone with an acrylic plate, a procedure that was completed 18 months after the initial operation. There have been no additional medical complications since the acrylic plate was fitted.

When John arrived at our clinic, he was required to undergo an independent neuropsychological evaluation before receiving treatment. Although John had undergone a limited neuropsychological evaluation six months after his first operation, an evaluation that had yielded 'no scores in the impaired range of functioning', the history of skull infection increased the chance that John had suffered brain damage in addition to that caused by the tumour and the surgery.

The results of the neuropsychological assessment were not encouraging. The psychologists who conducted the assessment concluded that John had 'mild to moderate cerebral dysfunction, right hemisphere worse than left'. A loss of function in the right half of John's brain was shown by 'lower scores on Performance IQ subtests than Verbal IQ subtests, markedly worse visual than verbal memory, slower fine motor speed with the left hand, and poorer coordination with that hand. [Note: John writes with his left hand.] Several tests tapping frontal lobe functioning [tasks involving planning] were also performed poorly. John's scores on tests of conceptual flexibility were well below expectations based upon his IQ subtest scores, and he had difficulty developing and maintaining effective problem-solving strategies on these tests. Scores on tests of visual attention were deficient; . . . verbal fluency was also impaired'.

The results of the neuropsychological assessment clearly indicate that John was showing symptoms consistent with brain injury. What is interesting, however, is that the neuropsychologists attribute not only John's cognitive and motor symptoms to the brain injury, but his emotional symptoms as well. Their report concludes: 'Although reactive depression might be expected following neurosurgery and a decrease in cognitive functioning, there is good evidence to suggest that the bulk of John's affective disorder can be ascribed to changes in brain function.'

History of the affective disorder

Prior to surgery, John had no personal or family history of emotional disorder, other psychiatric disorder or neurological impairment. To the contrary, John appears to have enjoyed a remarkably benign life — with just a few sparks of excitement thrown in to maintain a kind of balance — before the development of the tumour.

True, John's beginnings were less than auspicious. Born one month prematurely, he was not expected to live. But medical opinions are sometimes wrong, and so they proved to be in John's case, for not only did he live, he thrived. John describes a pleasant childhood and adolescence marked by a positive, if somewhat distant, relationship with his father, an assembly line worker, and a closer relationship with his mother, a building manager. School was not a problem for John, and he graduated from high school nudging a 'straight-A' average.

Following his school graduation, John continued his education, earning a science degree in chemistry before joining the armed forces. It was during his time in the forces that two memorable events occurred: the first was when he married Margaret, the second was when he was forced to eject from his crashing jet fighter. John's attitude to these two events can be deduced from the fact that although he resigned from the military, he and Margaret are still together.

The first recorded sign that John might be experiencing emotional problems came soon after his operation. It was during a routine bedside neurological examination that a surgeon first noticed constricted affect, an absence of emotional expression, in John's appearance. However, nothing was made of this symptom; John was discharged from hospital and before long he had returned to work.

Work was a problem. To begin with, the recurring skull infection meant that John frequently had to take leave from his duties, which meant that he quickly fell behind in his work, and was confronted with a growing backlog of chores each time he returned to his desk. The problem was complicated by the fact that John was finding the work itself difficult: his memory for recent events seemed to be impaired, he had difficulty concentrating and he made errors, sometimes serious errors. John's standard of work was clearly not what it had been.

Things came to a head some five months after his operation when John irretrievably lost some important data from his computer. The significance of this loss was due not only to the intrinsic importance of the data, but to what the mistake implied about John's post-operative capacity. John had always been something of a computer whiz, and so for him to make basic errors suggested that something was seriously wrong. John responded with what he calls a 'complete nervous breakdown'.

John stopped working and was referred to a psychiatrist for treatment. At the first psychiatric interview, John complained that 'I feel awful most of the time; I feel like everything useful is over. I can't relate to members of my family, I don't know where I stand with others'. John admitted that he had been feeling depressed for some time, indeed, ever since his return to work. He had been preoccupied with his work performance, and wondered whether he hadn't been trying too hard. But there were other symptoms besides the depressed mood and the concern about work; John was agitated, had difficulty concentrating, had difficulty sleeping, was often irritable or bored, appeared to have flat affect, and would have frequent crying spells. On the basis of these symptoms, and in the absence of any indication that John was experiencing hallucinations or delusions, the psychiatrist made a diagnosis of Major Depressive Episode, Severe, Without Psychosis. In making this diagnosis, he was formally indicating his opinion that the depression had not been caused by the brain injury; however, he hedged his bets by saying that 'organic brain syndrome was not completely ruled out'.

Initially, treatment consisted of a small dose of a common anti-anxiety drug, a standard anti-depressant drug and an occasional sleeping tablet. Although the psychiatrist detected some improvement in John's symptoms, he nevertheless decided that after two months of outpatient treatment, John needed a stay in hospital, a stay of ten days in all. The reasons for this hospitalisation and the treatment that occurred there are, unfortunately, a mystery.

Following hospitalisation, the anti-depressant medication was changed. But this treatment was no more effective than the first, and had the added disadvantage of causing a severe rash to develop over most of John's body. And so a third treatment regimen was established. This time both the anti-anxiety drug and the anti-depressant drugs were changed and the sleeping tablets were discontinued. At the same time, some three and a half months into the psychiatric treatment, John decided to switch to a new psychiatrist.

Treatment continued unmodified under the supervision of the new psychiatrist, who reported: 'Medication was continued at full strength' for about a 10-month period, following which it was 'phased out slowly over the next five months'. At the end of these 15 months of treatment, the clinician offered this opinion: John 'must be considered totally and permanently disabled as far as his ability to carry out his present job functions. The prognosis for recovery is poor, given the extensive trial period that has preceded this letter'. Some six weeks after this opinion was given, John arrived at our clinic for intake assessment.

Cognitive evaluation and treatment

John was not in great shape on evaluation day. In fact, not much had changed since he had first sought treatment for depression. Not only was his mood still depressed, he was uninterested in pretty well everything and almost incapable of experiencing pleasure. Nor did John present himself at his best: his face was without expression, his clothing was dishevelled, his speech slow and laboured, and his gait halting. He reported that he was still having trouble sleeping, especially in the morning, that his mood was always darkest at the start of the day, that he still had crying spells, had trouble making decisions, and that he suffered anxiety, especially when there was a risk of conflict. John admitted that he had withdrawn from most people and activities, but denied considering suicide as a means of escape.

John had another problem, too. Although he had been happily married for more than 20 years, strains had developed in his relationship with Margaret. The problem, John explained, was that Margaret couldn't understand his depression. She saw no reason why he couldn't return to his previous level of functioning, and so criticised him — rather severely, too — for not getting his act together. Alas, her well-meaning criticism only caused him to become more anxious, reinforced his sense of failure and increased his tendency to withdraw into himself.

As part of his initial evaluation, John completed several psychological tests. One of these tests, the Beck Depression Inventory (BDI) (Beck et al., 1961), is widely used to measure the severity of depression; John's score was 29, indicating that he was 'severely' depressed. A similar test for anxiety, the Beck Anxiety Inventory (BAI) (Beck et al., 1988) revealed that John was 'mildly' anxious. Finally, the Hopelessness Scale (HS) (Beck et al., 1974) is a measure of pessimism or how negative one expects the future to be; John scored 16, which suggested that he was extremely pessimistic about his prospects.

Apart from measuring symptoms, it was also important to discover something about John's beliefs. One of the assumptions of cognitive theory is that the symptoms of depressed people are self-sustaining because depressed people are interpreting their experience in a negatively-biased way. The negative bias is usually related to a series of unhelpful beliefs about how the world works. In cognitive theory, the unhelpful beliefs are known as 'dysfunctional attitudes', and the most common ones are included in a test called the Dysfunctional Attitude Scale (Weissman & Beck, 1978). When John rated his beliefs on this scale, it turned out that not only did he hold to a greater than usual number of unhelpful beliefs, his greatest vulnerability lay in his dysfunctional attitudes about work, achievement and his general competence — the areas most affected by the operation and its after-effects.

Treatment

After John had been assessed in our clinic, there was a six-week delay before his treatment started. This delay was necessary so that his neuropsychological status could be assessed. During these six weeks, John's condition worsened. As can be seen in figure 6.1 (see page 109), between intake and the first session, John's depression (BDI) score went up from 29 to 37, and there were also small increases in his pessimism (HS) and anxiety (BAI) scores.

In formal terms, treatment consisted of standard cognitive therapy for depression (Beck et al., 1979). Following the usual pattern, 50–minute sessions were held twice per week for the first two weeks, and on an approximately weekly basis thereafter. The treatment lasted 15 sessions, and 15 weeks had passed between the beginning of therapy and its end. The conclusion of therapy was a bit rushed because the therapist was due to move to another city.

Cognitive content

As I mentioned above, cognitive theory asserts that depressed people have a negative bias against themselves. One way that the bias shows itself is in the 'negative automatic thoughts' that typically preoccupy a depressed person. John's thinking included many of the automatic thoughts peculiar to depression, including: 'There is nothing to look forward to'; 'I can't do anything right'; and 'I'm a loser'. These thoughts also illustrate the unrealistic character of depressed thinking. Even if it were true that John had less to look forward to after his operation than he had before it, his saying that he had 'nothing' ahead of him was a gross overgeneralisation.

Besides these typical automatic thoughts, John also made many negative interpretations of his neurological condition, negative thoughts that were more specific to his own circumstances. For example, he would think: 'I'm not in control of anything any more'; 'My usefulness is limited'; 'I used to be good at this'; and 'Why can't I keep track of things anymore'? In general, John was alert to any possible sign of diminished competency and would interpret all such signs as indicating complete incompetency, complete loss of prospects and complete loss of worth.

It is important to emphasise that John's competency concerns were related to certain dysfunctional attitudes or unhelpful beliefs which he had held before he had become depressed. These attitudes, assessed with the Dysfunctional Attitude Scale at John's first visit to the clinic, included: 'People will think less of me if I make a mistake'; 'I must be a useful, productive, creative person or life has no purpose'; and 'If I am to be a worthwhile person, I must be truly outstanding in at least one respect'. The fact of neurological impairment had special meaning for a person who largely defined himself and his worth according to his level of achievement. For John, who was suddenly making mistakes, no longer useful to his company, and no longer an outstanding computer user, the unique combination of his beliefs and his circumstances was devastating.

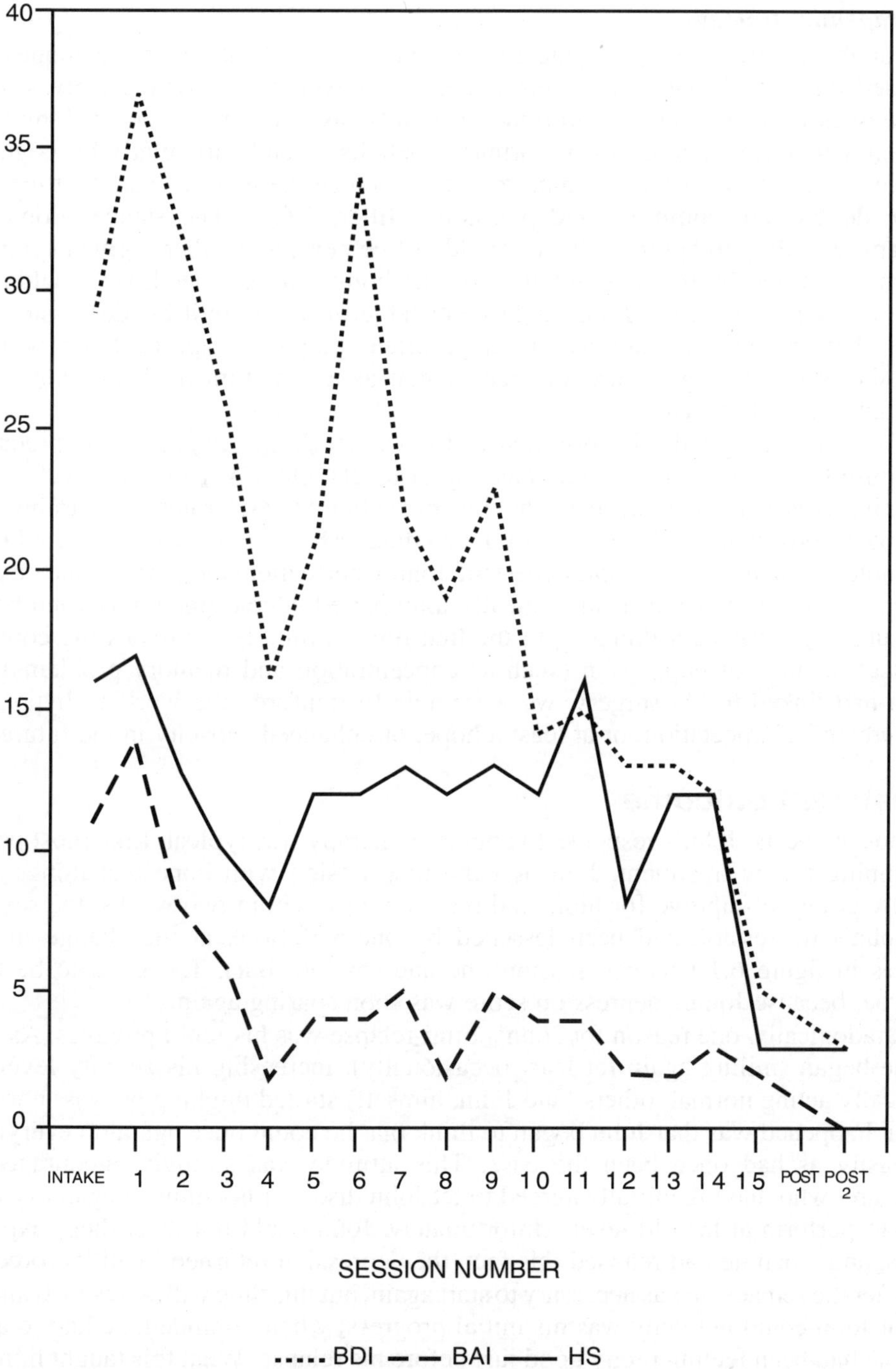

Figure 6.1: Beck Depression Inventory (BDI), Beck Anxiety Inventory (BAI) and Hopelessness Scale (HS) scores at intake assessment, at therapy sessions 1–15, and at 1-month and 15-month follow-ups

Therapeutic strategy

Although cognitive therapy typically involves the application of techniques like 'guided discovery' that aim to help patients discover things for themselves, these techniques were especially appropriate in John's case. As already noted, John had a tendency to attribute all of his performance deficits — and particularly his cognitive deficits — to his neurological impairment. Of course, he was unaware that many of these deficits are common to depression (Miller, 1975). The stance adopted in therapy was that, to begin with, we could not be certain whether a given symptom had been caused by the depression or by the brain injury. Indeed, we wouldn't be able to say for sure what John might be capable of doing until his depression was gone. Under these conditions, an appropriate empirical approach or working hypothesis was to regard any apparent deficit as a symptom of depression unless and until proved otherwise.

This working hypothesis permitted us to evaluate John's negative interpretations of himself at both cognitive and behavioural levels. On a behavioural level, John's negative bias was challenged by having him attempt tasks such as learning new computer programs that he had been avoiding. More cognitively, we could, for example, evaluate the appropriateness of John's perfectionistic performance expectations by asking whether neurologically unimpaired people (including John before his surgery) always get things right the first time. Similarly, by reviewing common clinical features of depression (such as concentration and memory problems) that John had linked to his surgery, we were able to reinforce the working hypothesis and create an expectation, or at least a hope, of enhanced capacity in the future.

Treatment outcome

In most respects, John's response to cognitive therapy was typical. Like most people beginning a new treatment, John left the first session with hope that things were finally going to improve for him. And they did, too: within two weeks, the severity of John's depression had been lessened by one-half (look at the change in BDI scores in figure 6.1 between session one and session four). Too good to be true? Maybe, because John's depression score was soon soaring again.

Paradoxically, one reason for John's mini-relapse was his rapid progress. As soon as he began smiling again (at least occasionally), increasing his activity level and basically acting normal, others (and John, himself) started thinking he was 'normal'. What happened was that John began to think that he could once again do everything as easily as had once been the case. This attitude was strongly encouraged by Margaret who, having initially agreed to let John discover his limits, began to expect him to perform at his old level. Unfortunately, John could not meet these expectations, and when he had realised this fact, the depression returned in all its force.

After the setback, it was necessary to start again, but this time with a fresh advantage. What John could not deny was his initial progress; when reminded, he had to agree that he had been feeling pretty good just before his relapse. What this taught him was that he was still capable of having something like a normal mood; in other words, whatever other effects the surgery might have had, it had not caused him to be permanently depressed. This fact provided a foundation for hope of further progress.

From the sixth session onwards, progress was more or less straightforward, even though there were two events that required John to make extensive use of the cognitive evaluation skills that he was learning. The first event was a neuropsychological consultation (between sessions seven and eight) that tended to undermine our working hypothesis by reminding John of the extent of his brain damage; the second event was the expiry of his notice period and the final loss of employment (after session ten). Apart from these two blips in the record, improvement occurred steadily and as can be seen in figure 6.1, treatment was ultimately successful. By the fifteenth session, there was complete remission of symptoms; John's depression, anxiety and hopelessness scores were all well within normal range.

Follow-up

Arrangements were made for John to complete the self-administered psychological tests and post them to me, one month and five months after treatment had ended. At the one-month follow-up (see 'Post 1' in figure 6.1), the test results indicated that the improvement in John's symptoms had been maintained. John's depression (BDI = 4), anxiety (BAI = 1) and hopelessness (HS = 3) scores all remained well within normal limits. Perhaps more significantly, most of John's unhelpful beliefs as measured by the Dysfunctional Attitude Scale were no longer in evidence. His score of 208 is actually lower than that of most non-depressed people, and suggests that John's longer term prognosis is pretty good. What is known for sure is that five months after the end of therapy (see 'Post 2' in figure 6.1), John's test scores still showed that all of his treatment gains had been maintained.

Implications

As a piece of evidence, the greatest strength of a case history is its usefulness in demonstrating that a hypothesis is false. This case study proves false the hypothesis that depressions associated with physical illness (including neurological problems) do not respond to psychological therapy. Of course, this result is not a surprise because other studies had already demonstrated the same thing (Larcombe & Wilson, 1984).

In the same way, this case study discredits the idea that depressions which are resistant to one form of biological therapy ought to be treated with another biological therapy. That approach clearly failed to work in John's case, and when it was tried had the added problem of causing him to develop a nasty rash. I don't mean to suggest that a psychological therapy, and cognitive therapy in particular, is necessarily the best alternative when an initial drug therapy fails; when drug therapies work, they are relatively cheap and can be very convenient. But this study does cast doubt on the view that the treatment-resistant patient must receive drugs, electroshock and augmentation with lithium carbonate or thyroid hormone.

Finally, this case study calls into further question the usefulness of the diagnosis of Organic Mood Disorder. Was John's depression caused by his brain injury (as the neuropsychologists believed) or was it a response to his new disability (as the first psychiatrist believed)? That is a question I can't answer, and I suspect that nobody else can, either. As John's case illustrates, there is no method for demonstrating that his depression was caused by one set of factors or another. If it cannot be shown that his depression did have a physiological basis, what is gained by pretending that it did? Certainly John's neurological condition is critical to understanding his case; if the tumour had never developed, it is extremely unlikely that the depression would have developed when it did. But to say that the neurological disorder is central to the case is a far cry from saying that the physical changes directly resulting from the tumour and/or the surgery and/or the skull infection were immediately responsible for changes in John's mood.

But if case studies are useful for 'disconfirming' hypotheses, they are not much help when it comes to making a positive contribution to knowledge. True, the present case suggests that cognitive therapy may be an effective treatment for some depressions associated with brain damage, but it provides no information about which such individuals might respond, or about why some of these individuals will respond to a psychological therapy when they have not responded to a biological one.

The function of this case study has not been to answer questions about depression so much as to raise them. And the questions raised by this case study are familiar enough: What causes any successful treatment of depression to be successful? What causes a usually successful treatment to fail in some cases, or a treatment which fails in most cases to be successful in a few? In other words, what are the mechanisms that underlie both the development and the remission of depression symptoms? And when it comes to answering this last question, all the knowledge that we have accrued about depression can come to seem something of a handicap. Knowing that treatments as diverse as cognitive therapy and electroconvulsive therapy are both effective treatments for depression, we are faced with the considerable puzzle of discovering their possible common mode of therapeutic action, or worse, their independent means of similarly affecting affect, behaviour and cognition. Perhaps it is not, after all, so simple as A→B→C.

Acknowledgements
I wish to express my thanks to John (a pseudonym) for consenting to have his case material published and for his cooperation in providing the follow-up data. David A. F. Haaga conducted the intake evaluation of the patient; E. Moss and B. Watson conducted the neurospsychological examination. Finally, thanks to Graham Davidson, Vic Illich and Michael John for their comments on drafts of this chapter and to Bogdan Kubicki for translation assistance.

Gina Geffen and Peter Butterworth
University of Queensland

7 Born with a split brain: the 15-year development of a case of congenital absence of the corpus callosum

The corpus callosum, an enormous bundle of nerve fibres linking the left and right halves of the brain, begins development in the early stages of foetal life. Crossing of callosal fibres between the two halves of the brain begins when the foetus is 12 weeks old and is completed soon after birth. Myelination of the corpus callosum, on the other hand, is only completed at puberty. Agenesis of the corpus callosum (ACC) refers to an absence of development of these neural pathways. The cause (or causes) of this failure is not understood at present although there may be a genetic influence. The case described in this chapter, James, has ACC. We describe the effects, studied over a decade, of absence of the corpus callosum on otherwise normal development.

The level of functioning of individuals with ACC varies enormously, ranging from apparently normal development, in which the defect may go undetected, to severe learning difficulties, seizures, visual handicap and gross motor control problems. ACC, however, is often associated with other brain malformations making it difficult to identify which clinical effects are specific to the condition. The frequency of occurrence within unselected hospital populations is between one and seven per thousand (Njiokiktjien, 1991). However, the actual frequency of occurrence of ACC and the deficits specifically related to it are difficult to calculate, as those without symptoms and those with only mild impairment are rarely diagnosed. James, for example, is a case who would not necessarily have been investigated. He was examined because at birth his head was somewhat larger in circumference (37 cm) than normal and continued to increase in size over the next eight weeks. A computerised tomography (CT) scan was conducted when James was 9 months of age which demonstrated ACC. This condition was confirmed when James was 13 years old by more precise Magnetic Resonance (MR) imaging.

Following the initial diagnosis, the doctors sought a source of support for James and his family. It was known that our neuropsychology laboratory had a specific interest in the functions of the corpus callosum and would therefore be suitable to measure the effects of the neurological abnormality on James' development, to counsel James and his family on the expected nature and rate of development, to design and implement remediation programs where applicable and to advise on academic and career decisions as needed.

The next section describes how the two halves of the normal brain are specialised for different functions and what their interconnections are. Further sections describe the problems James faced from kindergarten to high school and how he coped with them. We then describe results of testing intelligence and memory on five occasions between the ages of 5 and 15 years. Finally, we describe how the two halves of James' brain managed to interact without a corpus callosum.

Neuroanatomical and psychological background

Specialisation of the cerebral hemispheres

The two halves of the brain (more specifically, the cerebral hemispheres) are specialised for different functions. It is generally accepted that the left hemisphere is specialised for certain functions such as language, with the right hemisphere specialised for others such as the processing of spatial information. Although language and spatial perception functions are predominantly lateralised (that is, located) in each cerebral hemisphere, they are not exclusively so. Sensory input (visual, auditory, tactile and so on) and motor output (control of the limbs, for example) are crossed systems as each side of the body (for both sensory input and motor response) is controlled predominantly by the opposite (contralateral) hemisphere. Therefore, a touch sensation from the right hand is 'processed' by the left cerebral hemisphere and the motor output to initiate movement of the left foot occurs in the right hemisphere.

Since information from the senses and control of the limbs resides primarily in opposite cerebral hemispheres, transfer of information across the corpus callosum and other smaller interconnections is required to allow unified brain functioning. Individuals in whom the corpus callosum has been surgically cut to prevent the spread of epileptic seizures (so-called split brain subjects) are unable to transfer information across hemispheres. As an example, when objects are presented exclusively to the left visual field (which is processed by the right hemisphere), these patients are unable to name the object (this linguistic function being controlled by the left hemisphere). However, even these patients are generally indistinguishable from individuals in most everyday situations. This is because they can use behavioural strategies to get information to both halves of the brain. By making eye and head movements, objects can be viewed in both visual fields, thereby transmitting the information to each side of the brain.

The early identification of James therefore presented a rare opportunity to observe his development and to determine whether known functions of the corpus callosum were compromised. Would he show 'split-brain' symptoms? We studied the integration of information between the two halves of the brain, and the role of the corpus callosum in (a) the suppression of the activity of one hemisphere and (b) facilitation of information processing within each half of the brain. While deficits in James' performance will be related to the absence of the corpus callosum, we point out that he does have other brain abnormalities which may qualify the interpretation. Despite his neurological abnormalities, James seems to function at a normal intellectual level and is in the process of completing high school with the intention of future tertiary study. Cases such as James demonstrate the extent to which neural plasticity may compensate for abnormalities of structure.

Interhemispheric connections

The two cerebral hemispheres are interconnected by three compact bundles of fibres referred to as the forebrain commissures. By far the largest and most important of these commissures is the corpus callosum. A magnetic resonance (MR) image of a patient with an intact corpus callosum is presented in figure 7.1(a) viewed from the centre of the brain outwards. The corpus callosum is visible as a band of fibres (white) running across the top of the brain stem.

The most posterior portion of the corpus callosum transfers visual information while the transfer of touch information occurs across the central region of the corpus callosum (Ramaekers, 1991). The anterior two-thirds of the corpus callosum enables co-ordination of both hands. It probably also links the problem solving and planning functions of the left and right frontal lobes.

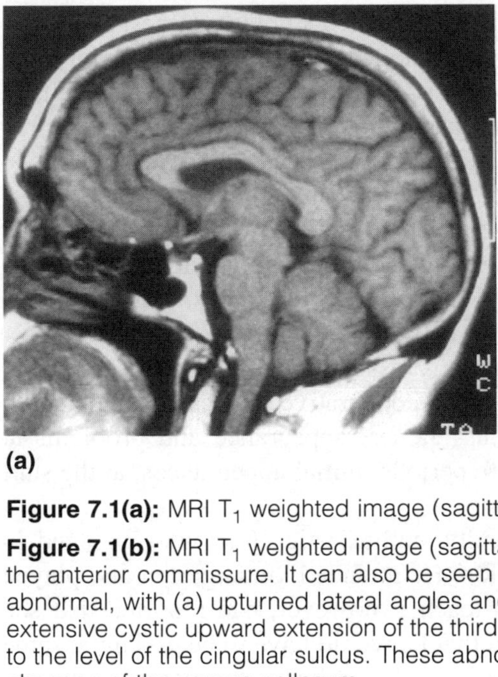

(a)

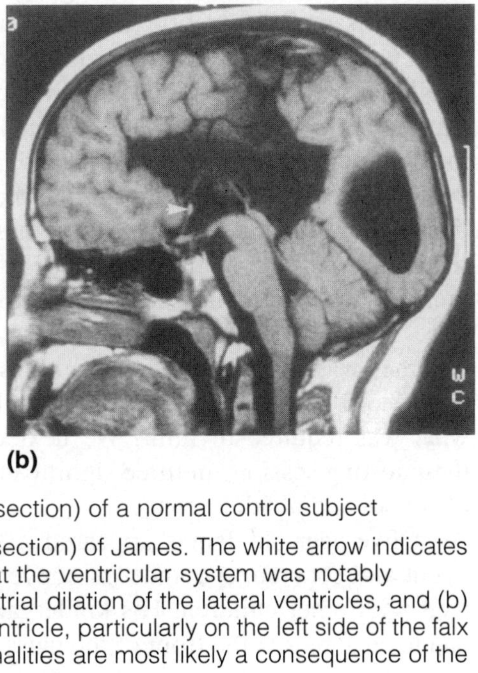

(b)

Figure 7.1(a): MRI T_1 weighted image (sagittal section) of a normal control subject

Figure 7.1(b): MRI T_1 weighted image (sagittal section) of James. The white arrow indicates the anterior commissure. It can also be seen that the ventricular system was notably abnormal, with (a) upturned lateral angles and atrial dilation of the lateral ventricles, and (b) extensive cystic upward extension of the third ventricle, particularly on the left side of the falx to the level of the cingular sulcus. These abnormalities are most likely a consequence of the absence of the corpus callosum.

An MR scan of James is presented in figure 7.1(b). While the anterior commissure could be visualised, neither the hippocampal commissure nor the corpus callosum was present. James also showed other brain abnormalities generally accepted as indicative of a brain without a corpus callosum. Within both hemispheres, regions (the occipital horns) of the lateral ventricles were dilated, with the left larger than the right; there was also considerable thinning of the posterior (visual) portion of the left hemisphere.

Course of development and general adjustment of James, a case of ACC

The study of James from childhood to adolescence allows a greater understanding of the role of the corpus callosum in normal development. Since James shows relatively little intellectual disability and no obvious sensory or motor problems, the plasticity of the brain in adapting to the absence of the corpus callosum also became evident.

In addition to observation and interview, James was given a number of psychological tests. To examine the effects of ACC on both between-hemispheric and within-hemispheric processing, a task of tactile finger localisation was given each time James was seen. Neuropsychologists have suggested that the corpus callosum is necessary for the normal lateralisation of function to a particular cerebral hemisphere. A dichotic monitoring task was, therefore, repeatedly used to find out which hemisphere was dominant for language function. As hand dominance is also related to lateralisation of function, this too was examined when studying James.

ACC has also been associated with cognitive deficits in the area of memory and intelligence. To identify possible memory deficits and the nature of such deficits, a learning test was administered to James on a number of occasions with a further memory test given when he was last assessed. Patients with ACC are thought to demonstrate unusual profiles on intelligence tests (Wechsler, 1967, 1974). To investigate this, James' intelligence was assessed on five different occasions. Previous research reports contained evidence of slow language development in ACC children, so we also administered the Illinois Psycholinguistic Ability Test at the age of 5.

James was formally assessed on these various tasks on five occasions, at ages of 5, 7, 8, 13 and 15. (He was always pleasantly cooperative and easily understood what was required of him.) We next discuss James' appearance and problems at these testing sessions in three significant life periods; initial appearances, at the start of school and at adolescence.

As a five-year-old James appeared a friendly, enthusiastic child who engaged in fluent and coherent spontaneous conversation. He attended kindergarten and played well with other children. His kindergarten teacher, however, had reported that she had to sit James at the front of the class and that he would have to be given the same instructions several times before he would attend. Similarly, his parents reported that he did not seem to concentrate at home. It was noted during testing that when concentrating, James would dribble, suggesting he was too preoccupied to swallow.

We recommended that James have his hearing professionally tested to rule out the possibility that a specific hearing problem was responsible for reports of inattention. His hearing, however, proved to be in the normal range. Our tests showed that James had difficulty sustaining his attention to long sentences. Consequently, he could not recall information presented early in the sentence. We recommended that short, clear instructions be used, preferably with visual examples. We also recommended that a speech therapist be consulted to help overcome comprehension and verbal logic difficulties that he exhibited with concepts such as 'why', 'alike', 'same', 'all' and 'except'. An occupational therapist had previously worked with James on his gross motor activities.

James was next assessed at ages 7 and 8, coinciding with his completion of the kindergarten grades of primary school. At this stage both James' mother and teacher showed concern at the difficulties he was experiencing. While he showed satisfactory (if not above average) ability on tasks such as reading and mathematics, James was having immense difficulties with fine motor skills. He was extremely poor at writing and drawing and avoided doing these if he could. James also showed deficits in tasks requiring the coordination of two hands such as putting on his shoes and socks, or putting his school gear away into his school bag. On all such tasks James was laboriously slow. By comparison, his younger sister easily completed many tasks which James found difficult. The two-handed tasks require the two halves of the brain to communicate so that coordination is possible. Therefore problems with such tasks were expected. Similarly, with packing of objects into a school bag, the hands move in and out of vision, and the object that a hand is holding, when out of sight, is perceived in only the opposite cerebral hemisphere. Thus, the task of packing or unpacking would have been difficult. The use of a hard case with a lid that remained open was recommended.

James' mother reported that he enjoyed video games and was able to sustain his attention for long periods while playing on them and, furthermore, that James and his father were highly competitive on such games. This seemed contrary to the initial assessment which concluded that James seemed to have difficulty sustaining attention.

James was also rather preoccupied with being correct and gaining approval. When faced with tasks which he found difficult he would show a reluctance to participate and withdraw or even not attempt them at all. Such withdrawal would also reduce the opportunities for James to practise and improve. A secondary problem was that neither his parents nor teacher could, with any confidence, set suitable standards of performance against which to judge James. His mother was unsure what level of performance she should expect and demand. For example, did James have genuine difficulties packing his school bag quickly before school in the morning or was he just being slow and lazy? It was of concern that James was often punished and kept in for detention during lunch time at school for his slow completion of the manual tasks listed above.

A meeting was arranged with James' mother and his teacher at which it was explained that the cause of his difficulties seemed to arise predominantly from poor processing of verbal instructions and difficulties coordinating his two hands. It was recommended that James be given training in tasks like tying his shoelaces and packing his bag and that these skills be taught as sequential units. Such practice should also be treated as a game. A reward system involving video games with his father was used to encourage practice on tasks he would try to avoid. In the meantime, we asked James' mother to buy him a pair of slip-on shoes that would not require two-handed coordination. A handwriting program that involved consistent practice was commenced. We also asked the teacher to use short, clear instructions to enhance James' understanding. We explained which tasks James found difficult and what the neurological basis for this was. We asked that on these tasks he should not be expected to perform at normal levels, but that progressive improvements in his own achievements be assessed and praised.

At age 13 and 15 James reported a series of migrainous-type headaches which were interfering with his learning. These headaches and associated anxiety and nausea appeared to be related to periods of pressure from school. A program of relaxation training was recommended and implemented. While James continued to exhibit occasional bursts of uncooperative behaviour and bad temper, such behaviour seemed as much the product of normal adolescence as an effect of ACC. His mother, nonetheless, was encouraged to implement behaviour management techniques in the home environment.

As when James first entered school, researchers from the neuropsychological laboratory consulted with the principal and teachers of his new high school. The aim was to help the school staff to gain an understanding of James' strengths and weaknesses and to ensure that unrealistic demands were not placed upon him. Equally important, the consultation ensured that his abilities were not underestimated thereby stifling the development of his potential.

James continued to show his greatest ability in mathematics, although his progress in English and his verbal skills in general were a cause of concern. Investigation, however, revealed that most of his poor results reflected a failure to submit assignments. This suggested his poor performance may, in part, reflect alterable motivational factors.

James had a strong desire for a career in meteorology, which required a tertiary education. Such a career remains a viable possibility and to help overcome possible motivational weaknesses, James was counselled as to what range of results he would have to attain to gain entry into the relevant course and what school subjects he would need as prerequisites. A period of work experience was also arranged in the local bureau of meteorology.

Cognitive abilities and achievements

Intelligence

James' scores on all subtests, as well as the verbal, performance and full-scale IQ scores on either the Wechsler Preschool and Primary Scale of Intelligence (WPPSI) or the Wechsler Intelligence Scale for Children — Revised (WISC-R) at the five ages are presented in table 7.1. While some researchers have argued that the usual acallosal patient has a low IQ, it is possible that in such cases the absence of the corpus callosum was but one feature of larger scale brain abnormalities, or the consequence of an acute neurological illness (for example, swelling of the brain following injury) that can cause brain damage. With advances in imaging of the brain, there is an improved rate of detecting ACC patients within the normal range of intelligence. The IQ profiles of acallosal patients do, however, generally show a greater distinction between verbal and performance scales than is usually expected (Chiarello, 1980). Put another way, although patients may show normal IQ scores on one of the IQ subscales (verbal or performance), the other scale is generally deficient.

Table 7.1: Scaled scores of Wechsler Intelligence Scales on James at five different ages (in years)

Subtest	5*	7*	8+	13+	15+
Information	11	6	17	11	11
Vocabulary	9	11	12	7	8
Arithmetic	10	14	17	18	12
Similarities	9	8	5	6	8
Comprehension	5	5	—	8	6
Sentences	8	—	—	—	—
(Digit Span)	—	—	13	15	12
V.I.Q.	92	92	102	100	94
Animal House*	11	7	—	—	—
Picture Completion	11	9	8	7	5
Picture Arrangement	—	—	11	9	8
Mazes	13	11	—	12	—
Geometric Design*	10	9	—	—	—
Block Design	12	10	9	9	10
Object Assembly+	—	—	8	8	5
Coding+	—	—	6	11	9
P.I.Q.	110	95	88	91	82
F.S.I.Q.	101	93	95	95	87

*WPPSI
+WISC-R

When James was tested on the WPPSI at ages 5 and 7 he showed a diverse profile (see table 7.1). His full-scale IQ was in the mid-average range, and at age 5, his performance IQ was significantly greater than his verbal IQ. As has been discussed, James had comprehension difficulties and his borderline score on the Comprehension subscale reflected this.

By age 8, although there remained a significant difference between verbal and performance IQ scores, it was now in the opposite direction. This seemed to reflect, however, James' superior arithmetic ability and general knowledge (Information).

Other verbal language subtests such as Similarities (which measures difficulties comprehending abstractions) remained at the borderline level.

At age 13, James' full-scale IQ score showed that he was performing at an equivalent level to 37 per cent of his peers. Again, very superior arithmetic abilities inflated his verbal IQ score. Finally, by age 15 his full-scale IQ was at the nineteenth percentile. His verbal IQ was again significantly greater than his performance IQ. Specific subscale deficits were interpreted as lack of attention to detail (Picture Completion), difficulty with abstract representations and slower than average fine hand movements (Object Assembly). These difficulties were consistent with the very child-like drawing that had persisted until the age of 15.

The table of IQ results does demonstrate a gradual decrease in full-scale IQ and shows several large drops in subscales between adjacent sessions (for example, Information and Vocabulary between 8 and 13, and Arithmetic between ages 13 and 15). These changes do not, however, reflect a decrement in performance but rather, as indicated by the stability of raw scores, James' failure to show the same level of developmental improvement as his age-matched peers.

As a gauge of James' weakness in verbal abilities, the Schonell Graded Word Reading Test was administered on the two latest testing occasions to ascertain his reading age. Reading age is calculated from the number of words a person can accurately read from a list of words organised so as to gradually increase in difficulty. At age 13, James' reading ability was equivalent to a normal child aged 11.6 years, while at age 15 his reading age was 12.4 years.

Auditory Verbal Learning Test (AVLT)

The AVLT was used to establish James' level of memory function as it enables measurement of several different aspects of memory (see Geffen et al., 1990). One list of words (list A) is read to the subject 5 times, with recall tested following each presentation. A second word list (B) is then read to the subject with recall of this new list and then the original (A) list (without presentation) subsequently tested. Finally, after a 20-minute delay, list A recall is again tested as is recognition of both lists A and B. From this process, measures can be calculated reflecting the rate of acquisition, effects of forward and backward interference among lists, the effects of word position, forgetting, retrieval of words, and approaches to memory tasks.

The consistent features of James' two AVLT tests were poor levels of acquisition and poor monitoring of recognition (misassignment of words to lists and a number of false identifications). James' results demonstrate inconsistency between the ages of 13 and 15. While at age 13 he showed poor primacy (low recall of items presented early in the list), at age 15 James' recency recall (items presented late in the lists) was poor.

An intact hippocampis is required for adequate storage of information in memory and it is possible that the absence of the hippocampal commissure, rather than the missing corpus callosum, is responsible for James' auditory verbal memory deficits. Similar memory deficiencies have, however, been demonstrated in an acallosal patient in whom the hippocampal commissure was present (Geffen et al., 1992). It seems, therefore, that the absence of the corpus callosum may prevent the storage of memories in both hemispheres. Even the memory traces within a single hemisphere may not be as precise as normal. Perhaps the corpus callosum facilitates information processing within each hemisphere. Thus, rather than being able to store and retrieve memory traces in both cerebral hemispheres, the absence of the corpus callosum may limit the process to a single hemisphere. It has also been suggested that the corpus callosum plays an important part in processing information (for example, sorting and storing items for subsequent retrieval, Ramaekers, 1991).

Other memory tasks

The evidence indicated James' difficulties lay in attending to and remembering verbal instructions and information. In contrast, he reported no difficulties with his everyday memory for pictorial and spatial material. The Wide Range Assessment of Memory and Learning (WRAML) was given to determine whether his memory difficulties were general. James' specific difficulties with verbal material were confirmed. In contrast, James' performance on the Visual Memory Index was above average.

James showed deficits in measures of intelligence, memory and learning which seemed specifically related to verbal material. This suggests the observed distinction between verbal and performance IQ measures of acallosal patients is representative of a generalised processing deficit affecting the verbal mode of presentation. The implication is that the corpus callosum has a role in such functions. An important consideration, though, are the other neurological abnormalities James demonstrated. His posterior left hemisphere is smaller than the right. In most individuals the left hemisphere is language-dominant and therefore these abnormalities of James' brain complicate our ability to explain the cause of his verbal insufficiencies. As will be seen, however, the localisation of James' speech in his left hemisphere was inconsistent over the course of development.

Sensori-motor functions of the corpus callosum

The corpus callosum not only transmits information between the two halves of the brain, it also plays a role in confining information to the specialised half of the brain, by inhibiting 'automatic' information transfer. We used a tactile test to investigate transmission of information and a listening test to examine whether James showed confinement of specialised speech information to one side of his brain.

Tactile inter-hemispheric transmission

The tactile finger localisation task allows comparison of between hemispheric (inter-) and within hemispheric (intra-) processing of tactile (touch) sensation. In this task, a blindfolded person sits with his or her elbows resting on a table and hands held up with fingers spread out. The tester then lightly touches a finger on one hand with a sharpened pencil point. The subject then has to indicate which finger was touched by touching that finger with his or her thumb. In the intrahemispheric (that is, within hemisphere) condition, the thumb of the same hand touched is used for the response (that is, the stimulus and response occur in the same, contralateral hemisphere). In the interhemispheric (that is, between hemispheres) condition the response is made with the opposite hand to the one stimulated. For example, if the experimenter touched the middle finger of James' right hand, he would respond by touching the middle finger of his left hand with his left thumb. The motor response is therefore controlled by the opposite hemisphere to that in which the initial touch was sensed, and thus an accurate response requires the integration of sensory and motor information from both cerebral hemispheres. Individuals with intact brains can do this task very well, whether responding with the same hand or the hand opposite to that touched. Patients with a severed corpus callosum can do the intra-hemispheric (same hand) task well, but perform at a chance level when required to respond with the other hand.

While normal subjects generally show near perfect performance on the within-hand conditions from an early age, the between-hands condition is less accurate until about 11 years of age. The nerve fibres of the corpus callosum are among the last of the cortex to mature, not becoming myelinated until beyond ten years of age. (Myelin is a fatty material laid about the nerve fibres as an insulator, enabling efficient conduction of electrical impulses and therefore efficient communication.) Gradual improvement with age on the inter-hemispheric transfer of information task is thought, therefore, to reflect the maturation of the corpus callosum enabling hemispheric integration (see figure 7.2).

Normal subjects do not show any hand differences in identifying which finger was touched. There is normally no advantage in localising the touch sensation in either the left or right hands in the intra-hemisphere condition, nor any advantage between the two halves of the brain (that is, the condition in which the stimulus is in the right and the response in the left hand is similar to the converse).

James' performance on the within hand, single finger stimulated condition was 10 per cent less accurate than normal children at age 5. By age 7, however, James was responding within the normal range with his left hand and by age 8 he had achieved perfect accuracy with both hands.

In contrast, James' accuracy when he responded with the opposite hand to the one touched remained much less accurate than age-matched control subjects (see figure 7.2). By 15 years of age James' ability to transfer information about touch between the two hemispheres resembled that of a normal 5-year-old. While there is some degree of integration in that the hemispheres are not entirely isolated, the results suggest that the mechanism by which James' brain has enabled the integration of information between the two cerebral hemispheres was inefficient and produced a significant developmental delay.

There are two possible mechanisms for inter-hemispheric (between hemispheres) transfer in the absence of the corpus callosum. One possibility is that the remaining cross-hemispheric pathways, such as the anterior commissure or sub-cortical pathways, take over the communication functions of the corpus callosum. Alternatively, the brain may compensate for the early absence of the corpus callosum by using enhanced ipsilateral sensory pathways, which lead from sensors to the hemisphere on the same side rather than the opposite side of the body. These uncrossed pathways are normally smaller than the crossed pathways and, in normal individuals, information from the crossed pathways is more strongly represented in the brain.

In a further abnormality, James showed an advantage transferring information from his left to right hand (left hand stimulated — right hand response) compared to transfer in the opposite direction (figure 7.2). There are two explanations for such an effect. Firstly, the result may indicate that the motor control of the left hand was less accurate than that of the right hand. This is unlikely given that James was left-handed. Alternatively, if the ipsilateral sensory pathways are highly developed, the greater accuracy of right hand responses may indicate that the left hemisphere is better able to detect stimulation of the left hand. James' ipsilateral pathways from his left hand to his left hemisphere may be more highly developed than the right ipsilateral pathways. Therefore, when his right hand was stimulated, James' right hemisphere would receive less precise information, and be unable to control accurate finger localisation with his left hand.

Figure 7.2 therefore demonstrates two points. One is that an alternative route for the transfer of information from within each hemisphere develops. While it is likely that other cross-hemispheric pathways develop, evidence supports the suggestion that the ipsilateral pathways are more highly developed in acallosal patients (see Jeeves, 1990) and James' pattern of results is consistent with such an interpretation. The second conclusion is that the alternative routes remain less efficient than the usual corpus callosum pathway in normal individuals.

Hemispheric specialisation

There is currently a debate about whether the corpus callosum is required to establish lateralisation of cerebral functions during development. According to one argument, certain cerebral functions are asymmetrical from birth, such as language, already lateralised in young children. There is a contradictory view, however, which suggests that from birth both hemispheres develop in parallel and that it is only at adolescence that lateralisation of function occurs. According to such theories, lateralisation can only occur following myelination of the corpus callosum, when the function in one hemisphere can suppress the development and duplication of similar specialisation in the opposite hemisphere. A conclusion of this theory is that acallosal patients will show more bilateral representation of function than normal individuals. Finally, bilateral representation has been proposed as an alternative compensation mechanism to overcome the inability of the two hemispheres to communicate.

An important consideration when studying cerebral organisation is handedness. Individuals who are left hand dominant are also thought to have a more symmetrical representation of cerebral functions and it has been proposed that left hand dominance is overly represented in the acallosal population.

Recent research has suggested that such proposals are erroneous (Jeeves & Silver, 1988). In the specific case of James though, during the early interviews he showed a left hand preference on tasks such as writing and drawing. On formal tests of handedness James was shown to be left hand dominant. James said he used his left hand to complete a number of everyday tasks (such as throwing a ball). Similarly, his left hand was quicker than his right on tasks of moving pegs (Peg-board Task) and putting dots in a series of bulls-eye targets (Marching Test).

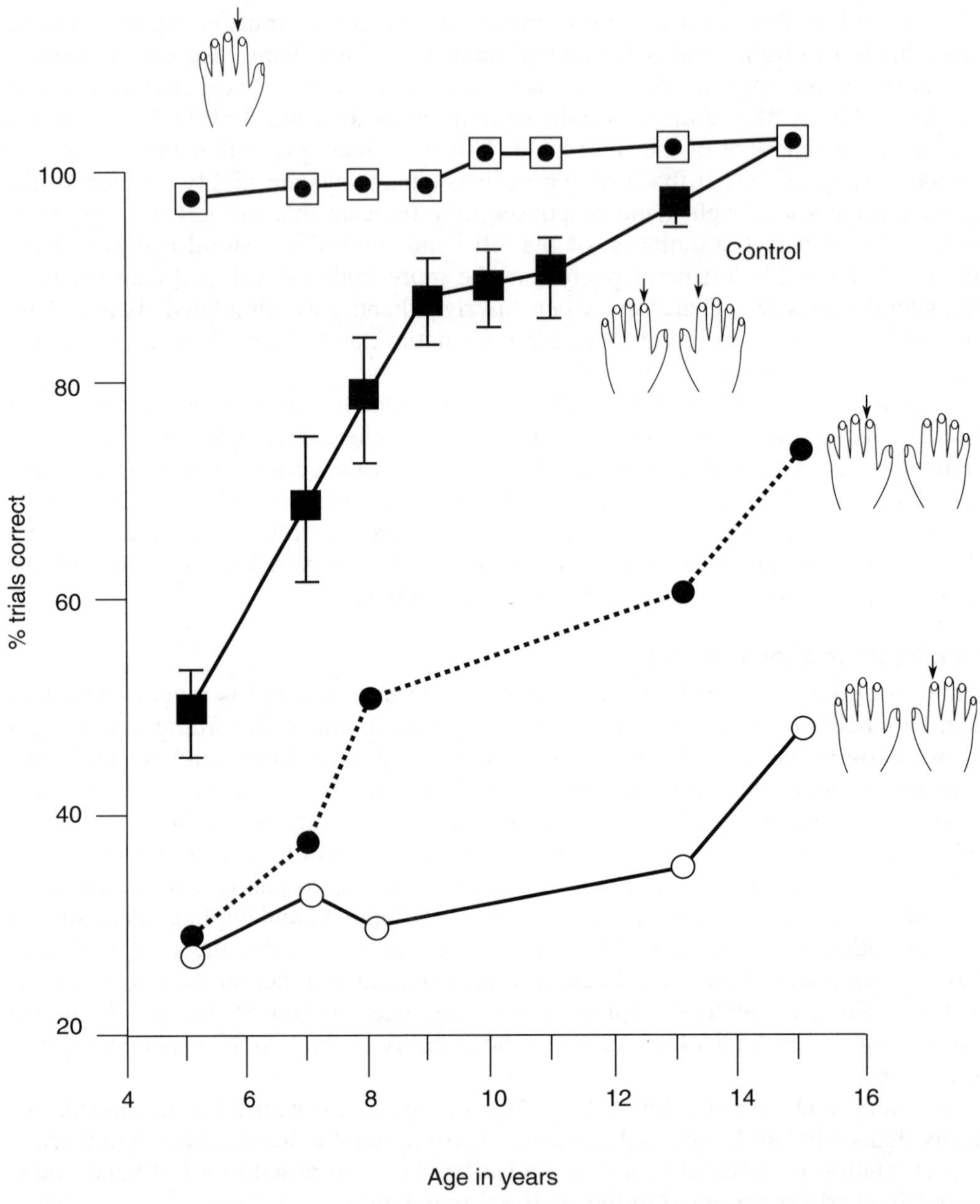

Figure 7.2: Accuracy on the tactile finger localisation task (as measured by percentage of trials correct). The top line demonstrates James' performance on the intra-hand conditions (left and right combined) showing performance at or near ceiling. The remaining lines compare the performance of James to that of age-matched controls on the inter-hemispheric task. The second highest line indicates control performance including standard error bars (both hands combined). The third line shows James' performance with left hand stimulated, right hand response, while the lowest line shows James' performance with his right hand stimulated and a left hand response.

To examine the lateralisation of function, James was repeatedly administered the dichotic monitoring task which identifies which hemisphere is language dominant. The dichotic monitoring task requires the subject to listen, via headphones, to a tape of paired words in which different words are presented simultaneously to each ear. Each time the target word, such as 'dog', is heard the subject must press a signal button. Most individuals show a right ear advantage. They respond to 20 per cent more target words in the right than left ear and are about 50 milliseconds faster at button presses to right than left ear words. The right ear advantage is interpreted as reflecting the stronger crossed pathways from the right ear to the language processor in the left half of the brain. Individuals who show a left ear advantage (only about 5 per cent of right-handers and 15 per cent of left-handers) have right hemisphere dominance for detecting words.

At 5 years of age, James showed a right ear advantage, detecting 35 per cent more targets in his right than left ear. This is consistent with lateralisation of language functions in his left hemisphere. Since his right ear advantage was within the normal range for 5-year-olds, it appears that normal lateralisation of speech perception functions can take place in acallosal cases.

While these early results tend to dismiss a role of the corpus callosum in lateralisation, James' dichotic monitoring task results at age 15 typify the uncertainty associated with interpretation of neurological disorders. At 15 years of age, James again demonstrated strong hemispheric lateralisation of language function, indicated by both speed and percentage of responses. This time, however, James showed a left ear advantage detecting 17 per cent more target words in his left than his right ear, indicating right hemisphere language dominance. Such changes of hemispheric dominance are unexpected.

It is tempting to conclude that such an unusual pattern of language lateralisation is due to the absence of the corpus callosum but such an interpretation is difficult to make. While it is unusual for right-handed subjects to change language-dominant hemispheres, such longitudinal studies have not been conducted with left-handed children. Left-handed individuals might also show inconsistent language laterality. We pointed out that James showed some other abnormality in the left parietal lobe that may have interfered with the maintenance of lateralisation. Witelson (1985) suggests that while hemispheric specialisation is present from birth, the corpus callosum may be involved in maintaining functional asymmetry.

Given the inability to efficiently transfer information inter-hemispherically, the change of language lateralisation to the right hemisphere would also have benefited James' writing ability. Being left-handed his right hemisphere would control his writing. With language lateralised in the same hemisphere that controlled writing, any need for inter-hemispheric transfer of linguistic information during writing could be avoided. It is possible that the development of his writing skills contributed to the change of lateralisation (as Curtiss (1985) suggests, language acquisition contributes to lateralisation).

It is, therefore, difficult to conclude from this case that the corpus callosum does contribute to hemispheric specialisation. Despite the change in hemisphere responsible for speech perception, the lateralisation of language was strong in both instances. This indicates that lateralisation of function can occur without a corpus callosum. Whether consistent lateralisation of particular functions requires an intact corpus callosum requires further longitudinal study of left-handed children with intact brains.

Conclusion

A striking feature of James is that despite being born without the corpus callosum he presents as a normal individual. The deviations from normal behaviour had to be carefully studied to be evident. Despite the presence of other brain abnormalities which may be responsible for his deficits, it can be concluded that James has difficulties with the inter-hemispheric transfer of information, bi-manual coordination (particularly when under pressure to perform quickly), fine motor control and fine sensory discrimination. These are features which have been noted frequently in other acallosal patients. In addition, James has mild impairments of verbal memory and verbal intelligence (and has outgrown attentional difficulties which were specific to verbal material). These are cognitive difficulties that have been reported in other ACC cases.

Our study of James confirms the role of the corpus callosum in the integration of information between the two hemispheres. However, its hypothesised role in the development of hemispheric lateralisation has not been supported. The consistency of lateralisation, for example, a right ear advantage, may require an intact corpus callosum.

Finally, James' case history shows that some compensation mechanism must develop to allow a form of inter-hemispheric (between hemispheres) communication. This compensation is not as efficient as the normal corpus callosum. The mechanism could either be the existing midline commissures (such as the anterior commissure or sub-cortical structures) or by the increased development of ipsilateral (that is, same sided) pathways. In everyday tasks behavioural strategies may also be utilised, such as rapid eye movements to ensure information is communicated to both hemispheres. It is through such strategies that acallosals manage to appear to function normally under all but the most controlling experimental designs.

Since James' condition was identified at such an early age there has been an opportunity for longitudinal, progressive assessment to be conducted regularly over a decade. While such assessment has obvious research benefits, the regular contact has also identified James' deficits and weaknesses (and also his strengths in daily living and learning). Such knowledge has facilitated the implementation of special programs and the adoption of various strategies to strengthen or overcome his various cognitive and physical deficits.

There are plans to continue the regular assessment of James in order to monitor his development. The outcome of such study may not only help to identify the functions of the corpus callosum, but may also be used as an example of the difficulties that occur in cases of ACC and how such problems may be managed.

Acknowledgements
Grants from the Australian Research Council and from the Julia Farr Centre Foundation (Inc.) to Gina Geffen supported this study and reporting of this case.

We are grateful to Mr Donald Simpson for referring this case and to Drs Lloyd Morris and Garry Le Quesne for their reports on the MR scan. Dr J. Nilsson and subsequently Ms G. Forrester shared responsibility with G. Geffen for counselling and intervention.

Sally Andrews, Philip B. Ward and Stanley V. Catts
Prince of Wales Hospital and University of New South Wales

8 Schizophrenia: understanding the processes underlying differences in symptoms and outcome

Schizophrenia has been recognised as a clinical syndrome for nearly 100 years yet its causes are still not fully understood. Difficulties in understanding the disorder are compounded by the fact that it is clinically heterogeneous — there is no single symptom that allows the diagnosis of schizophrenia and there are many different patterns of symptoms. This heterogeneity might indicate that there are many different causes of schizophrenic symptoms or that common causal factors can result in a variety of different symptom patterns.

Different theories of the causes of schizophrenia have led to differences in diagnostic practice. The *Diagnostic and Statistical Manual of Mental Disorders,* third edition (DSM-III) (American Psychiatric Association, 1980) and the *Diagnostic and Statistical Manual of Mental Disorders,* third edition, revised (DSM-III-R) (American Psychiatric Association, 1987) attempted to deal with this variability by imposing a classification scheme based on empirical criteria rather than aetiological theories of schizophrenia. The DSM-III-R criteria result in diagnoses that are reliable and that have some level of predictive validity regarding broad outcome, but that do not convey information useful to the development of more refined treatment procedures.

With the development of the *Diagnostic and Statistical Manual of Mental Disorders,* fourth edition (DSM-IV), the strengths and limitations of the existing diagnostic criteria for schizophrenia have been the focus of much discussion. Some of the diagnostic options being considered for DSM-IV represent major changes from those of DSM-III-R (Flaum & Andreasen, 1991). The first of these changes concerns the implications of including 'chronicity' (symptom duration) in the diagnostic criteria for schizophrenia; the second relates to the nature of the symptoms that define schizophrenia and how these symptoms vary between and within individuals during the course of the disorder.

This chapter first reviews historical changes in opinions of the causes of schizophrenia and how they have been reflected in diagnostic practice. This provides the context for a discussion of the DSM-III-R criteria, particularly with regard to duration and subclassifications into types of schizophrenia. Two case studies follow which illustrate differences in the pattern of symptoms within different individuals and the application of the duration criteria to distinguish between 'schizophreniform disorder' and schizophrenia. We then provide a brief example of research using cognitive psychophysiological approaches to investigate the cognitive processes underlying different symptoms of schizophrenia. Finally, we discuss how such a 'process-oriented' approach to understanding schizophrenia can contribute to the refinement of diagnostic and treatment procedures.

Issues in the diagnosis of schizophrenia

Historical overview

'Schizophrenia' was first defined by Kraepelin in 1896. He grouped together several disorders that had been described during the late nineteenth century, under the label 'dementia praecox' (mental deterioration which begins in adolescence). Kraepelin (1913) argued that dementia praecox had an organic basis that led to secondary psychological consequences reflected in 'a loss of inner unity of intellect, emotion and volition, in themselves and among one another' so that the person functioned like 'an orchestra without a conductor'.

Kraepelin's diagnostic procedures were controversial. Rather than being based on the aetiology of dementia praecox or on its physical pathology, he relied on its course and prognosis. Kraepelin reported detailed descriptions of the disease's characteristic features which included deterioration of the personality, usually beginning in adolescence, hallucinations, delusions and disorders of affect. In Kraepelin's descriptions, deterioration was the criterion that principally distinguished dementia praecox from other types of psychosis, but Kraepelin noted that 13 per cent of his patients made a short-term recovery. Although Kraepelin's observations provided a guide for diagnosis, he did not offer many objective diagnostic criteria.

Bleuler (1911) introduced the term 'schizophrenia' to refer to the 'split-mindedness' or splitting of psychic functions that he regarded to be the core feature of Kraepelin's patients. Bleuler argued against the term dementia praecox on the grounds that the disorder did not necessarily lead to deterioration and did not always start in adolescence. This shift from a deteriorating course to symptoms as the principal diagnostic criteria, considerably broadened the concept of schizophrenia, as did Bleuler's description of schizophrenic subtypes. Bleuler thought that the schizophrenias probably had an organic basis arguing that a purely psychological cause was conceivable, but unlikely — 'psychic events and experiences may release the symptoms but not the disease'. However, his major focus was on the psychological mechanisms leading to the development of symptoms.

Bleuler distinguished between primary symptoms produced directly by the disease and secondary symptoms reflecting the person's reactions to the psychosis and environment. The primary symptoms were summarised as 'the four As': autism (withdrawal), ambivalence, loosening of associations and blunting of emotional affect. The secondary symptoms included all of Kraepelin's clinical features — hallucinations, delusions (disturbed thoughts), catatonia (motor symptoms), somatisation (bodily changes) and changes in personality and some motor and memory functions, but Bleuler argued that the secondary symptoms could also occur in other disorders. What defined them as constituting schizophrenia is that they arose as a consequence of splitting or loosening of associations — 'the splitting is the prerequisite condition of most of the disease ... which gives the peculiar stamp to most of the symptomatology' (Bleuler, 1911). The form of the secondary symptoms was thought to reflect unconscious psychodynamic processes such as those discussed by Freud.

There are two critical differences between Kraepelin's and Bleuler's approach that have implications for defining schizophrenia. The first concerns the focus on empirical description as opposed to underlying process. Kraepelin relied on observable clinical phenomena while Bleuler emphasised underlying psychological processes. The second major difference arises from Kraepelin's emphasis on longitudinal criteria such as the deteriorating course of the disease which had an important influence on defining subtypes of the disorder.

While Kraepelin's approach dominated psychiatric practice in Germany and Great Britain, Bleuler's broader conception and his emphasis on underlying processes set the stage for developments in the United States. Further broadening of the construct was stimulated by Meyer (1917) who adopted a psychobiological approach which argued that each schizophrenic patient has a unique psychiatric disorder reflecting a combination of psychosocial and physical factors. This variety of influences led to a very loose conception of the disorder which was reflected both in variable diagnostic procedures, and a rate of diagnosis that was much higher than that obtained in Great Britain and Europe.

British psychiatrists adopted a much narrower view influenced by Jaspers' (1913) 'phenomenological' approach and by Schneider's (1959) attempt to translate Jaspers' ideas into diagnostic criteria. Jaspers cautioned against commitment to any causal theory whether organic or psychological and emphasised instead the need to describe as clearly as possible exactly what the patient believed and was experiencing. Jaspers' views inspired the existential school of psychiatry (for example, Maslow, 1968) and were the basis of Schneider's (1959) 'first rank symptoms' which attempted to define the characteristic features of the experience of schizophrenia in explicit objective terms. The 11 symptoms described by Schneider were selected empirically and included auditory hallucinations, 'thought disorder', delusions and passivity of feeling. They were not based on any causal theory and Schneider did not regard them as either necessary for a diagnosis of schizophrenia, or exclusive to this disorder. The first rank symptoms could be reliably described and identified and, therefore, were instrumental in providing clinicians with their first real diagnostic tool. They have been incorporated into the major diagnostic schemes including DSM-III and the DSM-III-R.

Jaspers and Schneider had essentially eschewed any specific theory of the aetiology of the disorder, but during the 1950s and 1960s an organically based view re-emerged in Europe, principally as a function of the introduction of anti-psychotic drugs and the realisation that certain drug-induced states appeared to mimic the symptoms of schizophrenia. In North America, the influence of behavioural psychology was reflected in theories emphasising disturbances in drive and motivation (for example, Mednick, 1958). Psychosocial factors also received increasing attention stimulated by epidemiological evidence of differential prevalence rates amongst different social classes (Hollingshead & Redlich, 1958) and investigations of the family background of schizophrenic patients which suggested high rates of psychiatric illness and marital discord (Lidz et al., 1957; Wynne et al., 1958). Simultaneously with these developments, the emergence of the study of information processing, stimulated largely by Broadbent's (1958) *Perception and Communication,* led to renewed interest and detailed investigations of the attentional disturbances that had been central to both Kraepelin and Bleuler's original conceptions of the disorder (McGhie & Chapman, 1961; Shakow, 1962; Venables, 1964).

Over the period from the 1930s to the early 1950s, the admission rate for schizophrenia at the New York State Psychiatric Institute rose from 20 per cent to 80 per cent, but it remained constant at about 20 per cent over the same period at the Maudsley Hospital in London (Kuriansky, Deming & Gurland, 1974). These differences in the diagnostic rate in different countries and their potential importance to the understanding of psychosocial influences on diagnosis combined with concern about the lack of reliability of available diagnostic procedures (for example, Beck et al., 1962), led to an emphasis on the development of standardised diagnostic criteria and assessment instruments. The use of the Present State Examination (PSE) in the US–UK project (Cooper et al., 1972) and the International Pilot Study of Schizophrenia (Carpenter, Strauss & Bartko, 1974) established the utility of standardised interview procedures and paved the way for explicit operational diagnostic criteria as a 'remedy for diagnostic confusion' (Kendell, 1975).

A number of diagnostic schemes were developed during the 1970s in an effort to increase reliability and provide a basis for comparability of research findings. This proliferation of diagnostic systems replaced the earlier confusion with a 'babble of precise but differing formulations of the same concept' (Brockington, Kendell & Leff, 1978). These developments culminated in 1980 with the publication of DSM-III and the consequent formalisation of a single set of diagnostic criteria that have been adopted by most clinicians within the USA and Australia. These criteria deliberately defined a narrow concept of schizophrenia to increase reliability of diagnosis.

The DSM-III-R criteria

DSM-III-R relies principally on Schneider's first rank symptoms of delusions and hallucinations to diagnose schizophrenia. Longitudinal criteria are also critical. Active symptoms such as delusions and hallucinations must have occurred for at least one week and symptoms, whether active, prodromal or residual, must have been present continuously for six months. The criteria also require evidence of deterioration of functioning since symptom onset. Thought disorder, which was central to Bleuler's approach, is of limited diagnostic relevance: it must co-occur with either delusions, hallucinations or blunted affect to be of diagnostic significance. The reduced importance of thought disorder in DSM-III-R occurred because of the incidence of this symptom in other disorders and because of difficulties in reliably defining the construct. Disordered thought can only be inferred from disorganised speech, so identification of this symptom must always be indirect (Schwartz, 1982). Further narrowing of the disorder is achieved by excluding cases with prominent affective symptoms. Simple schizophrenia was placed in a separate category, 'Schizotypal Personality Disorder', and individuals who show symptoms for less than six months are classified as having suffered from 'Schizophreniform Disorder', a classification included in 'Psychotic Disorders Not Elsewhere Classified' rather than with schizophrenia. Thus, DSM-III and DSM-III-R criteria ultimately define a Kraepelinian concept of schizophrenia with a deteriorating course and relatively poor prognosis.

Table 8.1: Diagnostic criteria for Schizophrenia

A. Presence of characteristic psychotic symptoms in the active phase: either (1), (2), or (3) for at least one week (unless the symptoms are successfully treated):
   (1) two of the following:
      (a) delusions
      (b) prominent hallucinations (throughout the day for several days or several times a week for several weeks, each hallucinatory experience not being limited to a few brief moments)
      (c) incoherence or marked loosening of associations
      (d) catatonic behaviour
      (e) flat or grossly inappropriate affect
   (2) bizarre delusions (that is, involving a phenomenon that the person's culture would regard as totally implausible, for example, thought broadcasting, being controlled by a dead person)
   (3) prominent hallucinations [as defined in (1)(b) above] of a voice with content having no apparent relation to depression or elation, or a voice keeping up a running commentary on the person's behaviour or thoughts, or two or more voices conversing with each other.

B. During the course of the disturbance, functioning in such areas as work, social relations, and self-care is markedly below the highest level achieved before onset of the disturbance (or, when the onset is in childhood or adolescence, failure to achieve expected level of social development).

C. Schizoaffective Disorder and Mood Disorder with Psychotic Features have been ruled out, that is, if a Major Depressive or Manic Syndrome has ever been present during an active phase of the disturbance, the total duration of all episodes of a mood syndrome has been brief relative to the total duration of the active and residual phases of the disturbance.

D. Continuous signs of the disturbance for at least six months. The six-month period must include an active phase (of at least one week, or less if symptoms have been successfully treated) during which there were psychotic symptoms characteristic of Schizophrenia (symptoms in A), with or without a prodromal or residual phase, as defined below.

(*continued over*)

Table 8.1: Diagnostic criteria for Schizophrenia (*continued*)

Prodromal phase: A clear deterioration in functioning before the active phase of the disturbance that is not due to a disturbance in mood or to a Psychoactive Substance Use Disorder and that involves at least two of the symptoms listed below.
Residual phase: Following the active phase of the disturbance, persistence of at least two of the symptoms noted below, these not being due to a disturbance in mood or to a Psychoactive Substance Use Disorder.
Prodromal or residual symptoms:
(1) marked social isolation or withdrawal
(2) marked impairment in role functioning as wage-earner, student, or homemaker
(3) markedly peculiar behaviour (for example, collecting garbage, talking to self in public, hoarding food)
(4) marked impairment in personal hygiene and grooming
(5) blunted or inappropriate affect
(6) digressive, vague, overelaborate, or circumstantial speech, or poverty of speech, or poverty of content of speech
(7) odd beliefs or magical thinking, influencing behaviour and inconsistent with cultural norms, for example, superstitiousness, belief in clairvoyance, telepathy, sixth sense, others can feel my feelings, overvalued ideas, ideas of reference
(8) unusual perceptual experiences, recurrent illusions, sensing the presence of a force or person not actually present
(9) marked lack of initiative, interests, or energy.

Examples: Six months of prodromal symptoms with one week of symptoms from A; no prodromal symptoms with six months of symptoms from A; no prodromal symptoms with one week of symptoms from A and six months of residual symptoms.

E. It cannot be established that an organic factor initiated and maintained the disturbance.
F. If there is a history of Autistic Disorder, the additional diagnosis of Schizophrenia is made only if prominent delusions or hallucinations are also present.

Classification of course. The course of the disturbance is coded in the fifth digit.
(1) Subchronic. The time from the beginning of the disturbance, when the person first began to show signs of the disturbance (including prodromal, active, and residual phases) more or less continuously, is less than two years, but at least six months.
(2) Chronic. Same as above, but more than two years.
(3) Subchronic with Acute Exacerbation. Re-emergence of prominent psychotic symptoms in a person with a subchronic course who has been in the residual phase of the disturbance.
(4) Chronic with Acute Exacerbation. Re-emergence of prominent psychotic symptoms in a person with a chronic course who has been in the residual phase of the disturbance.
(5) In Remission. When a person with a history of Schizophrenia is free of all signs of the disturbance (whether or not on medication), 'in Remission' should be coded. Differentiating Schizophrenia in Remission from No Mental Disorder requires consideration of overall level of functioning, length of time since the last episode of disturbance, total duration of the disturbance, and whether prophylactic treatment is being given.
(0) Unspecified.

The reliability and validity of the DSM criteria

The implementation of standardised interview procedures and clear descriptive criteria that characterised the diagnostic schemes developed during the 1970s dramatically increased the reliability of the diagnosis of schizophrenia.

However, different, equally reliable, methods of diagnosing schizophrenia can yield very different classifications (Endicott et al., 1982) reflecting differences in the underlying conception of the disorder and consequent weighting of symptoms. It is therefore necessary to establish the validity of these different conceptions.

Assessing the validity of psychiatric diagnoses is difficult, particularly for disorders such as schizophrenia where there are no clear external criteria for determining the presence of the syndrome. Most evaluations focus on predictive validity: how well diagnosis predicts the course of the illness. Clinical outcome studies have demonstrated that cross-sectional measures of symptoms at one point in time are poor predictors of outcome and that diagnostic schemes such as DSM-III that incorporate longitudinal variables like duration of illness are better predictors of both short- and long-term outcome (for example, Stephens et al., 1982).

However, one can question whether such evidence really constitutes a validation of the DSM-III-R criteria as much as a confirmation of the evidence that guided the development of these criteria. The scheme demonstrates validity with respect to the construct of schizophrenia it was designed to assess, but questions can still be raised about whether it divides patients into groups that differ in underlying aetiology. Is schizophrenia necessarily a deteriorating disorder? Or, more specifically, are the causes of a brief episode of schizophrenia from which the individual recovers with no evidence of deterioration (DSM-III-R schizophreniform disorder) different from the causes of the chronic deteriorating condition described by Kraepelin and formalised in DSM-III-R criteria for schizophrenia? This issue is highlighted in the two cases presented below.

Table 8.2: Diagnostic criteria for Schizophreniform Disorder

A. Meets criteria A and C of Schizophrenia.
B. An episode of the disturbance (including prodromal, active, and residual phases) lasts less than six months. (When the diagnosis must be made without waiting for recovery, it should be qualified as 'provisional.')
C. Does not meet the criteria for Brief Reactive Psychosis, and it cannot be established that an organic factor initiated and maintained the disturbance.

Specify: without good prognostic features or with good prognostic features, i.e., with at least two of the following:

(1) onset of prominent psychotic symptoms within four weeks of first noticeable change in usual behaviour or functioning
(2) confusion, disorientation, or perplexity at the height of the psychotic episode
(3) good premorbid social and occupational functioning
(4) absence of blunted or flat affect.

Heterogeneity of schizophrenia

Schizophrenia is clearly a heterogeneous disorder. The DSM-III-R delineates subtypes defined by different patterns of symptoms (Disorganised, Paranoid, Catatonic, Undifferentiated, Residual). Individuals with continuously prominent affective symptoms or with a short history of symptoms are excluded from the diagnosis of schizophrenia. Both affective symptoms and a short symptom duration are associated with a better long-term prognosis so these exclusions enhance the predictive validity of the diagnosis. However, the separation of 'schizoaffective' disorder and 'schizophreniform' disorder from schizophrenia implies a causal distinction which it not clearly justified on the basis of any other source of evidence apart from outcome. Even more problematically, the particular symptom clusters differentiated in DSM-III-R are difficult to reliably distinguish from each other and are not useful predictors of prognosis or treatment (Stephens, 1978). In this sense, the DSM-III-R symptom subtypes lack both reliability and validity.

An alternative, symptom-based, subtype distinction currently receiving attention is that between 'positive' and 'negative' symptoms (Andreasen, 1982). Positive symptoms are the behavioural excesses of schizophrenia: delusions, hallucinations and some sorts of thought disorder such as loosening of associations and inability to keep to a train of thought. Negative symptoms are the behavioural deficits: reduced expressivity of affect, impaired attention and impoverished abstract thinking. A symptom picture dominated by negative symptoms tends to be associated with a poorer premorbid history, a poorer outcome and a higher incidence of neurological dysfunction (Andreasen, 1990). The dichotomy between positive and negative symptoms has been consistently supported by factor-analytic studies, the results of which suggest at least three types of symptoms (Andreasen, 1990).

Recent discussions have combined the positive/negative symptom distinction with evidence of biological indices of heterogeneity. Crow (1980), for example, distinguishes between Type 1 and Type II schizophrenia. The former is postulated to result from a neurochemical abnormality and to be characterised by principally positive symptoms and a good response to antipsychotic drugs, while the latter is argued to reflect brain abnormalities and to be associated with negative symptoms and a poorer outcome. Murray et al. (1988) suggest that Type II schizophrenia may be a neurodevelopmental disorder arising from prenatal or neonatal brain injury and may be a separate disorder from Type 1 schizophrenia.

Case studies

The case studies presented below describe two individuals who were assessed and treated in the psychiatric unit at a major hospital in Sydney. Both showed the active psychotic symptoms of schizophrenia but their illnesses followed very different courses. The first, Mary A, responded quickly to neuroleptic medication and has remained symptom-free. Because her symptoms lasted for less than six months, her correct diagnosis is actually schizophreniform disorder. The second individual, Jenny B, suffers frequent symptom recurrences and some level of negative symptomatology even when she is relatively well. She has been diagnosed as suffering from schizophrenia. Mary and Jenny also differ in the relative prominence of positive versus negative symptoms, but only the difference in duration contributes to their differential diagnosis by DSM-III-R criteria.

Mary A: Schizophreniform psychosis

Mary A was a 29-year-old divorced female, living alone. She was a microbiology technician with a consistent work record who functioned at a high level in this occupation. She had been born overseas.

Her father was a minister of religion and a school teacher, and her mother was a medical receptionist. She attended school until the age of 17, obtaining matriculation requirements. Her perceptions of her childhood and family relationships were negative. She saw herself as the black sheep of the family because she could not accept the conservative values of her parents. She felt rejected by them, and critical of herself because she could not get on with them. She felt angry because of their apparent rejection of her lifestyle. Mary was a sensitive individual, rather introspective, and perceived by her female friends as self-centred and demanding, suffering extreme mood swings. Her relationships with men were particularly unstable and stormy. She took an overdose of alcohol and tranquillisers in the context of a heterosexual relationship break-up. At the age of 26 she married but divorced 12 months later. Mary emigrated to Australia 'to make a fresh start' two years before her assessment.

In Australia she quickly found work as a technician and made friends. She commenced an affair with a married man, which ended about five months prior to her first psychiatric hospitalisation. Four months prior to her admission she returned to her country of origin to spend the Christmas holidays with her parents. This visit did not go well and reinforced her perception of her parents as rejecting. On her return to Australia, three months before assessment, she became anxious and confused, and suffered disturbed sleep. She felt unable to cope and became emotionally labile, at times uncontrollably tearful. Her work performance deteriorated and her relationship with her employer became strained. Two weeks before admission, she became highly distressed and reported to her friends that she was possessed by demons and had lost her identity. During this period she was reported to be incoherent at times. She was fearful that she was going to die from a serious medical disease. Finally, she presented herself to the casualty department of the local general hospital with extreme feelings of inability to cope, tearfulness and suicidal thoughts. She was referred to the psychiatric ward for admission.

In assessment, Mary was neatly dressed and well groomed. She was overly dramatic in manner, with marked mood changes and a markedly confused, perplexed and fearful affect. She was tearful intermittently throughout the interview. Mary's conversational style was extremely vague. She was preoccupied with identity and family issues, saying that she was involved in 'self-analysis' and that her psyche had merged with that of her boss. She made frequent references to having a serious physical illness such as leukemia, cancer of the uterus or a brain tumour. She was convinced that she was about to die and, though she repeatedly requested reassurance on this point, could not be convinced otherwise. She said she had a 'phantom pregnancy' and needed an exorcism. She described fleeting suicidal thoughts and agreed to hearing voices in her head, but was unwilling to specify the nature of these. Formal thought disorder was present but variable. At times she was incoherent and at others relatively lucid. However, even when lucid she tended to address topics out of keeping with the questions being asked of her. Though perplexed and confused in affect, Mary was fully alert and attentive and there was no evidence of delirium. Flight of ideas was absent and there was no other evidence of an affective illness. Physical examination was normal; blood pressure, pulse and temperature were normal; urinalysis and a urine drug screen were negative.

Mary was admitted to the emergency psychiatric ward for assessment. For two days she was maintained drug-free, except for isolated doses of minor tranquillisers. During that time Mary continued to be disorganised and emotionally labile. Her condition seemed to fluctuate but her preoccupations remained constant. She said that she knew she was going to die but wanted to know why. She continued to believe that she was possessed by a demon. At one time she said that she had to find her 'dead twin brother' and that she needed a spiritualist. At another time she said that she was the twin of Jesus and possessed by a devil. Her extreme fear of death was continuous with frequent expressions such as 'I'm dying with each breath that I take, please put me to sleep'. On the third day of her admission, anti-psychotic treatment was commenced. Over the next week Mary improved rapidly and was able to be discharged from hospital 11 days after admission.

Mary was reviewed as an outpatient one week later and found to be much improved, but still showed mild signs of thought disorder and emotional lability. Her medication was increased. Mary took this increased dose for a few days, experienced drowsiness and stopped it without seeking medical advice. Psychotic symptoms re-emerged along with increased thought disorder and preoccupation with imaginary illnesses. She was significantly more disorganised. Her medication was changed and one month after discharge Mary was completely recovered. At follow-up six months after admission to hospital, medication was ceased. Six and twelve months after discharge Mary showed no evidence of psychosis. The diagnosis of schizophreniform disorder, with good prognostic features (DSM-III-R) was made.

Jenny B: Schizophrenia

Jenny B was a single 29-year-old woman who had been supported on disability benefits for five years. She was Australian-born and the third of seven children. Her parents were divorced when Jenny was about 13 years old. Thereafter the parents lived in the family home occupying separate rooms. The father previously worked as an office worker but when Jenny was about 9 years old, he became permanently unemployed and alcohol dependent. He displayed 'schizotypal' traits and was described as very isolated, preoccupied with peculiar ideas, having no friends and doing little more than 'potter' about the house. Apparently none of his children liked him and he did not assist with their upbringing. The mother commenced work as a clerk about the time the father became unemployed. She was a very reserved woman who likened herself to Jenny in personality.

Jenny had an avoidant and dependent personality, tending to avoid social contact, being easily hurt by criticism, and relying on important figures, especially her mother, to make everyday decisions. As a child she was always considered 'the odd one out', being quiet, unassertive and never a discipline problem. Adjustment problems emerged in adolescence and at about the age of 17 Jenny commenced seeing a psychiatrist in long-term supportive counselling. Jenny completed high school at the age of 18.

She did two years of a Bachelor of Arts course at a local university before dropping out to move interstate for 12 months where she did clerical work to save money for an extended overseas trip. At the age of 24 she returned to university for a further two years to complete her Arts degree. During this time she continued to see the psychiatrist, live away from home with a girl friend, and had her first steady heterosexual relationship lasting about 12 months. Jenny enrolled in a Diploma of Education course but early in the year there was a change in her behaviour, with marked social withdrawal which prevented her from attending classes. Jenny moved back home where she became even more withdrawn. She stayed in her room most of the time and only occasionally spoke to her siblings and mother. She did not attempt to contact friends. Associated with this withdrawal was marked restriction of day-to-day activities. Self-grooming and hygiene were affected. Jenny spent a great deal of the time lying on her bed or sitting staring into space. Occasionally inappropriate laughter and oddities in her verbal communication were noted. That year her psychiatrist arranged for a psychiatric assessment in hospital, when Jenny was 26 years old.

On admission, Jenny was very passive. She showed reduced spontaneous and expressive movements. She sat in a slightly unnatural or stilted manner, and movements were slowed. Long pauses sometimes occurred before Jenny answered a question. Her facial expressivity, expressive gesturing and vocal inflection were reduced. She was cooperative when general details were discussed; however, when items related to the possibility of a psychiatric illness were broached, Jenny became guarded and evasive, and her speech tended to be vague and circumstantial and occasionally difficult to follow. Jenny denied having delusions and hallucinations. Her affect appeared flat or blunted but she denied being depressed. Her physical examination was normal.

Jenny was admitted to an open ward and assessed drug-free in a variety of group activities. She was reluctant to be involved in such activities and remained emotionally withdrawn from staff and other patients. On occasions inappropriate grimacing and smiling, and giggling occurred without discernible cause. A trial of medication was commenced. She became more organised and motivated toward ward activities, and better able to express herself clearly. She was less socially withdrawn. Her tendency to smile inappropriately was reduced. Jenny was discharged improved but not recovered after two months in hospital. The diagnosis of schizophrenia, type unspecified, was made.

For the next two years Jenny was seen as an outpatient by a psychiatrist. She did not return to work or study. She alternated between living at home and having brief stays in bed-sitter accommodation. Her compliance with medication during this period was variable. She continued to show residual deficit or 'negative' symptoms of schizophrenia, as observed in hospital, particularly affective flattening and inappropriateness. Chronic mild formal thought disorder was evident, characterised by a tendency to make vague or 'woolly' statements reflecting imprecise or impaired abstract ability inconsistent with her educational record. Anti-depressant medication did not change Jenny's condition.

Two years after her first psychiatric admission, Jenny was re-admitted to hospital. She had a five-month history of non-compliance with medication and a two-month history of acute or 'positive' psychotic symptoms. These included the delusional belief that inconsequential events had particular significance to her (delusions of reference). She believed that people had been looking at her in an 'odd' manner and were making reference to her, and that she had heard people who did not know her calling out her name and making derogatory comments about her. She believed that a man, whom she could not identify, was following her and monitoring her behaviour with the intention of harming her. Prior to admission, Jenny had not coped with the demands of daily living, had not eaten properly and suffered disturbed sleep. She reported recurrent suicidal thoughts without any impulse or planning to act on them. In an interview, Jenny was noted to have poor eye contact and reduced emotional responsiveness. At times fatuous giggling inappropriate to the situation occurred. She was preoccupied with distressing thoughts that schizophrenia was a 'shared-reality', an idea she attributed to a social worker. She said this meant that the social worker wanted to harm her or threaten her. Formal thought disorder was evidenced by responses that were tangential to the question being asked.

Jenny's medication was recommenced. Her delusions and hallucinations settled, but Jenny continued to show impoverished abstract thinking, blunted affect and occasional inappropriate giggling. She was slowed in her movements and continued to show long latency in her responses to questions. Depressive mood and suicidal ideation ceased and Jenny was discharged to after-care halfway house accommodation, with arrangements for her to attend the occupational therapy program at the hospital several days a week. The diagnosis of chronic undifferentiated schizophrenia was made.

Following discharge from hospital, Jenny continued to be disabled by the deficit symptoms of schizophrenia. Variable compliance with medication continued and she occasionally considered suicide. Nine months after discharge Jenny was re-admitted to hospital for one month because of adjustment disorder with depressive features. A different medication was tried and Jenny was included in assertiveness training and cognitive therapy. After discharge from hospital, she joined a job retraining scheme. Three months later Jenny was re-admitted to hospital for two weeks. She became preoccupied with thoughts about her health and fears of dying. Her sleep had become disturbed. Several recent sources of stress, including a change of accommodation and her mother being out of the city, seemed related to the admission. Delusions or hallucinations could not be detected, but Jenny was almost mute with a frightened, perplexed facial expression. Other positive symptoms may, therefore, have been present. When she did speak she described 'loss of boundaries between herself and her environment', and distress arising from her inability to distinguish herself from the world. Hypochondriacal preoccupation was present, Jenny being constantly aware of her bodily sensations such as her breathing, her pulse and body parts that she was normally unaware of. Jenny's medication was increased slightly and she was discharged from hospital.

Three months later Jenny was again re-admitted with persecutory thoughts concerning her next door neighbour, and delusions of reference concerning the broadcast television. Deficit symptoms described on previous admissions were also present. After a further increase in medication, Jenny was discharged.

Case comparison

These two cases illustrate two major issues relating to the DSM-III-R diagnosis of schizophrenia. Firstly, only Jenny B received the diagnosis of schizophrenia. Though the two individuals showed similar symptoms during the acute stages of their illness, because Mary's symptoms were evident for less than six months, she is classified as having suffered from schizophreniform psychosis rather than schizophrenia. Secondly, there are differences in the pattern of symptoms demonstrated by the two individuals. Mary's symptoms were predominantly positive: fragmentary delusions, some hallucinations and signs of positive thought disorder. Jenny B initially presented with primary negative symptomatology including social withdrawal, deterioration in self-care and flattened affect but her later episodes have been characterised by more florid symptoms including ideas of reference, paranoid delusions and hallucinations in addition to inappropriate affect and negative thought disorder (poverty of speech and poverty of content of speech). It is, in fact, the history of negative symptoms listed as characteristic of prodromal and residual phases in DSM-III-R that allowed Jenny to be diagnosed with schizophrenia on her first admission.

The different diagnoses assigned to these individuals appear validated by their different outcomes. Whereas Mary appears to be completely recovered from the disorder, Jenny B has remained moderately to severely impaired and has suffered recurrent florid episodes. However, the different diagnoses are achieved entirely on the basis of the duration of symptoms. The symptoms experienced by the two women during florid episodes are similar, particularly with regard to the 'first rank' symptoms of delusions and hallucinations. Both also showed some evidence of positive thought disorder. Jenny B consistently showed more evidence of the negative symptoms of blunted and inappropriate affect. But the differential diagnosis is not achieved on these grounds, as DSM-III-R states 'the essential features of [schizophreniform disorder] are identical with schizophrenia, with the exception that duration … is less than six months'. That is, it is only because Jenny B recovers that she is not classified as suffering from schizophrenia.

At one level, these cases appear to justify the inclusion of duration as a criterion for the diagnoses of schizophrenia. The differences between these two individuals are in accord with the evidence showing that symptom duration is a good predictor of outcome (Stephens, 1978). However, accurate prediction does not reflect any theory or knowledge about the causes of the disorder and the reasons for the differences in outcome.

Reflecting this lack of understanding of the causes of the differences between the course of the two patients' illness, they received the same treatment: anti-psychotic medications. Different specific drugs were prescribed principally because of Jenny B's failure to continue to take tablets herself. Ultimately, when it appeared that she would experience recurrent episodes and fail to take medication herself, she was given injections of 'depot' medication. The modifications to Mary's medication were based on treatment response and side-effects of the drugs rather than assumptions about the specificity of drug effects for her particular symptoms.

Thus, the DSM-III-R criteria convey minimal information about the causes of differences in the particular patterns of symptoms shown by these two individuals. The criteria successfully 'predict' outcome, but without any understanding of the causes of acute versus chronic forms of the disorder.

To refine diagnostic procedures and improve treatment strategies we need more information about the basis of schizophrenic symptoms and the relationships of these symptoms to the course of the disorder. Theories of information processing drawn from cognitive psychology provide both a framework for understanding these relationships and a set of procedures for investigating them.

A process orientated approach to understanding the course of schizophrenia

Information-processing deficits and schizophrenia

Most theories of the cognitive deficit in schizophrenia have focused on the attentional deficits first described by Kraepelin and Bleuler. The general assumption is that schizophrenic symptoms result from an attentional dysfunction which leads to a breakdown in the selectivity of attention. A variety of different specific explanations of this breakdown have been proposed (Callaway & Naghdi, 1982; Frith, 1979; Hemsley, 1975; Venables, 1978).

An enormous variety of experimental tasks have been used to investigate attentional disturbances in schizophrenic populations. Nuechterlein and Dawson (1984) reviewed the results of this research not only in groups of patients who were actively psychotic, but also in people in whom florid symptoms had largely remitted, and in populations hypothesised to be at increased risk for the development of schizophrenia. They concluded that all three groups show attentional deficits in tasks that involve a 'high momentary processing load' — tasks which place heavy demands on attentional processes. The fact that deficits are evident in remitted and at-risk groups suggests that the abnormalities are related to the 'diathesis' (vulnerability) to schizophrenia (Zubin & Spring, 1977) rather than reflecting transient characteristics of the schizophrenic state.

Though this evidence underlines the importance of attentional disturbances in schizophrenia, it does not help to refine understanding of the precise basis of the cognitive deficit. Part of the difficulty in interpreting the evidence lies in the fact that there are a number of reasons why schizophrenics might perform more slowly and less accurately in attentionally demanding tasks: lack of motivation to undertake the task, difficulty in organising motor activity, or non-specific difficulty in fulfilling task demands. Although it is possible to control for some of these factors by using appropriate control conditions (Chapman & Chapman, 1973) it would clearly be an advantage to measure cognitive processes more directly in a manner that is less susceptible to the influence of motivation.

Brain event-related potentials (ERPs) provide such a measure. These electrophysiological measures are obtained by analysing brain electrical activity, the electroencephalogram (EEG), which is recorded using electrodes attached to the scalp while discrete stimulus events, such as tones, light flashes or mild shocks are experienced by a subject. When averaged across multiple presentations of the same type of stimulus, random fluctuations in the EEG tend to cancel out, and an 'ERP waveform' is obtained which consists of a series of positive and negative-going voltage deflections produced by the stimulus. This ERP represents the electrical activity that occurs during stimulus processing. Some of the deflections (bumps) in the waveform are present in the ERPs elicited in a wide variety of tasks and are systematically related to specific experimental manipulations. Such deflections are referred to as ERP 'components' and are assumed to reflect the operation of particular cognitive processes. Components are usually described in terms of their polarity (positive or negative), time of occurrence with respect to stimulus onset and distribution across the scalp. For example, a positive-going peak reaching maximal amplitude approximately 300 milliseconds post-stimulus and most evident at posterior scalp sites is referred to as P300 (positive 300).

The 'exogenous' components in the early part of the ERP waveform (approximately 100 milliseconds after the stimulus) are primarily sensitive to the physical characteristics of stimuli such as their intensity. Later, 'endogenous', components appear to reflect cognitive processes that vary according to the particular task the subject is engaged in while the recording is taking place (see figure 8.1, page 143).

ERP abnormalities in schizophrenia: P300

A number of ERP components have been investigated in schizophrenia (see Pritchard, 1986, for review). The component that has received the most attention is the P300. P300 has been observed in a wide variety of tasks but is typically investigated with auditory stimuli in which subjects must press a button whenever they hear a relatively infrequent 'target' tone amongst a background of other tones that differ from the target on a physical dimension such as pitch, intensity or duration. The ERP elicited by the target stimulus in healthy subjects is characterised by a large P300 which is absent from the ERPs for the background stimuli. The P300 shown by schizophrenic patients is dramatically reduced relative to that for healthy controls (see figure 8.2, page 145). A similar reduction in schizophrenics' P300 is evident in tasks using more complex stimulus such as words and sentences (Mitchell et al., 1991).

Reduced P300 amplitude is not specific to schizophrenia. This abnormality has also been reported in association with dementia, infantile autism, attention deficit disorder and alcoholism (see Pritchard, 1986, for review). Though P300 attenuation has also been reported in depressed populations, the evidence is equivocal. Any attenuation that is present appears to be less than in schizophrenic populations and to be normalised by tricyclic medication (Pritchard, 1986). By contrast, there is accumulating evidence that the P300 abnormalities in schizophrenia reflect an enduring disposition rather than a transient attentional disturbance.

A number of studies have found that the amplitude of P300 is reduced in the relatives of schizophrenics (for example, Friedman, Vaughan & Erlenmeyer-Kimling, 1982; Saitoh et al., 1984; but see also negative findings of Friedman et al., 1988) and in healthy subjects hypothesised to be at increased risk for the development of schizophrenia based on psychometric indices (for example, Simons, 1982; Ward et al., 1984; Josiassen et al., 1985; Miller, Simons & Lang, 1986).

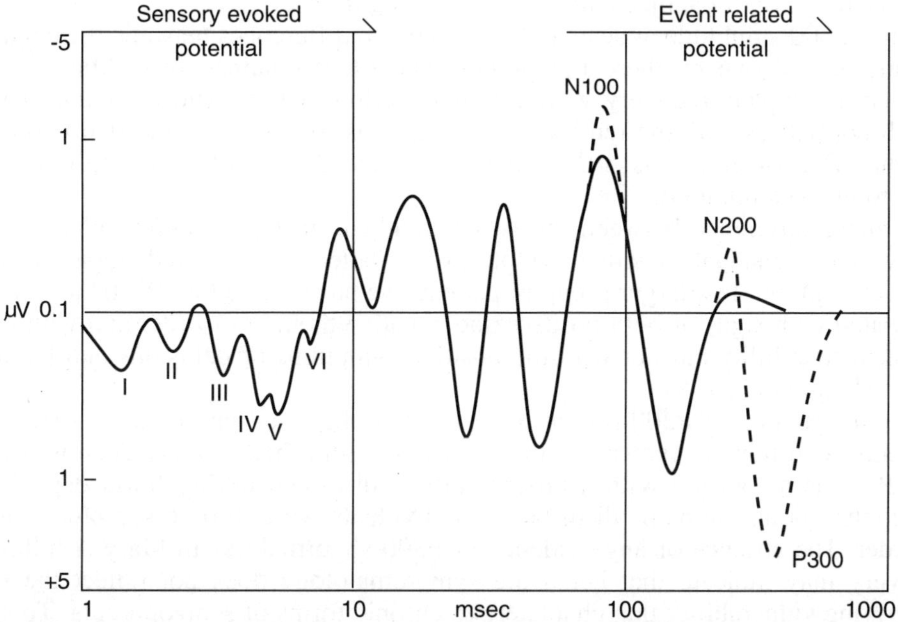

Figure 8.1: An example of idealised averaged waveforms elicited by simple auditory stimuli such as tones or clicks over the 1000 ms following stimulus onset. Deflections of the waveform in the first 10 ms (I-VI) are evoked by sensory characteristics of the stimulus. Later components appear to reflect endogenous processes that operate on the stimulus, thus the term 'event-related potentials'. Stimuli that must be attended to in order to make a decision and/or response (for example, dotted waveform) typically elicit a P300 component that is reduced or absent from the waveform for unattended stimuli (for example, solid line) and are also associated with enhanced N100 and N200 components (adapted from Hillyard, Picton & Regan, 1978).

Though one study has found evidence that patients who improve on neuroleptic treatment show a normalisation of P300 (Duncan et al., 1987), most longitudinal investigations have demonstrated that reduced P300 persists after remission of positive florid symptoms (for example, Kameyama et al., 1987; McPherson et al., 1991). This persistence is illustrated in the recordings obtained from Jenny B (see figure 8.3, page 146). Her ERPs reveal no clear P300 to target tones even though the recording was conducted when she was an outpatient and suffering only from residual negative symptoms — flattened affect and some impairment of abstract thinking. Given the absence of P300 when she was relatively well, it is most likely that her P300 was also reduced at the time that she showed florid psychotic symptoms. ERPs were recorded from Mary A on two occasions: at the beginning of her hospital admission when she was suffering prominent positive symptoms, and

5 months after discharge when she was completely recovered. On the first occasion when she was ill, the P300 elicited by the target tones was reduced relative to that typically shown by healthy subjects. By contrast, the P300 observed in the waveforms obtained following recovery is large and indistinguishable from that obtained from healthy control subjects in this task (see figure 8.2).

Thus, P300 amplitude appears to be sensitive to differences between the cognitive impairments shown by these individuals. The ERPs obtained from Mary A, who showed a complete recovery within a short period of time, show a reduced P300 which normalises with the remission of symptoms. By contrast, the P300 observed in Jenny B's waveforms is still dramatically reduced even when her florid positive symptoms have remitted.

A major difference between the two individuals in the remission phase is that Jenny B has residual negative symptoms — flattened affect and impairments in abstract thinking. In a larger group of patients we have found that P300 amplitude is correlated with signs of both positive and negative thought disorder and with attentional distractibility but not with the positive symptoms of delusions and hallucinations (Ward et al., 1991).

The attenuation of P300 shown by Mary A in the acute phase of her illness and by Jenny B following remission are consistent with a body of evidence indicating that P300 is associated with a process that is disturbed during florid episodes of schizophrenia and remains disturbed in individuals with chronic symptoms of the disorder. The absence of any evidence of P300 abnormalities in Mary A following recovery may indicate that her acute symptomatology does not reflect the same underlying vulnerability that characterises chronic forms of schizophrenia. This distinction is captured by DSM-III-R but only on the basis of the retrospective criterion of symptom duration.

The discussion so far does not address the issue of exactly what cognitive process is indexed by P300. There are many specific theories concerning the cognitive processes underlying P300 (for example, Pritchard, 1981; Polich, 1991). In general, these theories identify P300 with active attentional processes required to categorise a stimulus and make a decision about the required response. Some theorists assume that the major function of the processes indexed by P300 lies in updating of the 'hypotheses or models of the environment' (Donchin, 1979, page 66) that guide future behaviour. According to this view, schizophrenics' P300 abnormalities may reflect a failure to maintain an accurate model of the current environmental context that can serve as a basis for goal-directed behaviour.

P300 amplitude in normal subjects is correlated with measures of a conceptual thinking style referred to as allusive thinking (McConaghy et al., in revision; Ward et al., 1984; Ward, Catts & McConaghy, in press). Allusive thinking is reflected in a tendency to group objects more loosely and become aware of a broader array of relationships between objects (McConaghy, 1960). The fact that P300 is related to allusive thinking in healthy subjects and to negative thought disorder in schizophrenia suggests a relationship between some aspects of schizophrenic thought disorder and a mode of thinking also present in healthy individuals. The common feature of these two styles of thought may be a broader focus of attention perhaps arising from a failure to inhibit irrelevant associations (see Halgren, 1990).

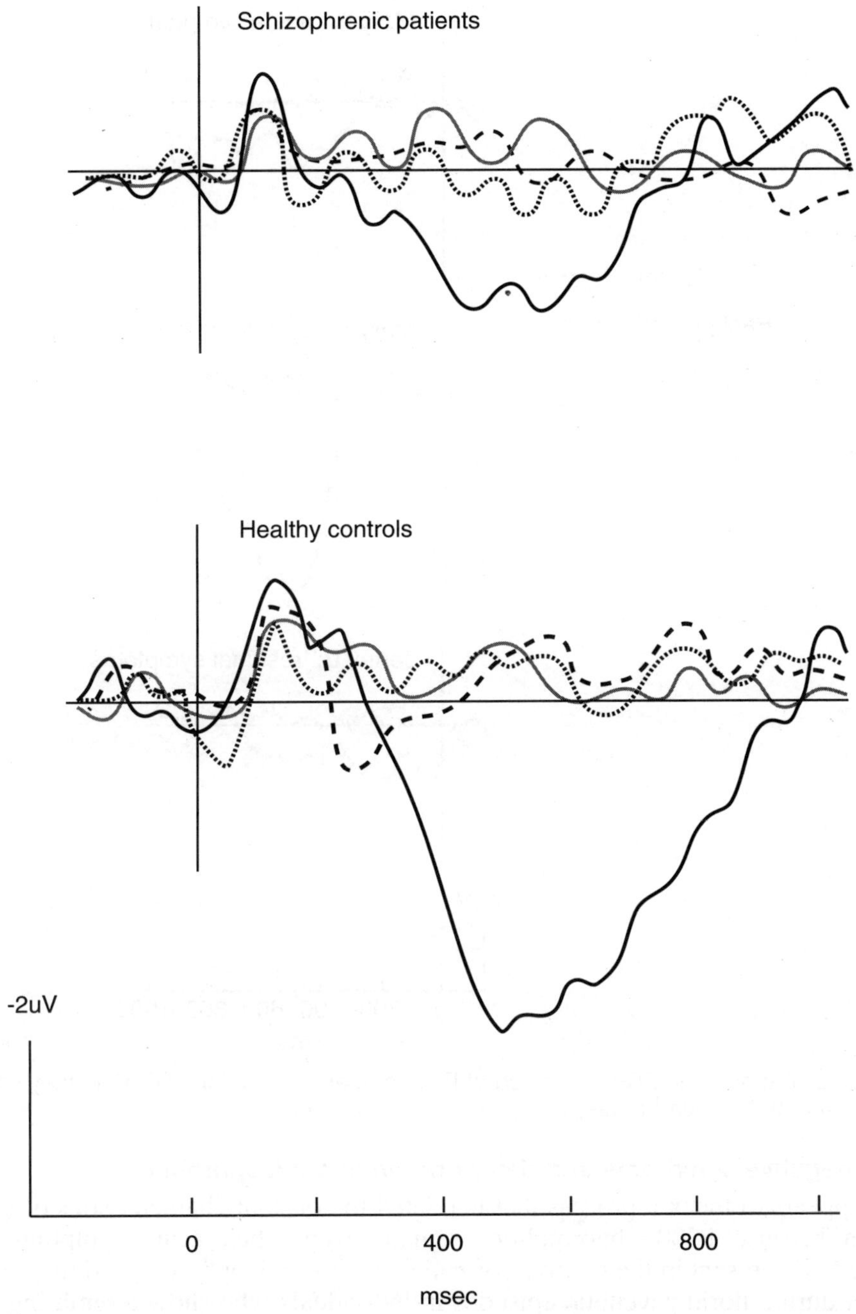

Figure 8.2: Averaged waveforms elicited by target (solid line) and background (broken lines) tones at Pz scalp site in a sample of schizophrenic patients and a sample of age- and sex-matched healthy control subjects. The major difference between the groups is that the amplitude of the P300 component is dramatically reduced in the schizophrenic sample (data from Ward et al., 1991).

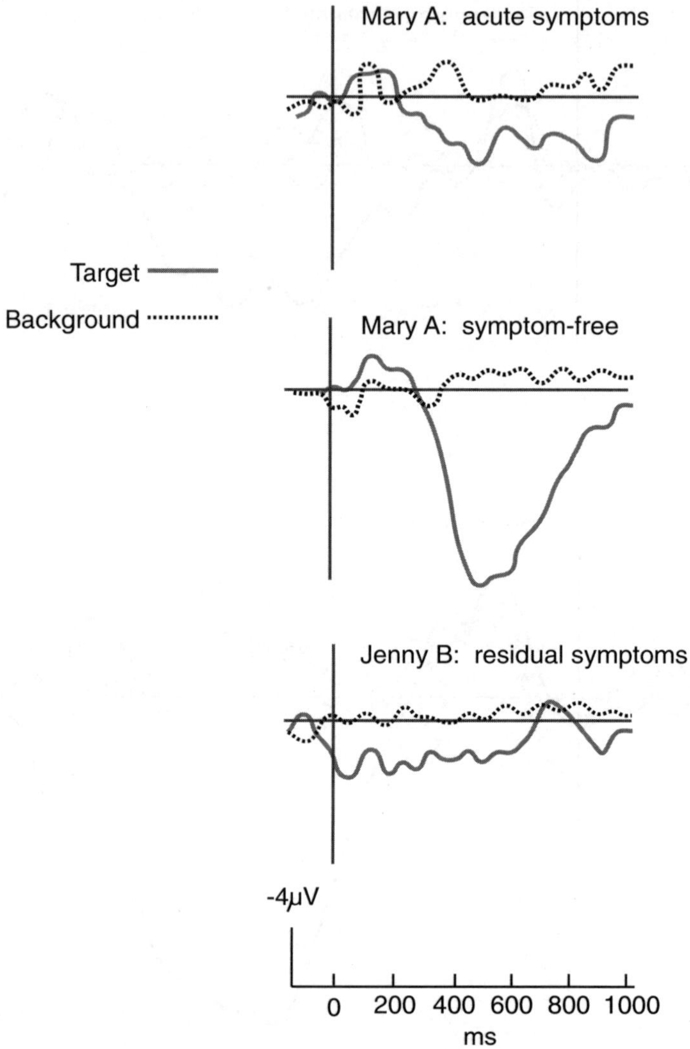

Figure 8.3: The average ERPs recorded at Pz from Mary A and Jenny B while they listened to target and background tones

P300, negative symptoms and deterioration in schizophrenia

P300 appears to index a process that is related to constant characteristics of schizophrenia because P300 abnormalities remain even when acute symptoms have remitted, are present in the relatives of patients with schizophrenia, and may only be evident during florid psychotic episodes in individuals who show a remitting rather than chronic form of the disorder. P300 appears to be related to symptoms of thought disorder and attentional disturbance but not to the first rank symptoms of delusions and hallucinations. This differential relationship is consistent with suggestions that positive and negative symptoms may reflect different processes or subtypes of the disorder (Crow, 1980; Murray et al., 1988).

The issue of the relationship between positive and negative symptoms is contentious. The distinction has its roots in the work of the famous neurophysiologist, Hughlings-Jackson (Berrios, 1985), who proposed a hierarchical model of central nervous system dysfunction whereby negative symptoms reflect the loss of 'higher' cortical functions. This loss facilitates the release of healthy lower centres, whose influence on behaviour is normally inhibited by the higher centres, and is reflected in positive symptoms. This model predicts that positive symptoms cannot occur in the absence of negative symptoms (Berrios, 1985), a view which conflicts with recent proposals that imply a dichotomy between positive and negative symptoms and identify them with distinct syndromes (Mackay & Crow, 1980). An alternative framework suggests that positive and negative symptoms are different reflections of a similar set of causal factors which interact with environmental stressors. Wing (1988) argues that either set of symptoms can become prominent in chronic patients with overly demanding environments leading to an exacerbation of positive symptoms and impoverished or under-stimulating environments resulting in the development of more negative symptoms. Some versions of this general framework have assumed that positive symptoms reflect an early response to the attentional disturbances underlying schizophrenia in which an attempt is made to interpret the multiplicity of stimuli impinging on the cognitive system, and that negative symptoms reflect a later protective response in which incoming information is inhibited to reduce cognitive overload (Bebbington & Kuipers, 1988). Such a view is consistent with a Kraepelinian concept of schizophrenia in which the stage of acute illness is succeeded by a defect state which steadily deteriorates.

In contrast to these suggestions that negative symptoms reflect a particular response to attentional dysfunctions or the later consequences of the deteriorating nature of the disorder, there is recent evidence that negative symptoms and associated abnormalities may precede positive symptoms and signal a subtype of schizophrenia with a relatively poor outcome. Some patients initially present with predominantly negative symptoms and only later show delusions and hallucinations. Jenny B, for example, showed such a symptom course. The presence of early negative symptoms is associated with a poorer outcome (Kolakowska et al., 1985) and these symptoms are better predictors of later social functioning than are florid positive symptoms (Wing, 1988). Negative symptoms have been demonstrated to be associated with evidence of structural brain abnormalities such as enlarged cerebral ventricles (Johnstone et al., 1976) and such enlargement has been found in first-admission cases of schizophrenia (Turner, Toone & Brett-Jones, 1986) indicating that they may precede the development of symptoms. It has been further argued that the prodromal symptoms of schizophrenia such as attentional disturbances, social withdrawal and reduced motivation and self-care might be regarded as early negative symptoms (Murray et al., 1988) in which case the well-established relationship between poorer premorbid functioning and poor outcome might be taken as further evidence that early negative symptoms reflect a deteriorating form of the disorder.

Murray et al. (1988) argue that the causes of this disorder may lie in the neuropathological consequences of perinatal brain injury. The incidence of obstetric complications is higher in schizophrenic than control populations (for example, Parnas et al., 1982) and a history of obstetric complications in people with schizophrenia is related to structural brain abnormalities in schizophrenic patients (Owens et al., 1985) and to difficulties in premorbid adjustment and early onset of schizophrenic symptoms (Lewis, Murray & Owen, 1988). Thus, in schizophrenic populations, brain injury consequent on obstetric complications is associated with poor premorbid adjustment, early onset and negative symptoms all of which are, in turn, associated with a relatively poor prognosis.

The association between P300 and negative symptoms, combined with the fact that P300 abnormalities persist in the absence of positive symptoms, implies that P300 may reflect cognitive processes related to those assumed to underlie the deteriorating form of the disorder. The evidence that P300 abnormalities also occur in the relatives of schizophrenics appears to conflict with the assumption that an environmental factor such as early brain injury plays a causal role. However, the effects of brain injury may interact with genetic factors. In fact, such an assumption seems necessary because the vast majority of individuals who suffer obstretic complications do not develop schizophrenia. While the site or timing of early brain injury may be critical determinants, it is also possible that obstetric complications only result in schizophrenia in individuals with a genetic disposition to the disorder. Consistent with this possibility, in families with a genetic risk to schizophrenia, a sibling who suffers obstetric complications has a higher probability of developing the disorder than siblings who have uncomplicated births (for example, Schulsinger et al., 1984).

The causes of positive symptoms

If negative symptoms are taken to reflect a neurodevelopmental disorder, what are the causes of positive symptoms? Do they reflect a distinct aetiology or are they a different response to the same causal factors? The fact that the majority of people with schizophrenia demonstrate both types of symptoms, albeit at different levels at different times, implies common causal factors. However, the existence of individuals such as Mary A who exhibit almost exclusively positive symptoms and do not demonstrate a chronic deteriorating disorder supports the possibility of distinct causal factors. A further possibility is that positive symptomatology reflects the influence of a 'final common pathway' which is involved in both acute and chronic forms of schizophrenia but reflects different underlying causes. The fact that even individuals like Mary who recover completely do show the cognitive abnormality reflected in P300 during the acute phase of the disorder is consistent with the existence of some common factor. However, in patients who recover, the attentional dysfunction indexed by P300 may be the consequence of some other cognitive deficit which is unrelated to the P300 abnormalities apparently associated with the disposition to schizophrenia.

Models of information processing provide relatively weak explanations of positive symptoms of schizophrenia, particularly delusions and hallucinations. The general interpretation offered by these models is that hallucinations and delusions reflect the fact that humans are active processors of information who attempt to synthesise and interpret incoming stimuli in the light of stored knowledge (Neisser, 1976). Thus, hallucinations are interpretations of the cognitive consequences of inadequately filtered stimuli and delusions are attempts to provide a coherent explanation of such disturbed perceptions (for example, Frith, 1979). However, such suggestions are very difficult to directly test and fail to provide explanation of other features of the experience of schizophrenia such as 'the spurious sense of significance' (Anscombe, 1987) or the loss of volitional control over behaviour (Frith, 1987).

In addition to these difficulties in defining the causes of first-rank positive symptoms, questions have recently been raised about the appropriateness of giving these symptoms the prominence that they have in DSM-III-R (Andreasen & Flaum, 1991). Many of these symptoms apparently occur for relatively brief periods of time in many people with schizophrenia. They also occur in other disorders, particularly the manic phase of bipolar disorder (for example, Carpenter & Strauss, 1974). In considering the implications of such evidence for the development of DSM-IV criteria for schizophrenia, Andreasen and Flaum (1991) conclude that 'they should not be given undue prominence or treated as the major criterion symptoms'.

Implications for diagnosis and treatment

Defining schizophrenia

The major emphasis in the development of the DSM-III and DSM-III-R criteria for schizophrenia was on achieving reliability of diagnosis. This resulted in an emphasis on positive first-rank symptoms to define the active phase of schizophrenia. The only negative symptom included as characteristic of the active phase is flat or inappropriate affect but other negative symptoms such as social isolation or withdrawal, blunted affect and negative thought disorder are listed as being characteristic of the prodromal or residual phase. The diagnosis of schizophrenia requires continuous evidence of symptoms from either class over six months including at least one week of active symptoms, but no diagnostic significance is attached to the relative balance of positive and negative symptoms.

The developers of DSM-III justified reliance on observable positive symptoms on the grounds that diagnostic reliability is a prerequisite for validity. If different clinicians and researchers adopt different definitions of schizophrenia, it is impossible to achieve meaningful communication between professionals or to accumulate evidence that will enhance understanding of the causes of the disorder. However, reliability does not guarantee validity — the fact that clinicians can agree that a set of individuals satisfy the criteria for schizophrenia does not establish that they are the 'right' criteria. Moreover, the scientific precision implied by high levels of reliability can disguise a lack of validity. If an inappropriate set of diagnostic definitions becomes cemented into clinical practice, progress in understanding and treating the disorder will be impeded.

The major criterion for determining the validity of a psychiatric diagnosis is its utility in making predictions about the course and treatment of the disorder. The major treatment used for schizophrenia is the class of anti-psychotic (anti-dopamine) drugs, which clearly reduces the acute symptoms of schizophrenia in most patients. Maintenance of anti-psychotic medication is associated with a reduced likelihood of relapse and rehospitalisation (see Johnson, 1988, for review).

In this sense, the diagnosis of schizophrenia does provide the basis for accurate treatment decisions. It is clear, however, that neuroleptic drugs are not equally effective for all individuals. Approximately 30 per cent of patients relapse within 2 years despite regular medication (although medication may delay relapse), and about 20 per cent of patients with chronic schizophrenia do not relapse and show equivalent levels of functioning with or without medication (Johnson, 1988). Current diagnostic criteria do not provide any basis for differentiating these subgroups.

Both by the inclusion of duration criteria and by the exclusion of individuals with continuous affective symptomatology, DSM-III-R ultimately defines a population with a reasonably homogeneous outcome. At least half of the individuals diagnosed as suffering from schizophrenia by DSM-III-R criteria will remain moderately to seriously impaired by the disorder (for example, Englehardt et al., 1982). However, this 'predictive validity' has been built into the diagnostic criteria. Prominent affective symptoms and a short symptom duration, often reflecting the absence of prodromal symptoms and in that sense better premorbid adjustment, are known to be associated with a better prognosis. Excluding such cases from the diagnosis guarantees a more homogeneous outcome.

Thus, while the DSM-III-R criteria for schizophrenia can be argued to demonstrate treatment and predictive validity, this does not establish the validity of the construct of schizophrenia defined by the criteria. The criteria define a relatively chronic deteriorating condition but this is not based on evidence that the causes of such a syndrome are different from the causes of schizophrenic symptoms in individuals who recover with minimal residual impairment. If the two syndromes do reflect different causal factors, then it may be possible to develop more tailored treatment procedures and to provide relatives and carers with more accurate information about likely prognosis.

Some of the options under consideration for DSM-IV involve changes to the duration criteria. The major modification suggested is to increase the period over which active psychotic symptoms must be present from one week to one month to increase compatibility with the International Classification of Diseases (ICD) diagnostic system, the tenth edition of which is due to appear at about the same time as DSM-IV. Field trials are currently considering the implications of increasing the duration requirement for active symptoms (Andreasen & Flaum, 1991). Even if this modification is adopted, the DSM and ICD systems will still differ because the ICD criteria do not require that some symptoms have been present for at least six months. Thus, many individuals diagnosed as suffering schizophreniform disorder in DSM-III-R are classified within the schizophrenia section of ICD-9. Though the possibility of dropping this requirement from DSM-IV was considered, it has been maintained in all of the options being field tested because of the strong relationship between symptom duration and outcome (Flaum & Andreasen, 1991).

This relationship is, however, not a validation of the differentiation and is, in fact, almost tautological. If an individual recovers within six months, they receive the diagnosis of schizophreniform disorder and if they retain residual symptoms or experience a recurrence they are diagnosed with schizophrenia. To render this distinction of predictive value so that it can be used to facilitate treatment planning, it is necessary to understand the different causal factors contributing to the course of the disorder. The case studies illustrate typical differences between both the course and symptom patterns associated with acute and chronic forms of schizophrenia. Mary A, who recovered quickly, showed primarily positive symptoms. Jenny B, who suffered a more deteriorating course, initially presented with primarily negative symptoms and these remained prominent in her behaviour throughout the course of the illness.

Defining the heterogeneity in schizophrenia

These considerations suggest that negative symptoms should be given a more prominent role in diagnosing schizophrenia and distinguishing between different subtypes of the disorder (Crow, 1980; Murray et al., 1988). DSM-III-R does distinguish between the two symptom groups in the sense that all of the symptoms described in association with the active phase of the disorder are positive except for flat or inappropriate affect. Other negative symptomatology is described as characteristic of the prodromal and residual phases. However, the two sets of symptoms are not distinguished when assigning diagnosis except that active symptoms must have been present for at least one week.

Most of the options being considered for DSM-IV increase the number of negative symptoms described, list positive and negative symptoms separately and abandon the association of negative symptoms with non-active stages of the disorder. Each of these changes increases both the emphasis on negative symptoms in diagnosis of schizophrenia and the implied centrality of these symptoms to the construct of schizophrenia. The changes reflect the recent accumulation of evidence demonstrating not only that these symptoms can be reliably assessed as long as they are clearly defined, but also that they are stable over time and highly correlated with each other suggesting that they might reflect common causal factors (see Barnes & Liddle, 1990, for review). Negative symptoms have also been found to be associated with brain abnormalities such as enlarged ventricles and with independent measures of cognitive impairment (see Marks & Luchins, 1990, for review). The findings regarding P300 and schizophrenia provide an illustration of such evidence. Thus, a variety of empirical evidence justifies a renewed emphasis on negative symptoms in DSM-IV, but a number of questions remain to be resolved regarding the nature and significance of these symptoms.

It is possible that there are different types of negative symptoms. Crow's (1980) description of Type II schizophrenia emphasises symptoms such as time disorientation and memory disturbances which are characteristic of organic brain dysfunction and thought to be immutable. The negative symptoms described in DSM-III-R such as blunting of affect and social withdrawal are psychological rather than organic in origin. While some researchers assume these symptoms to vary in response to both internal and environmental factors (Wing, 1988), others assume that such 'schizoid' traits are precursors of active symptomatology and reflections of early brain injury (Murray et al., 1988). Murray argues that the re-emergence of these features in the residual phase of the disorder is mistakenly interpreted as a sign of deterioration when it is consistent with behaviour prior to the active phase. A third class of negative symptoms that have received very little attention in formal diagnostic schemes, but are often extremely disabling for the patient and distressing for others, are concerned with lack of volition and motivation (Gubman, Tessler & Willis, 1987). Distinguishing between these differing views of the nature and significance of negative symptoms and their relationship to positive symptoms is critical to a full understanding of the causes of schizophrenia and is a major focus of much current research on schizophrenia (for example, Andreasen, 1990).

While more refined symptom descriptions will contribute to such understanding, an approach based on cross-sectional symptomatology alone is unlikely to allow accurate prediction of course and outcome. Attempts to make predictions from symptom patterns have a long history but have had little success (for example, Goldstein & Tsuang, 1988). Defining subtypes of schizophrenia in a manner that is useful for treatment requires a comprehensive understanding of the causes of different symptoms and their relative contribution at different stages of the disorder. That is, the precise descriptive approach advocated by Kraepelin must be combined with the emphasis on underlying psychological processes adopted by Bleuler.

Defining disturbances in cognitive processes

We briefly illustrated such an approach by describing the results of cognitive psychophysiological investigations of attentional processes as indexed by the P300 component of the ERP. Although these findings contribute only a small piece of the jig-saw puzzle of schizophrenia, it is potentially an important one. If P300 indexes a cognitive process that is associated with the vulnerability to schizophrenia, then further investigations of the nature of that process will contribute to a more detailed understanding of the disorder. Distinguishing the cognitive dysfunctions associated with the disposition to schizophrenia from transient deficits characteristic of florid episodes of schizophrenia is critical to accurate prediction and treatment of the disabling consequences of schizophrenia.

ERPs are a particularly useful means of investigating the cognitive deficits associated with psychopathological disorders both because they provide a dynamic measure of on-line cognitive processes and because they can be more directly linked to evidence regarding the biological dysfunction contributing to schizophrenia than gross measures of reaction time or errors. It is not possible to directly determine the neuroanatomical source of scalp-recorded ERP components, but the pattern of ERPs across different sites on the scalp does provide clues as to the areas of the brain that underlie different cognitive processes. When used in conjunction with the newer 'brain imaging' technologies such as Magnetic Resonance Imaging (MRI) and Positron Emission Tomography (PET) which allow precise localisation of the areas of the brain involved in performance of particular tasks, ERPs provide the opportunity to specify the neural mechanisms underlying cognitive processing and the manner in which they break down in schizophrenia (Andreasen, 1989).

Implications for treatment

Understanding the causes of differences in the pattern and course of schizophrenic symptoms contributes to treatment in a number of ways. Firstly, direct contributions emerge from a more precise understanding of the neurochemical disturbance reflected in schizophrenic symptoms. Current diagnostic criteria do not allow prediction of who will and will not respond well to medication or who does and does not require maintenance medication following remission of symptoms. Given this ambiguity, clinicians are likely to err on the side of caution in order to avoid risking relapse. Such a strategy is justified by the high relapse rates amongst patients who fail to take medication and the disruptive effects of relapse for both the patient and the community (Johnson et al., 1983). However, there are a range of side-effects associated with anti-psychotic drugs which interfere with the individual's functioning. These side-effects reflect the fact that the drugs in current use are not sufficiently specific in their effects. A more comprehensive understanding of the factors that differentiate individuals who do and do not recover following drug treatment would provide the basis for developing drugs which more selectively affect the neurochemical abnormality underlying schizophrenic symptoms and minimise disruptive side-effects. Such knowledge may also allow the development of drugs 'tailored' to particular symptom patterns.

Secondly, more precise knowledge of the causes of schizophrenia will contribute to the refinement of psychological treatments for the disorder. Psychological therapies have acquired a new importance in the treatment of schizophrenia because of evidence of an association between attributes of family interaction and relapse in schizophrenia: individuals diagnosed with schizophrenia who return to live with their family are more likely to suffer relapse if family members are high in 'expressed emotion' (see Leff & Vaughn, 1985, for review). Expressed emotion (EE) is assessed through the Camberwell Family Interview (Brown & Rutter, 1966) in which relatives' comments about the patient with schizophrenia are scored for the number of critical comments they make about the patient and for evidence of hostility and emotional over-involvement.

The relationship between high EE and relapse has been replicated in a number of studies, but interpretation of this relationship remains controversial. Some criticisms are methodological in focus and question both the generalisability of the results beyond the relatively chronic patients assessed in most investigations and the degree to which the results can be attributed to EE as opposed to correlated variables such as duration of illness (MacMillan et al., 1986). Others point to the difficulty in drawing any conclusions about the causality of the association between EE and relapse (Birchwood & Cochrane, 1990): do high EE relatives cause exacerbations of schizophrenic symptomatology or does high EE develop in relatives as a consequence of the distress and burden of living with a relative with schizophrenia? Further problems relate to the fact that most measures of EE combine critical comments, hostility and emotional over-involvement into a single index and ignore the possibility that they might reflect very different attributes of relatives (Koenigsberger & Handley, 1986). Resolving these issues is critical to understanding just why EE is associated with relapse in at least a subgroup of schizophrenic patients, but in the absence of clear-cut answers the existence of the relationship early points to the merits of treatments directed towards modifying relatives' attitudes or method of managing their ill relative.

A number of studies have demonstrated the effectiveness of 'psychosocial' treatment packages directed towards family members (see Tarrier & Barrowclough,

1990, for review). Relapse rates have been shown to be dramatically reduced in the 9–12 months following treatment but increased relapse rates at 2-year follow-ups suggest that these treatments delay rather than prevent relapse and therefore that long-term continuing intervention is necessary (Hogarty, Anderson & Reiss, 1987). More recent studies have attempted to establish which components of treatment packages play a critical role. Most programs include education in the nature and causes of the disease, medication and signs of relapse but such education does not, in itself, appear to affect relapse (Smith & Birchwood, 1987). Neither does the provision of general support or crisis intervention appear to reduce relapse (Hogarty et al., 1979). The programs have included a number of different techniques to reduce stress or facilitate problem solving and goal planning but it is difficult to determine the most important 'active ingredients' (Tarrier & Barrowclough, 1990). The crucial factor may be that the therapy brings about a change in relatives' EE level. Most direct investigations of this issue are consistent with the view that treatment efficacy depends on reducing relatives' EE (Bebbington & Kuipers, 1988).

The mechanism underlying the effects of EE on relapse remain unclear. The general assumption is that a high EE family environment acts as a form of psychosocial stressor. There is some evidence of changes in physiological arousal that are broadly consistent with this view (Tarrier et al., 1988), but systematic evidence is not available and there is no evidence of changes in arousal as a consequence of successful psychosocial treatment (Leff et al., 1982). Physiological arousal may, however, be an inappropriate measure of the stress associated with stressful environments. Responses to stress are cognitively mediated. Stressful environments may interact with an on-going attentional dysfunction to give rise to the symptoms associated with a relapse of schizophrenia. Relapse is most frequently defined as an exacerbation of florid symptomatology, so this view implies that the effects of stressful environments may act upon an existing attentional dysfunction to produce positive symptoms. Some negative symptoms might also be viewed as responses to either social overstimulation (Stevens, 1973) or to the poverty of the social environment (Wing & Brown, 1970). Different social environments might impose different demands. Day (1986) has distinguished between four types of 'toxic environments' that might influence the course of schizophrenia: cognitively confusing, emotionally intrusive, overly demanding and threatening or demoralising. These different types of environment might interact with the attentional and cognitive capabilities of the individual to determine course and outcome.

Again, a fine-grained resolution of these issues that can contribute usefully to assessment and treatment requires understanding of the cognitive disturbances underlying schizophrenic symptoms and how they respond to different environmental conditions. At the very least, the ability to accurately predict an individual's likely course early in the illness would allow relatives and other carers to adjust their expectations so that they can tread the fine line between creating a demanding and intrusive environment and failing to encourage the individual to reach his or her full potential.

Richard P. Mattick
National Drug and Alcohol Research Centre, University of New South Wales

9 Psychoactive substance dependence and associated states

Introduction

The seriousness of drug and alcohol abuse and dependence to the individuals who suffer their effects and to the general community has led to a dramatic increase in the level of international research on the nature and management of these problems. There is no doubt that the social and personal costs are huge. In terms of the economic burden on the Australian community, it has been recently estimated that for 1988 the financial cost of nicotine dependence was $6.84 billion, $6.03 billion for alcohol abuse and dependence, and $1.44 billion for illicit drug dependence — a total of $14.39 billion (Collins & Lapsley, 1991). This total figure represents the estimated minimum cost imposed upon the community, and it is a recurring annual cost in Australia.

Against this background of huge personal and societal costs to both individuals and society, the aim of this chapter is to attempt to provide an understanding of substance dependence, and of the current and foreshadowed international diagnostic criteria. Following this introduction, the area of psychopathology is expanded upon, using three case vignettes, — one of alcohol dependence, one of opiate dependence and one of nicotine dependence. Each is diagnosed using the *Diagnostic and Statistical Manual of Mental Disorders,* third edition, revised (DSM-III-R) (American Psychiatric Association, 1987), and the case conceptualisation and the intervention pursued for each case are then outlined. There is some overlap between the cases in terms of the types of psychological interventions that could be applied. The reader should be aware that some of the psychological interventions described in the case of nicotine dependence, for instance, will also be appropriate for other forms of substance dependence. The substance involved is less relevant than the individual's psychiatric and psychological state.

Because there is a description of three cases, the overall management of each case is dealt with in less detail than might otherwise have been possible. For each case, both psychological and somatic interventions are considered, as it is important to ensure that the role and the appropriateness of both types of intervention is fully understood. Psychological treatments for substance abuse are often only effective in the context of a somatic treatment (much as psychological interventions for schizophrenia are most likely to have a reasonable impact if the sufferer is already maintained on medication), or else their effectiveness is assisted by the use of a somatic intervention. The somatic interventions that will be discussed are generally some form of replacement therapy (for example, methadone replacing illicit opiate drugs, or nicotine being delivered by gum or transdermal (skin) patch rather than via a cigarette), but other (non-replacement) somatic therapies are considered as well.

It is worth noting at the outset that workers in the drug and alcohol field often frown on the use of medications or drugs in the treatment of drug dependence. This view appears to stem from a moral stance on their part rather than from therapeutic concerns. One encounters therapists, clinicians and workers in the drug and alcohol field who argue that the only appropriate goal in treatment is abstinence from all substances, and because of this stance they are resistant to the use of drugs in management. No doubt abstinence is the goal that we might prefer in the best of worlds, but the reality for many dependent individuals is that they require extra assistance to achieve the best outcome. If the assistance is in the form of a replacement drug which allows them to control their problem drug use with fewer negative effects, the benefits may outweigh the costs. This is true for opiates (Ward, Mattick & Hall, 1992) and also for tobacco (Mattick & Baillie, 1992).

Finally, in this chapter, the implications of the three cases considered are discussed in terms of the theoretical understanding of psychoactive substance dependence.

Conceptualisation and classification

Factors that determine use, abuse and dependence

Drug use, and dependence, is determined by both antecedent and consequent events and motivations. A complete account of drug use involves general societal factors which can be relatively distant from the actual drug use episode. These factors include legislation regarding the ease of availability and the use of psychoactive substances (for example, hours of opening of hotels, whether the drug is licit or illicit), as well as general societal pressures to use or not use, prohibitions on the permissibility of use (for example, of smoking in public places, or drinking outside private or licensed premises), and restrictions on age of use. At a more personal level there are factors that influence use such as peer group pressure, familial and parental drug use patterns, as well as early learning experiences, life events, initial drug use and genetic predisposition. Combined with these factors, the immediate antecedents of drug use, such as positive or negative expectations regarding the effect of the substance, as well as positive and negative mood states and withdrawal states, go together to determine the disposition of the individual to use a given psychoactive substance.

Drug use is often associated with both aversive, as well as reinforcing, consequences. The aversive consequences include the toxic and social effects of the use of the drug (for example, nausea and illness from intoxication, hangover after the drug effect has worn off, social embarrassment after intoxication) and a reduction in the drug effect after repeated administrations (that is, tolerance); with repeated abuse there may be a decrement in social functioning (for example, effects on the ability to work efficiently and to socialise). In the long term, organic damage and the more obvious physical results also have an impact on the continued use of the substance.

The mood-enhancing properties of drugs reinforce the use of psychoactive substances. These reinforcing effects can be part of the ability of the drug to produce a positive state, or they can result from the drug's ability to remove a negative state. For instance, amphetamines will allow a faster rate of work and are often used to enhance performance while continued use of nicotine will permit the dependent individual to avoid withdrawal. (The specific withdrawal symptoms associated with different compounds are outlined in Devenyi and Saunders (1986) and Goodman et al. (1990).) Alcohol augments social interaction and makes positive mood states even more pleasant for some individuals, but it also has the potential to remove negative states and to relieve withdrawal symptoms.

It would be inappropriate to attempt to determine the relative importance of these various factors on the uptake and continued use of drugs that affect one's psychological state. Space does not allow anything other than a brief consideration, and our current state of knowledge will not permit any clear statements about the importance of each factor. The single message that should be taken from this brief overview is that the use of psychoactive substances and, to a lesser extent, dependence on such substances are determined by a number of factors in ways that are not well understood as yet. However, an awareness of the range of factors potentially involved is important in clinical management.

Evolution of the classification of substance dependence and abuse

Until the middle of this century, drug dependence had largely escaped the attention of health professions as a distinct clinical phenomenon. It was subject to moral attitudes and judgements, and was considered to be a social aberration. Even when it came to be incorporated into the diagnostic nomenclature, drug dependence was considered to be a type of personality disturbance. Both the *Diagnostic and Statistical Manual of Mental Disorders,* first edition (DSM-I) (American Psychiatric Association, 1952) and the *Diagnostic and Statistical Manual of Mental Disorders,* second edition (DSM-II) (American Psychiatric Association, 1968) included dependence along with antisocial behaviour, sexual deviation and homosexuality as indicative of a personality disorder. Happily, the American approach was not taken up by those across the Atlantic who commenced the task of endeavouring to provide a view and an understanding of these problems which did not rely on moralising or judgemental stances.

Specifically, in the early 1950s, a number of World Health Organization Expert Committees undertook the task of attempting to provide a definition of drug dependence (Edwards, Arif & Hodgson, 1981). This early work set in train the efforts that have led to the development of the current international classificatory systems. Most particularly, the British psychiatrist Griffith Edwards has been prominent in conceptualising the phenomenon of drug dependence. He conducted his research on alcohol (Edwards, 1987), but his approach has now come to be applied broadly to all of the classes of psychoactive substance dependence, and it is reflected in the *Diagnostic and Statistical Manual of Mental Disorders,* third edition (DSM-III) and the DSM-III-R (American Psychiatric Association, 1980, 1987), as well as in the tenth edition of the *International Classification of Diseases* (World Health Organization, 1992).

Seven elements have been identified as indicative of psychoactive substance dependence. These are listed below with specific reference to alcohol, although the listing is equally applicable to other drug classes:

1. There is frequently a narrowing of the drinking repertoire. The non-dependent drinker (or other drug user) will vary the amount and type of drinking (or drug use) from day to day and week to week. With increasing dependence, the amount of the drug consumed becomes more stereotyped. The narrowing drinker tends to drink the same amount each day. Non-dependent drinkers will have more highly variable drinking patterns.
2. There is an increased salience of drinking in the life of the individual. With increasing dependence, alcohol takes precedence over other activities and concerns. The dependent drinker's history will show a progressively greater interest in drinking to the detriment of diet, health, financial, occupational, familial and social obligations.
3. There is an increased subjective awareness of compulsion to drink. The drinker will report having lost control over drinking, having difficulty in resisting the impulse to drink, being unable to stop drinking at certain times, or feeling constant cravings in the absence of alcohol. These reports all suggest a subjective experience of alcohol dependence.
4. There will be an increased tolerance to the effects of alcohol. Heavy drinking leads to an adaptation to alcohol consumption so that amounts which previously may have resulted in inebriation will eventually produce fewer obvious effects. While all heavy drinkers will show some tolerance, increased tolerance is also related to the level of dependence on alcohol. The dependent drinker often responds to tolerance by drinking more to achieve the desired effect. Tolerance may also be evident from the speed of drinking and the ability to consume large amounts without intoxication.
5. Repeated withdrawal symptoms occur. As dependence increases, the frequency and severity of withdrawal symptoms increases. In the case of alcohol withdrawal, these symptoms may include perspiration, tremor, anxiety, agitation, a rise in body temperature, hallucinations, disorientation and nausea.
6. There is relief from, or avoidance of, withdrawal symptoms by further drinking. The drinker may drink for relief from withdrawal or may maintain a steady alcohol level in order to avoid withdrawal.
7. Rapid reinstatement of dependence after a period of abstinence may occur. If the drinker has had a lengthy period of abstinence after which drinking was resumed, dependence is characterised by a rapid return to the pre-abstinence level of drinking and dependence symptomatology. This pattern may be evident from the history of drinking.

These seven elements are reflected in the DSM-III-R diagnostic criteria for psychoactive substance dependence which are presented in table 9.1 (see page 160). As noted by Edwards, Arif and Hodgson, 1981, drug dependence is best conceptualised as a syndrome that involves a behavioural pattern in which the use of a particular psychoactive substance (or a group of such substances) takes priority in the life of the individual. The notion of a syndrome means that there is a clustering of certain phenomena, without implying that all of the phenomena need to be present or present in equal intensity. Thus, not all of the seven elements need to occur in a given individual for dependence to be diagnosed. It is also notable that severity of dependence can vary from mild, to moderate, to severe, and the disorder may be diagnosed as in partial or full remission.

According to the American Psychiatric Association (1987), psychoactive substance abuse is a diagnostic category for maladaptive patterns of substance use that have never met the criteria for dependence. The criteria for the diagnosis are set out in table 9.2 (see page 161). This diagnosis is most likely to be applicable to individuals who have only recently started using psychoactive substances. It is also suggested that substance abuse is more likely to involve substances, such as cannabis and hallucinogens, that are less likely to be associated with marked physiologic signs of withdrawal and the need to take the substance to relieve or avoid withdrawal symptoms. The DSM-III-R provides some useful examples of situations in which this substance abuse diagnostic category would be appropriately applied. These are:

(a) a university student who binges on alcohol every few weekends, followed by a day or two of missing classes because of a hangover, but with no other symptoms or problems
(b) a middle-aged man who repeatedly drives his car when intoxicated with alcohol, with no other symptoms
(c) a woman who keeps drinking alcohol even though her physician has told her that it is responsible for exacerbating the symptoms of a duodenal ulcer, with no other symptoms.

More recently, the criteria have been combined into a single set that allows for a determination of dependence and abuse. This set of criteria is a draft in the forthcoming *Diagnostic and Statistical Manual of Mental Disorders,* fourth edition (DSM-IV) (Nathan, 1991), and it is set out in table 9.3 (page 161). The major change from the DSM-III-R approach is that the diagnosis of dependence requires the presence of either tolerance or withdrawal, rather than these symptoms being optional among a larger list as in the DSM-III-R. Physiological adaptation is required. Psychological dependence alone is insufficient to allow the diagnosis to be made. This approach is a marked departure from that developed by Edwards, Arif and Hodgson (1981), although it was the approach taken in the DSM-III (American Psychiatric Association, 1980) and it will be some time before we will be able to tell whether this proposed alteration has improved our understanding and treatment of these problems.

Under the draft set of criteria, substance abuse is no longer a residual category, but is diagnosed based on a set of distinct and specifiable behaviours. Indeed, the psychoactive substance abuse criteria described by Nathan (1991) are quite different from those set out in the DSM-III-R. Under the DSM-IV draft criteria, 'abuse' can be based on the presence of symptoms that under DSM-III-R were taken as indicative of 'dependence'. Moreover, under the DSM-IV proposals, the three examples of substance abuse discussed earlier (the university student, the middle-aged man, and the woman) would not meet criteria.

Table 9.1: The DSM-III-R diagnostic criteria for psychoactive substance dependence

A. At least three of the following:
(1) substance often taken in larger amounts or over a longer period than the person intended
(2) persistent desire or one or more unsuccessful efforts to cut down or control substance use
(3) a great deal of time spent in activities necessary to get the substance (for example, theft), take the substance (for example, chain smoking), or recover from its effects
(4) frequent intoxication or withdrawal symptoms when expected to fulfil major role obligations at work, school or home (for example, does not go to work because hungover, goes to school or work 'high', intoxicated while taking care of his or her children), or when substance use is physically hazardous (for example, drives when intoxicated)
(5) important social, occupational or recreational activities given up or reduced because of substance use
(6) continued substance use despite knowledge of having a persistent or recurrent social, psychological or physical problem that is caused or exacerbated by the use of the substance (for example, keeps using heroin despite family arguments about it, cocaine-induced depression, or having an ulcer made worse by drinking)
(7) marked tolerance: a need for markedly increased amounts of the substance (that is, at least a 50 per cent increase) in order to achieve intoxication or the desired effect, or a markedly diminished effect with continued use of the same amount.

Note: The following items may not apply to cannabis, hallucinogens or phencyclidine (PCP):
(8) characteristic withdrawal symptoms
(9) substance often taken to relieve or avoid withdrawal symptoms.

B. Some symptoms of the disturbance have persisted for at least one month, or have occurred repeatedly over a longer period of time.

Criteria for Severity of Psychoactive Substance Dependence:

Mild: Few, if any, symptoms in excess of those required to make the diagnosis, and the symptoms result in no more than mild impairment in occupational functioning or in usual social activities or relationships with others.

Moderate: Symptoms or functional impairment between 'mild' and 'severe'.

Severe: Many symptoms in excess of those required to make the diagnosis, and the symptoms markedly interfere with occupational functioning or with usual social activities or relationships with others.

In Partial Remission: During the past six months, some use of the substance and some symptoms of dependence.

In Full Remission: During the past six months, either no use of the substance, or use of the substance and no symptoms of dependence.

Table 9.2: The DSM-III-R diagnostic criteria for psychoactive substance abuse

A. A maladaptive pattern of psychoactive substance use indicated by at least one of the following:
(1) continued use despite knowledge of having a persistent or recurrent social, occupational, psychological, or physical problem that is caused or exacerbated by use of the psychoactive substance
(2) recurrent use in situations in which use is physically hazardous (for example, driving while intoxicated).
B. Some symptoms of the disturbance have persisted for at least one month, or have occurred repeatedly over a longer period of time.
C. Never met the criteria for psychoactive substance dependence for this substance.

The DSM-IV Options Task Force (Task Force on DSM-IV, 1991) outlined similar approaches to that presented by Nathan (1991), but they retained as an option the DSM-III-R approach adding a scheme to 'subtype' individuals as displaying or not displaying physiological dependence. It is clear that the presence of physical indices of dependence is taking on a more prominent role in the classification of a dependent state. Whatever the ultimate form of the DSM-IV, this emphasis will be reflected somehow.

Table 9.3: Proposed DSM-IV criteria for substance abuse and dependence

A. Psychoactive substance abuse involves a pattern of repeated problems with the substance as indicated by at least two of the following:
(1) substance taken in larger amounts or over a longer period than intended
(2) persistent desire or unsuccessful efforts to cut down or control substance use
(3) a great deal of time spent on activities necessary to obtain the substance (for example, visiting multiple doctors or driving long distances) or take the substance (for example, chain-smoking)
(4) continued substance use despite knowledge of persistent or recurrent social, psychological or physical problems caused or exacerbated by the use of the substance (for example, daily cigarette smoking despite knowledge of a heightened risk of lung cancer, cocaine use despite cocaine-induced depression, or continued drinking despite an ulcer made worse by alcohol consumption)
(5) recurrent substance use resulting in inability to fulfil major role obligation at work, school or home (examples include (a) repeated absences or poor work performance related to substance use, (b) substance-related absences, suspensions or expulsions from school, and (c) neglect of children or household responsibilities because of substance use)
(6) recurrent substance use in situations in which it is physically hazardous (for example, driving an automobile or operating a machine when impaired by substance use)

(*continued over*)

Table 9.3: Proposed DSM-IV criteria for substance abuse/dependence (*continued*)

(7) important social, occupational, or recreational activities given up or reduced because of substance use; or
(8) recurrent substance-related legal or interpersonal problems (examples include substance-related arrests and traffic accidents, and physical fights related to substance use).

B. Psychoactive substance dependence involves, additionally, one or both of the following:
(1) tolerance, defined by (a) the need for markedly increased amounts of the substance in order to achieve intoxication or desired effect, (b) markedly diminished effect with continued use of the same amount of the substance, or (c) evidence of the ability to function adequately at doses or blood levels of the substance that produce significant impairment in a casual user (for example, consuming a fifth of whiskey or its equivalent per day); or
(2) evidence of withdrawal, characterised by a withdrawal syndrome observed after reduction or cessation of substance use or in response to a challenge with an antagonist.

Comorbid psychiatric states

It would be remiss to not mention the importance of concurrent (or comorbid) psychiatric disorders in those suffering from substance abuse or dependence. Comorbid psychiatric disorders are frequent among those who abuse or are dependent on psychoactive substances, and the prevalence of these disorders is higher than in the general population (Regier et al., 1990). Frequently co-occurring diagnoses are depressive disorder, personality disorder (especially antisocial personality disorder) and anxiety disorders. Clinically it is most important to be aware of the possibility of a comorbid psychiatric disorder and to deal with it in treatment. Dealing appropriately with comorbid states enhances the outcome for the drug or alcohol problem.

Case 1: Alcohol dependence with comorbid psychiatric conditions — the case of the nervous drinker

Social and drug use history

Gary is 33 years old. He is manager of a hardware shop with a staff of six. He is reasonably well educated, having completed high school, and has above-average intellectual abilities. He is sexually impotent, has memory problems and is faced with the loss of his marriage and probably his job. He has been drinking steadily at an excessive rate for about 15 years, since he left school. He first started drinking at 16 years of age when he was introduced to hotels by his school mates. He would tag along with the group and initially did not enjoy the taste of alcohol. He gradually developed the 'taste' for it, and by the time he was 20 he was drinking daily, although not excessively at that time. He did not become drunk very often, although he would usually be somewhat merry. Typically at that time he drank about 4 or 5 cans (or schooners) of beer a day, a level that placed his consumption above the cut-off for harmful drinking according to the Australian National Health and Medical Research Council (Pols & Hawks, 1987). He met and married his wife when he was 23 years old, and they put off having a family so that they could 'establish themselves financially'.

Over the years, as his drinking increased, he became quite tolerant to the effects of alcohol. He rarely appeared to be drunk to others and apart from the increasing severity of the memory problems he was not obviously affected. These memory problems were affecting his work performance, and on several occasions over the past six months he had forgotten to place orders for hardware goods and other supplies, and this had led to trouble with the general manager of the hardware chain that he works for. His impotence had provided increasing problems with his wife, who wished to start a family.

Gary visited his general practitioner for advice. He showed some signs of excessive consumption that raised his doctor's 'index of suspicion' that he may be drinking excessively. These signs were dilated facial capillaries (telangiectasis), 'blood shot eyes' (conjunctival injection) and coating of the tongue, which, taken together with his memory problems and impotence, were strongly suggestive of excessive alcohol intake. Further investigation, using biological markers of alcohol intake, was also undertaken by his doctor. These were found to be above normal range, confirming the GP's suspicion of alcohol problems.

Gary again visited the general practitioner to obtain the results of the tests, and after some discussion he admitted to drinking quite heavily, providing the following information. He took his first drink in the morning, usually at home. He rose before his wife to get to work early (by 7.30 a.m.), and because of this he said that his wife did not notice his morning drinking. Whether or not he got a drink at home, he would typically take a couple of cans of beer with him to work. These he drank on the train he caught to work, and he usually consumed them before he arrived. Through the day he would drink about eight cans of beer at the rate of one every hour or so, depending on the work load. He attempted to hide his drinking from the customers and employees by using strong breath freshener. In the night at home he would drink another five to eight cans of beer, falling asleep by 10.00 p.m. He essentially followed this pattern of drinking seven days a week. He was never obviously drunk, but during his waking hours he drank consistently. On some days he could consume up to two dozen cans of beer, although this was a rare occurrence. If he failed to have an early morning drink, or if he did not drink through the day he suffered trembling hands, perspiration and nausea.

Gary also suffered from two comorbid psychiatric disorders. He explained to his general practitioner that his 'serious drinking started ten years ago after a heavy night with my work mates'. The day after that heavy drinking session he found that he was hung over and was visibly shaking and suffered continuous diarrhoea, so much so that at work he was heading to the toilet every few minutes during the early part of the morning. Some of his friends at work laughed at him because of his shaking and he became very self-conscious about doing everyday things in front of them. Subsequently he gradually developed an extreme awareness of being observed carrying out normal activities in the presence of others. Initially, he was slightly aware of writing in front of others, for fear that he should shake and others might notice. This fear gradually grew to the extent that he found a number of routine activities including eating, drinking and writing very difficult. He told the general practitioner that he had always been shy, and had avoided social activities generally. If he had to be involved in social activities he had always found that the use of alcohol assisted him to cope.

DSM-III-R diagnosis

Gary's primary diagnosis was alcohol dependence. He also had a social phobia and an avoidant personality disorder. His physical disorders involved liver dysfunction and symptomatic impotence. He was under some social stress (arguments with wife, problems at work due to memory failure) and his highest level of functioning in the past year indicated moderate difficulties.

Conceptualisation and treatment

Conceptualisation

Gary was severely alcohol dependent. He had a high tolerance to the effects of alcohol, and he experienced withdrawal symptoms on those occasions when he went without alcohol for a prolonged period. The most appropriate initial treatment approach for Gary was detoxification in an in-patient detoxification facility, or else detoxification at home under the supervision of his general practitioner and possibly with the assistance of his wife. Thereafter his abstinence from alcohol had to be maintained, his drinking-related problems addressed, and the comorbid psychiatric disorders dealt with to maximise the probability of continued abstinence. It was not thought that the option of 'controlled drinking' was appropriate in this case because of his high level of physical dependence, the presence of cognitive impairment and liver dysfunction, and because he had not shown signs of control over his drinking to date (cf., Heather et al., 1991).

Initial intervention

Alcohol withdrawal and the alcohol withdrawal syndrome is of major significance in the clinical management of physically dependent drinkers. This fact is due to the danger to life that the alcohol withdrawal syndrome has for the sufferer. Individuals who are physically dependent on alcohol are likely to go into withdrawal 6–24 hours after the last drink. In some individuals this withdrawal syndrome is short-lived and inconsequential, in others it increases in severity over the first 48–72 hours of abstinence and some individuals will progress to delirium tremens (the 'DTs'), an acute organic brain syndrome that is life-threatening. The level of alcohol intake is the most important single determinant of the occurrence and severity of an alcohol withdrawal syndrome. In Gary's case it was likely that he would suffer a severe withdrawal syndrome if he abruptly ceased consumption.

The signs and symptoms that are indicative of the onset of the alcohol withdrawal syndrome include those that are related to autonomic nervous system hyperactivity. Specifically, the signs and symptoms of the alcohol withdrawal syndrome include:

- increased body temperature
- increased pulse rate (tachycardia)
- increased respiration rate
- increased blood pressure (hypertension)
- nausea and vomiting
- tremor
- sweating
- agitation and anxiety
- tactile disturbances (for example, pins and needles, itching, burning, numbness, crawling sensations, 'electric fleas') including tactile hallucinations
- auditory and/or visual disturbances including hallucinations.

Home or ambulatory detoxification was an option in Gary's case. However, as his wife worked and was unable to assist in the process, in-patient detoxification was chosen in a medical detoxification facility. Usually, admission to such detoxification facilities would be based on meeting at least one of a set of specific criteria. These criteria include:

- a history of severe withdrawal symptoms or episodes, such as seizures, recurrent withdrawal fits, delirium tremens (the DTs);
- the probability of imminent marked alcohol withdrawal, or else the presence of a marked withdrawal state;
- concurrent psychiatric or medical disorders, such as depression, suicidal ideas, chest infection, pneumonia or an inflamed pancreas;
- a home environment that is unfavourable to successful detoxification; or
- a lack of a home detoxification service.

Gary was admitted on the following day and detoxification proceeded, using adjunctive sedative medication. Specifically, Diazepam, a benzodiazepine tranquilliser, which is widely used in medicated detoxification from alcohol, was chosen. Unlike chlormethiazole (which is an alternative medication), it has a long half-life (of 18–40 hours) and the half-life of its biologically active metabolite, desmethyldiazepam, averages 2–5 days. Diazepam is therefore sometimes given in a loading dose, after which a further dose is usually unnecessary. However, in Gary's case it was given on an interval basis, as an initial IV injection of 10 mg Diazepam, followed by two further doses over the next half-hour. During his time in the inpatient detoxification facility, Gary was introduced to the notions of Alcoholics Anonymous. He was not particularly engaged by the ideas espoused, and refused to attend any AA meetings after he was discharged some 4 days after his initial admission.

Secondary intervention: Disulfiram

Gary required help to maintain the abstinence that he achieved through the detoxification process during the critical short-term period upon return to his daily activities. He then needed a range of interventions to assist him to maintain abstinence in the longer term. After detoxification Gary was seen on an outpatient basis. He was referred to a drug and alcohol team comprising a psychologist, a psychiatrist and a social worker. He attended with his wife. After an assessment by the team, it was decided that Gary required an initial period on the drug Disulfiram, during which time he needed an intensive outpatient intervention using basic counselling techniques and specific cognitive-behavioural interventions. These specific interventions were needed to deal with the danger of relapse. He also needed to learn the skills to assist him to cope with life without drinking.

Research indicates that oral Disulfiram has a positive effect on treatment outcomes but only when it is provided to the client under supervision (Mattick & Jarvis, 1992). Disulfiram acts by inhibiting the action of enzymes in the metabolism of alcohol. The results of ingesting alcohol while on a Disulfiram treatment regimen are unpleasant. They include flushing, dizziness, nausea and vomiting, irregular heart beat, breathlessness and headaches. The aim of Disulfiram was to aid Gary to avoid drinking alcohol through ensuring his awareness of the unpleasant side-effects that would occur. Disulfiram treatment is not an aversive therapy per se, rather it produces immediate rather than delayed negative consequences for drinking. It has been argued by some that Disulfiram is better considered a behavioural intervention, rather than a medical procedure (Heather, 1989). The use of Disulfiram is likely to be effective for the first three to six months of treatment. Disulfiram was an appropriate treatment for Gary as:

- he wished to abstain from alcohol
- he accepted that there was a need for an external control on his drinking
- he displayed no serious medical or psychosocial contraindications
- he was prepared to be supervised in the daily dosing of the medication.

The therapist explained the effects of Disulfiram to Gary. Discussion of the negative effects of Disulfiram when alcohol was taken is an important part of the therapeutic strategy because Gary's anticipation of its effects would greatly enhance its effectiveness as a deterrent against drinking. The therapist also discussed motivation and supervision of dosing with Gary. Gary needed to understand supervised Disulfiram as a useful strategy to assist in the maintenance of the choice of abstinence. Supervision of Disulfiram dosing is likely to have a marked impact on compliance with the prescribed regimen, and to subsequently markedly improve the ability of this intervention to stop drinking.

Supervision can present problems for some clients. First, it might be difficult to organise. The client needs to be prepared for public disclosure either with the therapist or some other person who is chosen to supervise. Although Gary's wife was an obvious choice for supervision, she initially objected that this approach placed the responsibility for the drinking (inappropriately) on her shoulders. She had learned through long bitter experience that she could not control Gary's drinking. The therapist acknowledged that she could not be expected to control the drinking and emphasised that her responsibility as supervisor was simply to observe Gary taking the Disulfiram. This process has been argued to be extremely important as a cooperative method for rebuilding lost trust, and it should not be construed as a coercive checking-up operation by any of the parties involved.

Secondary intervention: Cognitive-behavioural therapy

Once Disulfiram dosing was under way, a psychotherapeutic intervention involving a number of interventions was undertaken. The counselling style advocated was one that is not aggressively confrontational, but one that allows an interaction between the therapist and Gary. Basic counselling skills are valuable for developing rapport and dealing with Gary's distress and ambivalence about treatment goals. By carefully listening to Gary and then communicating understanding of what Gary was feeling and of the experiences and behaviours which underlie those feelings, the therapist indicated acceptance of Gary and contributed to a mutual working relationship. This was coupled with an open and honest explanation of what treatment would entail. By showing positive regard for Gary, the therapist could help to reduce distress and distrust and foster his motivation to become actively involved in the treatment. It has been suggested that the following three stages are useful in the understanding of the structure of counselling:

- identifying and clarifying problem situations and unused opportunities
- goal-setting, or developing and choosing preferred life scenarios
- action, by moving toward and achieving the preferred scenario.

Additionally, there is consistent evidence that skills training helps to reduce alcohol consumption in both the short and long term (Mattick & Jarvis, 1992). Skills training techniques (for example, communication skills training, stress management procedures, assertiveness training, social skills training and relaxation training) are advocated as techniques for assisting clients with alcohol problems or dependence where assessment suggests the need for such intervention. Skills training has been linked to relapse prevention as advocated by Marlatt and Gordon (1985) and may help clients to deal with high risk situations. Alternatively, the training might help to compensate for skills deficits which have led to the use of drinking as a coping strategy. In Gary's case skills-based approaches seemed very appropriate given his comorbid psychiatric disorders.

Monti et al. (1989) have recently produced a useful clinical guide to the management of alcohol problems. This guide discusses a number of strategies including those listed below. It is noted that there is some overlap in the techniques, however, there is sufficient difference in procedure and purpose to divide them into separate sections:

1. *Drink refusal skills training.* In this procedure the drinker is taught to say 'no' to offers of alcohol or pressure from others to drink. The aim is to provide the drinker with the strategies to do this in a confident fashion without hesitation and without making excuses. The emphasis is on speaking directly to the person making the offer, suggesting alternatives to alcohol, dealing with the pressure to drink in an appropriately assertive fashion, and not feeling guilty about refusing. Additionally, drink refusal skills training can be used in conjunction with behavioural self-management to assist the client to deal with situations in which alcohol is present.
2. *Assertive training.* In this procedure the client learns that he/she has the right to express personal opinions and feelings, to request that other people change behaviour which affects the client and to accept or reject other people's requests. Underlying this approach is the development of self-respect and respect for the rights of others.
3. *Social skills training.* In this procedure the client learns to listen and to communicate effectively, to give and receive compliments and criticism, to refuse unwanted requests, to communicate non-verbally and verbally, to talk about personal feelings and communicate in intimate relationships, and to build a

social support network. This procedure may be of special value to the client who uses alcohol as a social 'lubricant'.

4. *Relaxation training.* In this procedure the client learns techniques for inducing relaxation which might include deep muscle relaxation, relaxing imagery, and letting go of physical stress.
5. *Stress management skills training.* In this procedure the client learns how to use relaxation in stressful situations, to manage stressful moods such as anger and to be aware of, and manage, negative thinking.
6. *Problem solving therapy.* In this procedure the client learns to recognise when a problem exists, to develop a range of solutions which can be applied, to select the most promising course of action and to assess the effectiveness of the selected approach.
7. *Relationship enhancement therapy.* This procedure includes specific communication skills such as assertiveness, giving and receiving criticism, expressing positive feelings and active listening. The intimate relationship could present special problems such as communication about sexuality, and this should be dealt with.

Monti et al. (1989) recommend that the skills be taught within a group context in which co-therapists model the behaviours and group members role-play the application of the skills to personal situations. Others have provided evidence that programs based on social skills training and cognitive restructuring are more effective when presented in groups (cf., Mattick & Jarvis, 1992). Gary was likely to benefit from drink refusal, social skills and relaxation/stress management training, as well as relationship enhancement therapy.

Skills training can be used with clients aiming at moderation or at abstinence. Several approaches may be appropriate for the one individual. The intervention which is chosen should be relevant to the client's needs. Training in social skills and other coping skills will require some commitment on the part of the client as these methods are enhanced when the client actively participates in therapy and continues to practise outside therapy. It is inappropriate to train a client in skills in which that client is already adept. This is consistent with the research that suggests that relaxation training may only contribute to reductions in drinking for those clients showing high anxiety, and not those showing little or no anxiety (an unsurprising but notable result).

Intervention for comorbid states

Gary had a serious anxiety disorder present, that stemmed in part from his drinking, but which also probably stemmed from his avoidant personality disorder. His social phobia may have predisposed him to relapse. The social phobia may be treated through a reasonably structured and time-limited cognitive-behavioural approach (the basic approach has been outlined elsewhere — Mattick & Peters, 1988; Mattick, Peters & Clarke, 1989), which was also likely to assist with his drinking through allowing him to develop skills to alter his habitual perceptions that others think negatively of him and notice his anxiety. However, as noted recently, a large proportion of those clients who go through such a structured approach will not improve sufficiently, and it may be that his avoidant personality disorder would benefit from a longer intervention over a period of months (Mattick & Newman, 1991).

Long-term follow-up

Gary succeeded in attaining and maintaining abstinence for a period of six months after the end of the daily Disulfiram dosing and the psychological intervention. During that time his relationship with his wife improved markedly, as did his self-esteem and general mood. He was also successfully treated for his social phobia, although he still has quite marked concerns over the opinions that others might have of him, and he remains essentially 'shy' and unsure of himself in social situations. He is happier at work and performs his duties more efficiently. He did return to drinking on two occasions when he decided to 'test' himself to see if he could drink 'just a little' with his mates. He became quite drunk on both occasions, but the threat from his wife that she would leave him 'for good', and the realisation of his own lack of control over drinking, convinced him that abstinence from all alcohol is the only appropriate goal for him.

Case 2: Opioid dependence — the case of the reluctant heroin dealer

Social and drug use history

Tony is a 27-year-old small-time heroin user/dealer. He has lived in a de-facto relationship for the past 18 months. He lives in an inner city suburb in shared rented accommodation where the other occupants are heroin and multiple drug users. He has never worked in full-time employment, and is in receipt of unemployment benefits. He left school early, just before his fifteenth birthday. He had not completed junior secondary school at this time, and he had often been truant from school. He also left home at that time. He had run away from home on three prior occasions for varying lengths of time, stealing food to eat, or shoplifting goods to sell in order to purchase food.

His mother was a heavy drinker as was his stepfather, and they were frequently in conflict. He was often subjected to physical beatings from his stepfather who was also verbally and physically abusive to his mother. After leaving home, he found his way to 'squats' (derelict housing used for accommodation) in Sydney, where he found shelter and some company with other adolescents slightly older than himself. Although he had used cannabis and alcohol occasionally prior to this time, it was about then that he started to use a variety of psychoactive substances including alcohol, quite frequently. He also became involved in petty crime, including frequent shoplifting and the occasional burglary with more experienced youths.

By the age of 17 Tony had developed a heroin habit, and occasionally for the next year or two he worked as a male prostitute in the city to support this habit. He soon stopped this work and instead he started to deliberately enlist and 'steer' potential customers to a dealer, also assisting in the physical transfer of the drugs and the cash. For this activity the dealer gave him heroin, as did some of the customers, which helped him to maintain his heroin habit without prostituting himself. He was also using 'pills' regularly. These he would purchase from other users, or occasionally he would attend an inner city medical centre renowned for the ease with which it was possible to gain a prescription for the drugs. He smoked cannabis regularly, but by this time he tended to avoid alcohol, unless he was short of supplies of other drugs. He also smoked about 30 cigarettes per day.

By 22 years of age Tony had started in dealing himself, as a user/dealer. He did not purchase heroin from the 'ounce' dealer who supplied him. Rather he would do 'home deliveries' for a dealer on his motor cycle, being given between 15 and 30 grams of 10 per cent pure heroin each day, and addresses to deliver to. This delivery run allowed him a regular supply of heroin. He would 'cut' the heroin with glucose to 'make good' the amount that he would keep for himself. Typically, in the early days he would keep 1 gram of the 10 per cent pure heroin for himself, divide it into quarter 'weights' and inject three or four times per day — prior to breakfast, at lunch, at dinner time and late in the evening. This use equated to approximately 100 milligrams of pure heroin per day. By the time he was 27 years old he had built this habit until he was using three or four weights (grams) per day, still approximately 10 per cent pure, or about 300 to 400 milligrams of pure heroin per day (cf., Dobinson & Poletti, 1989). He was quite tolerant to this amount of heroin. He would also store heroin away to ensure that he had a steady supply, and so that occasionally he could shoot up extra. His habit at that time was equivalent to a cost of $900 to $1200 per day, although he was not required to finance this directly as his courier work ensured a steady supply.

If Tony missed out on injecting for some reason he would soon develop opioid withdrawal symptoms. Even on waking, before his first dose of opiates, his body would ache and feel stiff, he would experience stomach cramps, notice his heart pounding, have hot flushes, feel miserable and depressed, tense and occasionally panicky, and he would have a strong craving to use opiates. He would always inject within an hour of waking up. By this time he had recognised that his opiate use was out of control, and he had come to worry about his use and was increasingly wishing that he could stop.

Tony had been unhappy since he was quite young, after suffering the physical and psychological rejection and abuse from his mother and stepfather. Despite having escaped that environment, his depression and unhappiness had increased over the past three or four years as a consequence of his realisation of the extent of the drug problem. He also was aware of the gulf between his lifestyle and the lifestyle that he would like to have, and that caused him significant anxiety and depression. His unhappiness manifested as quite low self-esteem, feelings of hopelessness about the future, low energy and sleepiness, and a poor appetite. This poor mood was a chronic state for Tony, and escalated on occasion into a major depressive disorder.

Tony first came to the attention of the health system when he was admitted to an inner city hospital casualty department unconscious from an apparent drug overdose. At this time he had been using illicit drugs regularly for 10 years. His dealer of four years' standing had been arrested by the police, and because of this his regular supply of heroin suddenly dried up. He had a small reserve supply of heroin, but this was gone within a week, and he was forced to buy heroin from other dealers and to attend general practitioners' surgeries in order to get scripts for sedative and hypnotic medications, although he increasingly found it difficult to meet his substantial needs in these ways. He also commenced drinking alcohol heavily. His de facto wife was also affected by the sudden loss of supply and she and he fell out over the issue. Some three weeks after his dealer had been arrested he took 15

Rohypnol tablets (a short half-life tranquilliser used as a 'sleeping' pill) and he had injected the contents of ten Normison capsules (temazepam, another 'sleeping' pill), as well as drinking a third of a bottle of gin. He lost consciousness and was taken by his flatmates to the hospital accident and emergency department.

In the accident and emergency department, he received an injection of Flumazenil which is used to offset the effects of the sleeping medication (Hunkeler et al., 1981). He was roused within five minutes of the administration of this drug. At this time he was still affected by the alcohol that he had consumed and his blood alcohol content was measured as 0.12 per cent. He subsequently became drowsy again and was admitted overnight for observation and tests. While he was in the hospital, he was screened for a number of diseases, including the human immunodeficiency virus (HIV). He was subsequently diagnosed as suffering from chronic hepatitis B and hepatitis C, which are common infections among injecting drug users (Strang & Farrell, 1991) and which resulted from sharing 'fits' (injecting equipment) with his de facto wife and flatmates. He was generally in a poor state of health, being malnourished, and because of his hepatitis he was at risk of developing cirrhosis and cancer of the liver in later life.

After one day in hospital under observation he was visited by a psychologist who works as a drug and alcohol counsellor in a hospital-based service. At this time Tony was suffering quite severe withdrawal symptoms, and the hospital staff who had become aware of his drug dependence were reluctant to prescribe any medication to relieve these symptoms, a feature of the failure of the general health care system to know how to cope with the drug-dependent individual.

DSM-III-R diagnosis

Tony was diagnosed as Opioid Dependence, Dysthymia, Primary type, with early onset. He also had a conduct disorder in childhood and an antisocial personality disorder. He was suffering from hepatitis B and C and was under considerable stress. The global assessment of his functioning in the past year indicated serious symptoms were present.

It is worth noting that although Tony met the DSM-III-R diagnostic criteria for antisocial personality disorder, he did not deserve the diagnosis. The DSM-III and the DSM-III-R place a heavy emphasis on behavioural criteria when making this diagnosis, a feature that has been criticised recently (Gerstley et al., 1990). The DSM-III-R is in marked contrast to the approach taken in the *International Classification of Diseases* (World Health Organization, 1992) which emphasises attitudinal and cognitive factors. Likewise, under the earlier Research Diagnostic Criteria (Spitzer, Endicott & Robins, 1978) from which the DSM-III partly derived, he would not have received the diagnosis, as these earlier criteria required the presence of markedly impaired interpersonal relationships and that the antisocial behaviours be independent of the substance abuse.

It is also worth noting that Tony had had a dysthymic disorder for many years, and that this was a primary diagnosis which was not due to his substance use, but which stemmed from the rejection and emotional abuse that he experienced prior to the age of 15 when he lived with his mother and step-father. Tony had no doubt that his dysthymia had been fuelled by the chaotic and anxiety-producing lifestyle that he had been involved in for some years. The diagnosis of dysthymia had important treatment implications for his management.

Conceptualisation and treatment

Conceptualisation

Tony was severely opiate dependent and he had a long history of illicit drug use. He had shown tolerance and withdrawal symptoms. He had not sought out treatment voluntarily, but rather had it thrust upon him by circumstances. The most appropriate initial treatment approach for Tony was methadone maintenance with ancillary counselling as needed. After his maintenance dose had been achieved and he was stabilised, his comorbid psychiatric disorders needed to be addressed to maximise the probability of continued abstinence from illicit drugs and from injecting. Tony required a 'fast-track' admission to a methadone maintenance program. The alternative of drug-free intervention on an outpatient basis, in a residential therapeutic community or from a self-help group (such as Narcotics Anonymous) was not likely to appeal to him at that stage. Neither was he likely to be able to cope with the regimen of a residential community or the lack of constant structure of a self-help group, and he was very likely to leave and to quite quickly relapse to injecting (Mattick & Hall, 1992). Given his high tolerance and dependence on opiates, ongoing injecting was likely, and this would continue to expose Tony and others to the risk of infection with diseases that are easily transmitted when injecting equipment is shared (hepatitis and HIV). Methadone maintenance has been shown to be associated with a reduced risk of infection with these diseases (Ward et al., 1992).

Treatment

The drug and alcohol counsellor who spoke to Tony in hospital discussed the options with him, and Tony made it clear that he really did not wish to go on to a methadone program. He said that he knew that 'it gets into your bones, and rots your teeth', and he also complained that he knew he would 'have to be watched while I piss in a bottle every day', a humiliating experience that he did not wish to be subjected to. He was, however, acutely aware of the need to do something about his heroin and other drug use, and that it was going to be difficult to afford to maintain his habit now that his supply was gone. He discussed the option of detoxification but realised that even if he did detoxify from opiates successfully, he would find it difficult to stay away from using them. He grudgingly agreed to an assessment in the methadone clinic attached to the hospital, and was seen the same day in the hospital ward.

Tony commenced methadone that day, starting on 40 milligrams in divided doses under observation to detect sedation, and to preclude the dangers associated with over-dosage. His dose was increased to 65 milligrams over the next 10 days at a rate of 5 milligrams every two days. By this time he was out of the hospital, back in his share accommodation.

Tony's dysthymia had been present for many years, but with the loss of the focus of his life — opiates and his de facto wife — he was more depressed than usual. He was also still complaining of daily withdrawal symptoms, especially in the morning when he most missed his usual injection. His complaints at the methadone clinic led to his dose being gradually increased to 110 milligrams of methadone per day over the next six weeks. He was in a state of psychological disarray, and it took him some three months to start to feel 'normal'.

After this period of three months he attended the methadone clinic daily and had a dozen brief counselling sessions with a nurse counsellor. He had not received any psychiatric assessment nor had he been seen by a clinical psychologist. He was in need of an intervention for his dysthymia. At this time he was still using heroin at least once a week, and smoked cannabis almost daily. His drinking had increased somewhat, and he used tranquillisers often to help him sleep, or else to augment the effect of other drugs. He was found to be using drugs by routine urine testing (urinalysis) conducted by the methadone clinic. This brought him to the attention of a psychiatrist who threatened him with expulsion from the program unless he ceased all illicit drug use. After some discussion with the prescriber it became apparent that there was an affective disorder that heightened the likelihood and frequency of use of psychoactive substances. The psychiatrist arranged for an assessment for treatment of the depression with a clinical psychologist from a nearby mood disorders clinic, however, neither Tony nor the staff of the clinic were interested in the prospect of treatment. He went to the assessment, but was told that he should 'get clear of the methadone' prior to intervention for the depression. Again this shows the failure of the general health care system to understand or be willing to assist 'drug addicts'. Tony stayed on the methadone program for a further 18 months without any intervention, beyond the occasional (and important) general counselling provided by the nurse dispensers at the clinic and by the prescriber. There were psychologists and a social worker attached to the unit but they and Tony did not achieve an ongoing therapeutic relationship.

Tony was repeatedly detected as having used illicit drugs during this 18-month period. The recognition that in Tony's case initial abstinence or reduction in drug use is followed by repeated relapse had forced the methadone clinic staff to focus their attention on methods of maintaining abstinence. The general approach taken to this problem, which has been promoted through the work of Marlatt and Gordon (1985), is termed 'relapse prevention'. Evidence from the areas of smoking cessation and opiate dependence suggests that relapse prevention may be beneficial in the treatment of drug dependence. The work of Marlatt and George (1984) has demonstrated an association between relapse and specific situations or mood states, especially negative mood states. There is a substantial relapse rate, even among opiate-dependent individuals who maintain abstinence from illicit drugs for up to a year. Withdrawal symptoms are an important potential determinant of relapse, especially in the short term, and because of this methadone doses should be adequate to ensure that symptoms do not occur (Ward, Mattick & Hall, 1992). In the longer term other factors have been found to be associated with a return to drug use. The factors most frequently associated with relapse include: (a) negative emotional states such as frustration, anger, anxiety, depression, boredom; (b) interpersonal conflicts associated with relationships such as marriage, friendship, family members or employer-employee relations; and (c) social pressure to use drugs, either of a direct nature where the individual is persuaded to use, or of an indirect nature by simply being in the company of others who are injecting or using.

The relapse prevention methods described by Marlatt and Gordon (1985) are separated into two classes: specific intervention strategies and global self-control strategies. The overall goal of the specific intervention strategies is to teach the user to recognise and cope with the high-risk situations that might precipitate a lapse, and to modify the reaction to a lapse so that it does not develop into a full-blown relapse. The first step taken was to assist Tony to recognise those particular high-risk situations that might precipitate a relapse. Typically this would involve reviewing a list of common relapse situations, identifying those that are likely to cause difficulty for the individual, and devising methods to either avoid these situations or cope with them without using opiates. In addition to reviewing typical high-risk situations, the assessment of idiosyncratic risk situations can highlight the situations (and skills deficits) associated with use. High-risk situations, whilst important, have been overemphasised in that there is a failure to recognise that users often relapse in unexpected situations.

Tony was encouraged to initially avoid the high-risk situations. The next step in the procedure involved teaching him alternative coping responses that might be used in the face of these situations. Marlatt and George (1984) noted that a number of areas should be covered, including assertiveness, stress management and anger management (cf., Monti et al., 1989). Practice of coping responses should be performance-based and personalised to the drug user.

The procedures are also designed to deal with the 'lapse' or slip back into drug use. Tony's reaction to such lapses was viewed as crucial. Marlatt and George (1984) have suggested that a single lapse can result in a complete return to drug use because the drug user sees the lapse as an indication of powerlessness over the drug in question. Relapse prevention, therefore, taught Tony to view a lapse as a temporary return to drug use and not as a complete failure. Moreover, there is an emphasis on learning from the events preceding the lapse and making strategic plans for limiting future lapses. A final part of the approach is the encouragement of global lifestyle changes through encouraging the development of recreational activities and behaviours that are incompatible with drinking alcohol.

Intervention for comorbid states

Tony's dysthymia was eventually treated with an approach based on procedures utilising cognitive-behavioural principles. Although it was a chronic condition it was not thought appropriate at this time to intervene with anti-depressant medications. If a psychological intervention did not bring about a resolution of the problems then other approaches would need to be considered. The dysthymia usually improves with psychological intervention, although the disorder remains present and occasionally becomes more severe and predisposes to alcohol abuse.

Long-term follow-up

Tony was maintained on methadone for a period of 4 years during which time his use of illicit drugs continuously declined until he is now rarely involved with any drugs other than cannabis or alcohol. He has moved out of share accommodation in the inner city to a suburban flat, and has started to work as a tyre fitter at a local tyre shop. At about this time, he was detoxified from methadone over a six month period and although he had significant fears of life without methadone, he succeeded in attaining and maintaining abstinence for three months thereafter. He lapsed twice, followed by a further period of one year on methadone. He again withdrew from methadone, but he remains abstinent. Occasionally he will use tranquillisers but this use is not a problem for him in his life.

Case 3: Tobacco dependence — the case of the happy smoker

Social and drug use history

Alice is 37 and has been smoking tobacco for a period of almost 20 years. She has enjoyed smoking over this time although occasionally she has considered quitting, particularly when she was pregnant with her three children who are now 14, 11 and 9 years old. She did cut down during pregnancy but still smoked daily.

She lives in a happy relationship with her children and her husband, who is a non-smoker but who has never really pressured her to quit. She smokes her first cigarette with breakfast, within an hour of rising in the morning and this is a cigarette that she would hate to give up. She smokes 25 cigarettes per day, avoids non-smoking areas in public places, and even smokes when she is ill in bed. According to one validated measure of nicotine dependence she is best considered to be quite severely dependent on nicotine (Heatherton et al., 1991).

She does not wish to stop smoking but has been advised that her workplace is to go 'smoke-free' in a few months time. She and her co-workers have been told by the management that they should try to become involved in a smoking cessation clinic so that the transition to not smoking at work is eased. She spoke to her general practitioner about the possibility of stopping, and she asked him about whether hypnosis could 'cure' her. He told her that she could try it, although there was no evidence that it has a unique or specific effect (cf., Mattick & Baillie, 1992). He advised that she seek assessment at a smokers' clinic at a major teaching hospital.

DSM-III-R diagnosis

The primary diagnosis is nicotine dependence. No developmental or personality disorders are present nor are there any physical disorders or conditions. She is not under any special stress and a global assessment of functioning in the past year indicates serious symptoms are absent.

Conceptualisation and treatment

Conceptualisation

Alice is not highly motivated to cease smoking tobacco. She has smoked happily for many years and she is only seeking help because of the introduction of a smoke-free policy in her workplace. She does not wish to stop smoking, but rather she wishes to be stopped. She is also highly dependent on nicotine, and she has not gone without daily smoking for two decades. She will require an assessment of her motivation to quit along with a motivational intervention to enhance her desire to successfully cut down. She will then require an intervention comprising nicotine replacement and psychological procedures to maximise her likelihood of successfully quitting and maintaining abstinence. In summary, for Alice's situation it is important for the smoking clinic staff to:

- determine whether she wishes to quit (stage of change)
- provide an intervention to heighten her motivation to quit
- personalise the health effects of smoking
- provide firm advice to quit smoking straight away
- provide a booklet containing self-help material
- set a quit date (if she is motivated to quit)
- identify social support for Alice from family or friends
- assess her nicotine dependence and advise her on the correct use of nicotine gum
- identify high-risk relapse situations and explain relapse prevention, including the identification of alternative strategies
- organise a follow-up visit or some other form of follow-up/referral.

For a variety of reasons, the following procedures are not likely to be useful for Alice: hypnosis, acupuncture, sensory deprivation (including 'float tanks'), aversion treatments, cue exposure and response prevention, and stress management per se (that is, extensive relaxation, meditation or breathing control training, which are seen as distinct from training smokers in brief techniques that might be useful in coping with high-risk situations).

Intervention

Pre-treatment assessment to select the intervention(s) to be used is important. The first area to assess is the level of motivation to actually cease smoking; the second is the level of dependence on tobacco (nicotine). It is obvious that even the most efficacious intervention will be ineffective if the individual is not keen to change or to quit. A prominent and influential model of motivation to cease use has been developed by Prochaska and DiClemente (1984, 1986), who provide a simple discovery procedure for determining the 'stage of change' of the drug-dependent individual, which may allow the tailoring of specific interventions to motivate the smoker to quit. Similar models have been put forth by other workers in this field (for example, Raw, 1986).

According to the model, readiness for change is conceptualised as involving four stages:

- a pre-contemplative stage, during which the user is not considering quitting
- a contemplative stage, during which the user becomes more aware of the costs of dependence and the benefits of quitting, but is ambivalent about quitting and does not act
- an action stage, during which the user will engage in active attempts to cease or reduce use
- a maintenance stage, which occurs after quitting has occurred, but during which the user may relapse and return to an earlier stage.

Recently, DiClemente et al. (1991) have subdivided the contemplation stage into contemplation and 'preparation'. The distinction between these stages is that preparation involves seriously considering a quit attempt in the next six months, planning to quit in the next 30 days, and having made a 24-hour quit attempt in the past year. The contemplation stage now involves considering a serious quit attempt in the next six months without the other aspects of the new preparation stage. The model proposed by Prochaska and DiClemente is at present supported by correlational data in terms of the predictive validity of the model in the context of smoking (Prochaska & DiClemente, 1986; DiClemente et al., 1991), although further research is required to demonstrate the utility of using the model to match users to specific interventions.

Because of the recentness of the stages-of-change model, there are no validated instruments available for clinical use. However, one simple method for assessing the stage of change of a smoker (for example) is simply to discuss the issue. This may be the most useful way for workers in this field to determine appropriate strategies for a client. Two questions that might prove useful are: 'How interested are you in quitting now?' and 'Do you feel that you ought to quit, or do you really want to?' Alternatively, the worker has two options: (a) to let the smoker self-select the stage of change; or (b) simply raise the issue with the smoker by asking: 'How do you feel about your smoking at the moment?' Responses may vary from the pre-contemplative (not ready to stop) responses such as 'I'm happy being a smoker', 'I enjoy smoking', 'I'm not interested in stopping'; through to (b) the contemplative (unsure about quitting) responses such as 'I'm thinking about stopping', 'I'm not sure if I'm ready at the moment', 'I'm interested in weighing up stopping'; to (c) the action-oriented (ready to quit) responses such as 'I want to stop now', 'I may need some help', or 'The disadvantages of smoking outweigh the benefits for me'. The responses made by the smoker may indicate a need for a motivational intervention (particularly for the ambivalent 'contemplator'), methods for which are outlined below. Alice responded to these questions by stating that she was happy with her smoking and that she really did not wish to stop, placing her in a pre-contemplative stage of change.

The recent emphasis placed upon the stage of change of the smoker has been paralleled by the development of 'motivational interviewing' or motivational enhancement therapy. Motivational interviewing is a technique that is thought to be particularly useful for working with smokers experiencing ambivalence (or conflict) about their behaviour and its cessation. The goal of motivational interviewing is to elicit the smoker's concerns and reasons for change. Within the principles of the procedure, the style of the interview and the role taken by the clinician are thought to be critical. For example, while many clinicians may attempt to motivate a smoker to quit by using a direct confrontational approach, this appears to be inappropriate (Miller, Sovereign & Krege, 1988). Motivational interviewing instead utilises non-directive counselling skills, such as open-ended questions and reflection of the smoker's concerns. However, the procedure is paradoxically directive, as it systematically steers the smoker towards motivation for change. This is achieved by using selective reflection and reinforcement of the smoker's concerns about smoking and reasons for wanting to quit, and by seeking to amplify the discrepancy between the smoker's personal goals and current smoking behaviour. The technique avoids confronting smokers who deny that smoking is a health problem, yet again it is paradoxically confrontational in that it aims to create self-confrontation within the smoker. Confrontation is seen as a goal of motivational interviewing rather than a style.

Thus, the technique is essentially one of reflective listening to assess the stage that the smoker has reached in terms of quitting. If the smoker is at the contemplation stage, the interview is aimed to assist the smoker to consider the benefits and costs of quitting and of smoking, leading to a decision to quit. If the smoker is at the pre-contemplation stage, the interview is aimed to provide non-judgemental objective information that will assist in moving the smoker into the contemplation stage and beyond. The worker may ask the smoker 'What do you enjoy about smoking?', and draw the responses out from the smoker, balancing the information on the positive aspects of smoking with questions like 'What are the negative aspects of smoking?'. Miller (1983) originally postulated three general processes through which motivational intervention may achieve its effects: affirmation, awareness and alternatives. Miller, Sovereign and Krege (1988) have set out the general characteristics of this form of intervention in the context of problem drinking.

Following from these earlier descriptions, Miller and Rollnick (1991) have recently further outlined five broad clinical principles that underlie motivational interviewing. These principles are: (a) express empathy; (b) develop discrepancy; (c) avoid argumentation; (d) roll with client resistance; and (e) support the client's sense of ability to change. The expression of empathy refers to an attitude of acceptance and respect for (rather than an identification with) the smoker, and involves reflecting the smoker's own concerns about smoking. The notion of developing discrepancy is aimed at clarifying with the smoker important life goals and exploring the consequences of continued smoking that conflict with those goals. Avoiding argumentation is seen as critical to the process of motivational interviewing, as such argumentation is likely to produce a defensive attitude in the smoker, and puts the interviewer and the smoker at odds when they should be working in a cooperative manner. The technique of rolling with resistance is obviously related to avoiding confrontation, and involves inviting new perspectives if resistance is met.

To design an optimally effective intervention to enhance motivation, one would use strategies that would promote awareness of the risk associated with smoking and offer the smoker acceptable and effective behaviour change alternatives within a generally accepting and empathic atmosphere.

Personalising the adverse health effects of smoking is a way of educating and motivating Alice to quit. Indeed, smokers are often advised to quit in a discussion of health risks. The feedback of health risks may provide medical information on health status or effects from smoking by using measures of carboxyhaemoglobin (blood carbon monoxide level), lung function (spirometry), or else may simply occur through a discussion of cardiac, vascular, pulmonary or other smoking-related disorders and symptoms. The use of the procedure is supported by limited but impressive empirical evidence from controlled research trials (for example, Risser & Belcher, 1990).

A further step that should be taken in this context is the offer of nicotine gum which, if accepted, requires instruction on the correct use of the gum. Alice should also be provided with a general intervention to reduce her risk of relapse as discussed for an earlier case in this chapter (cf., Mattick & Baillie, 1992).

Long-term follow-up

Alice was able to abstain successfully while she was using nicotine chewing gum, and her abstinence was generally maintained for a year after the intervention. She relapsed at a Christmas party after having a few drinks, but she regained abstinence soon thereafter with the re-application of the procedures that she learnt.

Implications for the understanding of substance dependence

The disorders that are subsumed under the labels psychoactive substance abuse and dependence are often continuous with normal behaviour. They should not be considered to be under markedly different forces from those that lead many non-dependent persons to use psychoactive substances. They serve a function in the life of the individual, and unlike many other psychiatric disorders which are entirely aversive to the sufferer, there are benefits to the user from the use of these substances, even if there are significant negative effects.

In this sense it should be recognised that these disorders are appetitive disorders and that because of this there is a need to determine the reasons for use and for cessation. Motivational interviewing is a procedure that was designed to assist the drug user to make an evaluation of the role of drug use in his or her life — to increase the likelihood of cessation. It does this by ensuring that the reasons for cessation are 'owned' by the user, not imposed by the therapist. Relying on this approach to enhancing motivation alone, however, is insufficient to be confident that changes will occur and remain in place.

Clients will often benefit from replacement of the substance that they are dependent on, and this avenue of treatment must be one that responsible therapists retain in their response to drug dependence. Coupled with intervention to minimise the risk of relapse, and to build skills that may assist in resisting temptation and high-risk situations, replacement therapies have an important role to play.

Additionally, the onset, course, severity and maintenance of dependent states can be markedly affected by the presence of comorbid psychological states. The presence of depressive symptomatology is frequently found in association with dependence on those drugs that have serious effects on lifestyle (such as alcohol, opiates and other illicit drugs). This should not, however, be taken as a suggestion that psychoactive substance dependence cannot occur without other contributing psychological problems. Clearly the best example of dependence unfettered by psychological problems is provided by the 3 million dependent tobacco smokers in Australia. They do not generally smoke because of depression, anxiety or aversive emotional states.

The disorders are relapsing. Despite the fact that all of the cases described were more or less successful in the long term, a large proportion of drug-dependent individuals will fail in their effort. It will be through careful continued research and the link between research and clinical practice that the outcome for these individuals will be enhanced (cf., Mattick & Ward, 1992; Miller, 1987).

Peter C. Birrell
University of New South Wales

10 Psychophysiological disorders: hypertension and angina

In recent decades there has been an increasing awareness of the influence of psychological stressors on the precipitation and exacerbation of a wide range of physical illnesses. The terms 'psychophysiological disorder' or 'psychosomatic disorder' have been used to highlight those physical diseases where it has been thought that psychological factors play a major causal role in initiating or maintaining the physical pathology. The growing realisation that psychological conditions can affect physical health has resulted in a tendency among some psychopathologists to drop the use of the term 'psychophysiological disorder' on the grounds that all physical diseases may be influenced to some degree by psychological states.

Thus, whereas the *Diagnostic and Statistical Manual of Mental Disorders,* second edition (DSM-II) (American Psychiatric Association) in 1968 had a diagnostic category Psychophysiological Disorders, the *Diagnostic and Statistical Manual of Mental Disorders,* third edition, revised (DSM-III-R) (1987) has suppressed the term and asked clinicians instead to make a judgement about the presence of a 'psychological factor influencing a physical condition' and to note the physical condition itself. Many psychopathologists prefer to retain the term 'psychophysiological disorder', as have Davison and Neale in the latest (fifth) edition of their textbook *Abnormal Psychology* (1990). The virtue of the traditional usage is that certain physical diseases in which psychological stress plays an especially important role can be highlighted. Moreover, the DSM-III-R decision simply to note 'psychological factors affecting physical condition' can lead to arbitrary decisions, especially given the rather vague criteria outlined in the full DSM-III-R text.

In Australia there is an important additional reason for retaining the emphasis on psychophysiological disorders in relation to cardiovascular diseases in particular. In 1988, the Australian National Heart Foundation released a major and influential report on stress and cardiovascular disease in the *Medical Journal of Australia* which concluded that stress could not be regarded as a risk factor in coronary heart disease (CHD) and other cardiovascular diseases (Stress Working Party, 1988). The report spelt out the behavioural implications for intervention in its conclusions. The report's authors did not believe that stress should be included in the lifestyle risk factors that should be targeted behaviourally. The findings and conclusions of the National Heart Foundation's report run counter to the consensus of international opinion and this fact was pointed out almost immediately (Birrell & Lovibond, 1988). Nonetheless, the view has spread among Australian cardiologists and general practitioners, as a result of the Heart Foundation's report, that 'stress' is not an important risk factor and that all efforts should, as the report recommended, be focused on modifying 'the established risk factors' such as high serum cholesterol levels, cigarette smoking, hypertension (or high blood pressure) and a sedentary lifestyle.

As a consequence, there has been a recent marked decline of attention in Australia to stress management of patients with 'established risk factors' such as hypertension, in spite of overwhelming evidence that psychological factors worsen the disease. Moreover, the role of psychological stress in provoking and exacerbating attacks of the coronary syndrome, angina pectoris (pain produced by inadequate circulation to the heart), which is so obvious to any careful clinician, has been given less emphasis, while the drug and surgical management of angina has become for many the exclusive focus. Significantly, less than 12 months before the Australian National Heart Foundation report was released, a major American cardiological journal, *Circulation*, published by the American Heart Foundation, issued a special supplement: *Conference on Behavioral Medicine and Cardiovascular Disease* (1987). The supplement noted the importance of psychological and behavioural influences in diseases of the heart and blood vessels and the need for behavioural intervention to supplement or even replace conventional pharmacological and surgical treatments.

Hypertension and angina

Hypertension refers to high blood pressure, a condition in which a person's arterial blood pressure is higher than adequate and desirable levels. Blood pressure is usually measured at the brachial artery just above the elbow. Here, in adult Caucasians, pressures during the pumping cycle of the heart (systole) of between 120–140 millimetres of mercury (120–140 mm Hg) and during the resting cycle of the heart (dia–stole) of between 70–90 mm Hg are considered to be within the normal range. A systolic (pumping) blood pressure of 145 mm Hg or more or a diastolic (resting) blood pressure of 95 mm Hg or more (if found on repeated occasions) would suggest at least mild hypertension. Consistent readings of 160/100 mm Hg or greater would establish the presence of mild but definite hypertension. Blood pressure is measured traditionally in millimetres of mercury. The clinician uses an instrument called a sphygmomanometer, which incorporates a mercury column; the height of the mercury is determined by air pressure in a cuff placed around the arm of the individual whose blood pressure is being measured. By pumping up the cuff and listening to the arterial blood movement through a stethoscope, the clinician can determine (a) the cuff pressure which blocks flow of blood during systole, hence yielding the upper or systolic blood pressure and (b) the cuff pressure which is insufficient to block even the arterial blood flow during diastole, hence yielding the lower or diastolic blood pressure.

Untreated hypertension is an insidious disease which produces pathological changes in the walls of blood vessels resulting in arteriosclerosis (hardening of the arteries and small arterial branches) and damage to various organs, especially the kidneys. The major disease end-point risk of hypertension is cerebrovascular accident or stroke, a leading cause of death and disability in Australia. In stroke, a vessel supplying the brain bursts or is blocked and consequently brain tissue normally supplied with oxygen and nutrients by the blood vessel dies (infarcts). Once the kidneys are damaged by the elevated blood pressure, the disease accelerates because the damaged kidneys release a pressure-raising hormone which preserves, in the short term, the filtering function of the kidneys, but which leads to yet greater and spiralling damage.

The most common form of hypertension, essential hypertension, is conventionally said to have an as yet unknown distal aetiology (long-term causation), although the proximal (immediate) cause of the disease has been known for decades — namely, constriction of the peripheral arterial system due to increased tension in the smooth muscle walls of the blood vessels (hence the term hypertension). The risk factors for the disease are also well known: family history, obesity, excessive sodium intake (especially sodium chloride or table salt), sedentary lifestyle and stress. Almost all authorities agree that these risk factors worsen existing hypertension, but not all are agreed that each risk factor is involved in the distal aetiology of the condition. Nonetheless, there is widespread agreement that dramatically reducing, or better still, eliminating the behavioural risk factors will greatly improve a patient's blood pressure, even restoring it to the normal range. A good outcome is most likely when the patient is in the mildly to moderately hypertensive range. In spite of the widespread international support for behavioural lifestyle change as a treatment modality, the majority of Australian hypertensives are medically managed with a variety of anti-hypertensive drugs.

Angina pectoris (angina of the chest) is a condition associated with a suffocating pain in the chest and is one of the classic coronary heart disease end-points. The pain, which may spread to the shoulders and arms, is brought about by lack of sufficient oxygen-containing blood being delivered to the heart through one or more branches of the coronary artery, the artery which directly supplies the heart muscle itself with fresh blood so that it can continue its pumping activity. In angina patients, the coronary artery is partially blocked in one or more places by cholesterol-rich atherosclerotic 'plaques'. At rest, enough blood gets through the narrowed artery or its branches to satisfy the heart's oxygen needs. But if the heart is subject to higher work demands and begins to pump more vigorously, the narrowed coronary artery cannot meet the heart's needs and the resulting hypoxia (reduced oxygen supply) gives rise to the angina symptoms. The pain subsides when the heart becomes less active or the sufferer takes medication which dilates the coronary artery, allowing more blood to reach the heart.

The long-term cause of angina is blockage of the coronary artery or its branches by cholesterol-rich deposits — this slow-developing process is called coronary atherosclerosis. In severe cases at least one branch of the coronary artery may be more than 90 per cent blocked. Angina patients are at risk of two potentially fatal forms of coronary heart disease: myocardial infarction (or heart attack) and cardiac arrhythmias. In myocardial infarction the artery becomes completely blocked, usually by a blood clot (or thrombus) forming at a particularly obstructed point in the artery. No blood gets through and the area of the heart muscle served by that branch of the coronary artery begins to die. Angina can also lead to disturbances of the rhythm of the heart's beat. In the worst case, the heart's rhythm can be so disrupted that no effective pumping takes place and unless the arrhythmia is immediately corrected the patient will die.

The near or proximal cause of angina is almost always physical or psychological stress. Even patients who avoid physical exercise stress so as not to place excessive demands on their heart are at great risk of angina attacks being provoked by psychological stress. Any source of emotional over-arousal puts angina patients at some risk. Even an argument with a spouse can cause the nervous system to stimulate the heart and to release stress hormones such as adrenalin which further stimulate the heart, producing pain. Anxiety, conflict and worry can have the same effect. Not even during sleep are angina sufferers spared. A disturbing dream can bring on an angina attack and the patient will awake from the nightmare with the savage pain of angina as the rapidly beating heart demands more oxygen than the partially blocked coronary artery can supply. Modern sleep research has shown that many angina attacks occur during Rapid Eye Movement (or dream) sleep and that the risk of an anginal attack during a dream is directly related to the arousal the dream produces. Moreover, the incidence of disturbing dreams is closely related to daytime stress patterns (see Dream Anxiety Disorder in the DSM-III-R (American Psychiatric Association, 1987)).

To sum up, hypertension and angina pectoris are two psychophysiological disorders which, once diagnosed, are known to be profoundly influenced by psychological factors in the patient's life, especially environmental stressors. The management of psychological stress is an essential part of the treatment of patients suffering from hypertension and angina. What is often not realised is that the two conditions frequently coexist in the same patient. This fact should not be surprising as high blood pressure is an established risk factor in coronary atherosclerosis and, hence, angina. The frequent concurrence of the two syndromes, especially in middle-aged individuals, raises important issues of clinical management.

Case study

Kevin Marshal is a 49-year-old dentist who maintains two professional suites: a prestige office in Sydney's central business district in Macquarie Street (an area highly sought after by health professionals) and rooms in one of Sydney's eastern suburbs close to where he, his wife Margaret and their two teenage children live. In recent years, Kevin has spent rather more than half his work time in the city practice, but was still determined to maintain his suburban rooms where he had initially built up his reputation and had many loyal, mainly lower-middle class patients, including whole families. Kevin had leased his city surgery after the family had returned from five years sojourn in England. There, Kevin had joined a group practice with several other Australian dentists in an outer London suburb and had also taken specialist courses in paediatric orthodontics.

It was now seven years since he had returned to Australia and much of his current work in his city Macquarie Street suite was in orthodontics. Since graduating in dentistry from Sydney University in 1967, Kevin had worked exceptionally long hours. Since his entry into a city-based semi-specialist practice the hours had become even longer and there was the pressure of shuttling between his two work sites, with their quite dissimilar clientele and demands. Kevin countered his wife's arguments that he should concentrate on his city practice by pointing out the very substantial mortgage and other financial commitments the family had incurred. Owning a house in Sydney's eastern suburbs was very expensive and the couple's two sons went to a highly rated private school with substantial tuition fees. The economic recession had affected his city practice more than his suburban work. He believed he needed the suburban work to make ends meet.

Margaret, who had met Kevin when she was his dental nurse and still helped out in the suburban practice, knew that much of what he said was true; but for some years she had been troubled by her husband's pattern of overwork and was herself willing to see their lifestyle modified to make things less demanding for Kevin. One thing that worried Margaret was that Kevin had virtually no social interests or hobbies, other than the occasional dinner party which she organised and his rather reluctant attendance at their boys' school functions. He seemed to live for his work (or as he often said to her) 'I have to work to live'. He was not even involved to any significant extent in professional society matters, although he arranged to attend regular workshops and conferences given by local and overseas experts on orthodontics. Margaret had noticed that in recent years he always seemed very tired when he returned home in the evening, and when she worked with him at his suburban practice he often seemed exhausted and irritable.

In the previous six months her concern had escalated. One day while working on a child in the city practice, Kevin developed chest pains. Like many health professionals, he did not have regular medical checkups, and he believed that he had always enjoyed robust good health. He boasted that he had only taken one week off for illness since he had graduated and that had been for an attack of influenza in the family's first winter in London. He was aware that his father, a retired high school principal, had been treated for hypertension for several decades, but surprisingly Kevin had not had his own blood pressure taken for at least several years and then only for an insurance examination.

On this occasion, the chest pain was so severe that he had to reschedule the patient and, at his receptionist's insistence, he went across the road to the Sydney Hospital Casualty Department. He expected a long wait, but as soon as he reported his symptoms he was ushered into a curtained cubicle where a nurse asked him to take off his shirt and he was wired up to an electrocardiograph (ECG), a machine that records the electrical activity of the heart muscle. The nurse also wrapped a sphygmomanometer cuff around his upper right arm. The junior resident who came in just as the casualty nurse was taking Kevin's blood pressure glanced at the sphygmomanometer column and the ECG tracings. After a brief conversation with the nurse, he took Kevin's blood pressure himself several times and in the interim asked him about his chest pains. The resident then called a more senior colleague.

'Am I having a heart attack?' Kevin asked, now thoroughly anxious. The senior registrar did not answer immediately but examined the ECG tracings with great care. 'Do you still feel the chest pain?' Kevin replied that he did; in fact, after subsiding in his surgery the pain was now almost as intense as it had been when he had been operating on the child. The registrar asked the nurse to give Kevin some medication to place under his tongue. Almost immediately, the sense of pain and pressure in his chest decreased. 'I've given you anginine, Mr Marshal, as you aren't getting enough blood to your heart and the anginine will dilate the blood vessels and relieve the symptoms. I gather you are a dentist from across Macquarie Street, so I expect I can be fairly sharp and to the point with you. We will confirm the diagnosis with an exercise ECG and with an X-ray of your coronary artery tree in the next few days, but I'm pretty certain that you were having an angina attack. In answer to your question, you definitely are not having a myocardial infarct, if that's any immediate comfort. However, at least one, probably several, of your coronary artery branches are severely clogged up — hence the angina. The resting ECG we are taking here was revealing signs of myocardial circulatory insufficiency, but that is gone now that the anginine seems to be doing its job. Hence the need for the further tests, especially the angiographic X-ray. I don't think there is any immediate risk of arrhythmia, but we'll watch you here for an hour or two.'

The registrar paused, 'There's a second matter, Mr Marshal, your blood pressure is too high. In fact, probably as a consequence of the pain and anxiety, the first readings were very high systolically — that has come down a bit now, but your readings are still well above normal. Are you hypertensive?'. 'My father is, but I haven't had my pressure taken for a while', Kevin replied. 'What is it now?' 'About 165/110 and it's the diastolic reading which worries me. As you know, the diastolic resting pressure is much less susceptible to transient elevation — so I suspect we'll find you have moderate hypertension. Were you doing anything physically demanding when the chest pain came on?' 'No, I suppose I was rather tired and was getting exasperated with the child I was working with. To tell the truth I was really quite angry with the patient and her mother as they hadn't complied with my instructions about her wearing her teeth bands.' 'Do you often get angry like that in your work?', the registrar asked. 'Of course', Kevin responded, 'but you can't afford to show it, can you?'.

The follow-up tests with a consultant cardiologist confirmed that Kevin had hypertension and angina. The coronary angiography (an X-ray of the coronary artery blood supply) revealed a moderate degree of atherosclerotic obstruction in two branches of his coronary artery. The cardiologist advised that conservative treatment was in order — by-pass surgery was a future option. 'We can use medication for both conditions but your blood pressure is labile (i.e., it varies somewhat from day to day) as it often does with mild to moderate cases, and it seems to be affected by your work and emotional states. Your angina attack was linked to emotional factors, not physical overload. I personally think it is very important that you learn to control your levels of anxiety and stress.' The cardiologist hesitated for a moment, 'The National Heart Foundation has suggested we downplay the role of stress in cardiovascular disease, but 30 years of practice has convinced me that stress can be critical in the management of angina and also hypertension. Consequently, I'd like you to see a clinical psychologist at the university Psychology Clinic who has had a great deal of success in this area. I will continue to see you, and until we re-evaluate the situation in the light of your response to whatever program Dr Saunders prescribes, you will continue with the medication for your blood pressure and angina'.

Conceptualisation and treatment

Dr Saunders, to whom Kevin was referred, specialises in health psychology, especially the application of behavioural change principles to cardiovascular risk factors, including stress. He knew from experience and research studies that cardiovascular diseases are markedly influenced by psychological factors. Moreover, Dr Saunders believes that not only stress but also other behavioural factors in physical diseases need to be dealt with in a multi-focused or integrated approach. Simply attempting to correct high levels of stress by, say, relaxation training was, in Dr Saunders's opinion, naive and unscientific. All aspects of the patient's life which could contribute to modifying stress should be incorporated into the stress reduction program. Thus, physical exercise, a balanced diet, and time management were significant components of a properly balanced behavioural program (see Lovibond, Birrell & Langeluddecke, 1986). In stress management, the various elements interacted synergistically to produce a more marked effect than any component alone. Behavioural intervention, by influencing physical fitness, nutrition and body composition, also contributed to the reduction of load on the cardiovascular system and, in appropriate circumstances, would lead to lower blood pressure and reduce the symptoms of other cardiovascular conditions such as angina. Dr Saunders often found that many patients who initially presented with mild to moderate symptoms no longer required standard medication and became symptom-free after participating in a behavioural health program, as long as they continued to implement the behavioural regimen recommended for them.

Before Kevin's first visit to the university clinic, Dr Saunders perused the referral documents and found that stress apparently was the big factor. Kevin was not high on the other standard cardiovascular risk factors, except for an unfavourable balance between the 'good' high-density lipoprotein (HDL) cholesterol and the 'bad' low-density lipoprotein (LDL) cholesterol. The excessive amount of LDLs and Kevin's rather low HDL levels had doubtless played a long-term role in the coronary artery atherosclerosis which put him at risk of angina. Fortunately, the aerobic exercise and dietary components of Dr Saunders's program would help to lower Kevin's stress and to balance his cholesterol levels. If the latter did not respond to behavioural intervention, the cardiologist had suggested a trial of one of the more recently introduced cholesterol-lowering drugs which also, importantly, altered the HDL/LDL ratio. Kevin was a trifle overweight and certainly not aerobically fit. Dr Saunders anticipated that the behavioural management program would deal with these problems in as much as they interacted with stress reactivity to exacerbate Kevin's hypertension.

Dr Saunders's first session with Kevin was devoted in part to establishing rapport between himself and his patient and to discussing the concept of stress and its role in Kevin's life. In particular, Dr Saunders explained the dangerous 'habituation' phase of the stress response as it had been outlined by the distinguished Canadian stress researcher, Hans Selyé (1976). In the 'habituation' phase, the individual becomes so apparently adapted to stressors (the environmental stimuli which provoke the stress response) and to the stress response itself, that he or she tends to ignore the telltale signs of over-stress. In this phase, too, the stressed individual often adopts modes of interacting with his or her environment — both with situations and with people — which are stress provoking. For example, irritability, fatigue and emotional lability (easily shifting mood), which are part of the pattern of chronic stress, lead the stressed person to interact negatively with others, often developing hostility, anger and verbal aggression. The negative responses they receive from others act as further stressors. The poorer attention span and impairments of concentration and memory which also are signs of chronic over-stress can, by occasioning poor judgement and decision making, lead to further stress, including interpersonal tension.

'Kevin, now that we have discussed the nature of stress, especially chronic stress, do you see any patterns of stressors in your life?' Kevin responded to Dr Saunders's question with more than a hint of exasperation in his tone, 'Really, this whole notion of stress is something new to me. Sure, as Margaret is always telling me, I work long hours and I often feel tired, but doesn't everyone? Why should dealing with a moderately difficult patient and her mother suddenly bring on angina and lead to my being diagnosed as hypertensive?'

Dr Saunders had heard this type of response often. Even with highly educated health professionals who found themselves suddenly in the position of being patients, it was quite commonplace to meet with this denial of the presence and effects of chronic emotional pressure.

'Kevin, you had reached a point in your coronary atherosclerosis, a threshold if you like, where soon the imposition of some physical or psychological stressor would provoke the symptoms of angina. As to your blood pressure, many factors, including probably a genetic predisposition, have made you hypertensive. But we know that once someone has essential hypertension, stress triggers elevation of blood pressure and generally exacerbates the condition. Put another way, I am confident that when we have carried out a behavioural analysis of the stress patterns in your life, and if we implement an integrated stress management program, we should bring your blood pressure back to normal and greatly reduce your risk of angina attacks. All aspects of the program will help. The exercise regime I want you to start on will not only have a direct effect on your stress reactivity, but, together with the dietary component of the program, will work in other ways physiologically to help your hypertension and angina.'

Kevin now asked a question which had been troubling him since the first angina attack some three weeks before. 'Look, what I want to know is whether my so-called stressful lifestyle caused the angina and the high blood pressure — my cardiologist is decidedly cagey on the subject.'

Dr Saunders smiled at this reminder of the recent National Heart Foundation controversy. 'In my opinion, the scientific evidence would suggest a larger role for chronic stress in the long-term aetiology of hypertension than in the long-term aetiology of atherosclerosis of the coronary arteries. However, even in the distal causation of atherosclerosis, stress probably plays a role in many cases. But, I must stress, once the patient has demonstrable hypertension and symptomatic angina, stress becomes most definitely a major causal factor in the progress of the diseases.'

Dr Saunders realised that, valuable as such discussion was, it was characteristic of patients such as Kevin that the therapy sessions could easily be sidetracked into 'scientific' discussion which kept both therapist and patient away from the current patterns of behaviour, thought and emotion that needed to be dealt with.

For their next meeting Dr Saunders asked Kevin to monitor daily any events, personal encounters and environmental stimuli at home and at work about which he felt negative. He gave Kevin special self-monitoring sheets to help him organise his homework. 'I want you to pay special attention to anything that makes you feel tense, hostile, irritable or overly tired.' Dr Saunders also asked Kevin to monitor the pleasant and relaxing episodes in his life. Before Kevin left the clinic Dr Saunders asked him to complete several psychometric tests which measure levels of perceived tension and anxiety and estimate a person's hostility, anger and verbal aggression. Although his cardiologist had placed Kevin on anti-angina and anti-hypertensive medication, Kevin had experienced three anginal episodes since the initial trauma in his city surgery. Dr Saunders noted with interest that two of these attacks had occurred in his city workplace and one had been triggered by a discussion with his wife, Margaret, after the last patient of the day had left his suburban practice. 'What were you discussing, Kevin?' 'Oh, just the same old issue — Margaret thinks I should concentrate on the city orthodontic work and that I'll feel less exhausted with a shorter working week. But I pointed out for the hundredth time that I'll just have to work more hours in Macquarie Street — that's if I get enough referrals anyway. At least the local practice pays a lot of our bills and, to tell the truth, is more reliable than the prestige city practice.'

Dr Saunders also noted that the pattern which emerged in the hostility, anger and verbal aggression tests administered to Kevin was one which many researchers had recently identified in people with a disposition to coronary artery disease and to hypertension, in particular labile hypertension (where there are transient peaks in an overall elevated blood pressure). This pattern was one marked by hostility or 'anger-in' (see Dembroski et al., 1985 and Siegman, Dembroski & Ringel, 1987).

At their next meeting the following week, Dr Saunders and Kevin began by going over the completed monitoring sheets. 'You seem to be reporting a lot of suppressed anger and irritability both at work and at home. Am I correct?', Dr Saunders asked. 'Do you think the pattern was much the same before you were recently diagnosed, or do you feel that it is largely a reaction to finding yourself with two major cardiovascular conditions?' He asked the question partly to see what insight Kevin may have gained as a result of careful self-monitoring. Dr Saunders knew that the psychometric tests he had administered at the previous session indicated (as had Kevin's clinical history) that Kevin possessed marked traits of hostility and tension. These traits were unlikely to be consequences of his recent cardiovasular diagnoses.

'Well, I have to admit how surprised I was by the number of times I found myself writing down feelings of suppressed anger and general tension', Kevin replied. 'In dentistry we are always dealing with anxious and often reluctant patients, but I thought I was quite detached. I thought it was only the patients who didn't do what I'd asked them to do that got under my skin. And I thought that was pretty rarely. It's the "hostility", as you call it, that I seem to be showing at home as well as at work that worries me.'

'You mean your reactions to your discussions with Margaret and the boys', Dr Saunders interjected. 'Yes', said Kevin, 'I get very angry inside — I suppose that's part of what you mean by hostility — but I notice that I've long ago given up expressing the bad feelings outwardly'. 'Did you ever express your negative emotions very much — I mean both explosively and also constructively — by commenting that you feel angry with the person or situation?' 'No, not really', Kevin replied, 'I hate fights, and in my profession we were always taught to never, ever lose our tempers with patients, particularly in the surgery'. Dr Saunders felt both relief and pleasure that Kevin had been able to express this important insight.

'One of the planks of our multi-focused management of your condition will be to teach you what we call cognitive strategies for dealing with what an American colleague has referred to as "anger-in", that is, unexpressed hostility and anger. In the United States the very high incidence of hypertension among Afro-Americans has been linked to this behaviour pattern.' Dr Saunders was referring to work carried out by Harburg and his associates (see, for example, Harburg & Hauenstein, 1980) and many other investigators who had found that frustration and unexpressed passive anger arising from unavoidable environmental stressors seemed to be linked with the initiation and progression of essential hypertension in Afro-Americans.

'I see you and Margaret have decided to make a decision about your two practices.' 'Yes, although Margaret doesn't particularly like the idea — she never visits Macquarie Street and maybe that's why she sees it through rosy spectacles, plus the fact that it makes me a mid-city "specialist" — I think I could move my orthodontic work to the suburban clinic. I would still get the referrals and I would avoid a lot of hassle. If the ordinary work got too much, I think I would take on an assistant. I'd like you to talk to Margaret, Dr Saunders.'

'Well, I'm very happy to see both of you together, but it is vitally important that with a bit of coaching from me, you are able, in my presence initially, to express to her your strong feelings and your resentment at what you see as her resistance to changes which will benefit your health and the well-being of the whole family. Is that okay?' 'Yes, that's fine, and a bit of a relief really', Kevin responded. 'I suppose the "coaching" as you call it is part of what you referred to as the cognitive behaviour therapy part of the treatment.' 'You're right, it is, and in your case a very important part. I also want Margaret, and perhaps the boys too, involved in your exercise program. The monitoring sheets reveal not only that you haven't got very far with starting this aspect of the program, but that there's little time left for recreation of any sort in your daily life.' 'I suppose I've become a work machine over the years and, if anything, Margaret has encouraged me by all the pressure to keep the city practice, although she's always saying how worried she had been by my fatigue, even before the angina attack. You know, after my Saturday practice hours, I just crash on the weekend except for compulsory visits to relatives and things like that.'

Dr Saunders gave Kevin a copy of a book by Dr Chandra Patel, a British pioneer in multi-focused behavioural intervention against cardiovascular disease. Patel (1989) has had much success treating the stress element in hypertension and her techniques are widely used by both psychologists and medical practitioners in Great Britain. 'You will find Dr Patel's book a useful adjunct to the Behavioural Change Program Manual I have already given to you. As well as seeing me on a weekly basis for another couple of months, I want you to join one of our Behavioural Health Program groups where you will be taught many of the skills I want you to master. Your progress on behavioural risk factors such as fitness level, body weight and general stress reactivity will be measured objectively at fortnightly intervals. Margaret may like to join the group also.'

Dr Saunders had, by now, a reasonably clear picture of Kevin Marshal's specific and general health problems. With Margaret's cooperation, which in the event was readily forthcoming, he was sure that Kevin's stress levels could be dramatically modified. All aspects of the program would play their part, but as Kevin had such a marked disposition to passive hostility and suppressed anger, changing his mode of emotional expression was very important. Contrary to what was often taken for granted in textbooks, relaxation training was not the essential key — certainly not in Kevin's case. In fact Dr Saunders knew that teaching Kevin a relaxation technique (for example, meditation) without dealing with his personality profile and without implementing other aspects of the program, such as exercise, would yield very little benefit. But as part of the overall treatment strategy, the relaxation tape which he had given to Kevin and which Kevin used on a daily basis for about twenty minutes, was useful.

Later adjustment

Kevin made excellent progress in the first two months of Dr Saunders's program. Kevin and Margaret agreed to consolidate the practice in their suburban surgery. As he expected, he received enough referrals for his orthodontic work from colleagues. In fact, to preserve a mid-week half-day break (Kevin and Margaret decided to begin golf lessons), Kevin was negotiating to have another dentist join the practice. By week eight of the program, Kevin's blood pressure was 130/80, well within the normal range, and his cardiologist had, on trial, reduced his medication dramatically. He had had no more angina episodes, and was jogging 4 km at least four times each week.

After the initial two months, Dr Saunders asked Kevin to return in four months (or earlier if there were any problems). A few weeks before his scheduled visit Kevin telephoned to say that he needed some help in dealing with his new assistant. Again, it was a matter of relative inability to express negative thoughts and emotions. Following a few sessions with Dr Saunders, the new skills he had learned in the first two months of intervention had been generalised to the specific problem. However, it was clear that Kevin might need 'booster' sessions of this type for some indefinite period. He was not particularly adept at transferring cognitive skills to new situations. Dr Saunders organised a regular meeting at three-monthly intervals. Nonetheless, nothing as serious as the problem with the new colleague emerged and overall Kevin made continued progress. Very importantly, he was showing new insight into factors which in the past he had ignored or denied.

At a two-year follow-up Kevin's cardiologist was extremely pleased with his patient's general health. The atherosclerosis in his coronary artery had not progressed, and his excellent fitness level and much reduced stress reactivity had eliminated most of the risk of anginal attacks. His blood pressure without medication was now 128/76. The cardiologist thought a coronary by-pass operation was unnecessary and would only be considered if there were untoward future changes in the condition of his coronary artery tree. The only medication he kept Kevin on was a small dose of aspirin every day. A major recent American trial had shown that in patients with proven coronary atherosclerosis, the equivalent of about half an aspirin tablet each day reduced by about 50 per cent the risk of a thrombus (or clot) forming in the coronary artery and myocardial infarction occurring.

Aetiological considerations

Kevin Marshal's case, in which two cardiovascular conditions, hypertension and angina, coexisted, and where the diagnosed conditions were clearly being maintained and aggravated by psycho-emotional factors, highlights the critical importance of distinguishing between distal and proximal aetiology in psychophysiological disorders. The overwhelming evidence of the influence of environmental stimuli and personality traits on the proximal (near or immediate) causation of elevated blood pressure in hypertensive patients and of anginal attacks in patients with coronary atherosclerosis makes it mandatory to attend to the role of stressors and stress reactivity. Clinically, this response would be demanded even were it the case that there was no evidence of a distal role for 'stress' as a causal determinant in either essential hypertension or coronary atherosclerosis. To play down the causal influence of psycho-emotional factors is foolhardy in the extreme. At worst, the patient is put at unnecessary and even mortal risk and any management regime is rendered less effective.

As it is, there is growing evidence of a causal role for stress in the long-term aetiology of cardiovascular disease. In any case, there is more than sufficient reason to retain for particular physical pathologies the term 'psychophysiological disorder' if only to highlight situations where there is a special need to consider stress as a cause and stress management as a treatment focus. The current classificatory arrangements of the DSM-III-R fail in this respect and leave far too much room for ambiguity and the personal bias of the individual diagnostician.

J. Christopher Clarke
University of New South Wales

11 The nature and treatment of panic anxiety and agoraphobia

Introduction

The subjects of this chapter are agoraphobia, its relation to panic disorder and the optimal treatments for each. Agoraphobia is the most disabling and most prevalent of phobic disorders and is the complaint of 50–80 per cent of all those who seek clinical assistance for phobic disorders (Mathews, Gelder & Johnston, 1981; Marks, 1987). Prevalence figures vary from 6 per 1000 (Agras, Sylvester & Oliveau, 1969) to 20 or more per 1000 in Australia (Clarke & Wardman, 1985). By these estimates the number of agoraphobics in Sydney alone would lie somewhere between 20 000 and 60 000. Typically agoraphobia strikes females (the ratio to males is approximately 3:1 (Marks, 1969)) and has a sudden onset following the occurrence of a panic reaction. The age of onset is usually the early twenties, although there is another smaller peak in the distribution in the late thirties.

The term agoraphobia was coined in 1871 by the German psychiatrist Westphal to describe a condition he observed in four cases (interestingly, all four were male). The term 'agoraphobia' translated literally means a 'fear of the agora' (the market place in ancient Athens). Westphal chose the term because his patients all reported a fear of open spaces. A closer reading of Westphal's classic monograph on the subject (see Boyd & Crump, 1991) reveals that the patients also feared being alone, especially if they had to go out alone, experiencing intense physiological arousal during trips into 'danger areas'. Had these matters received closer attention agoraphobia might not for so long have been conceived of as only a 'fear of open spaces'. This misinterpretation could perhaps also have been perpetuated by its seeming complementary status to claustrophobia which truly is a fear of confined spaces.

As noted earlier, agoraphobia is the most disabling phobia encountered in clinical practice (Marks, 1969, 1987). Equally, there is little dispute as to the link between the development of panic attacks (sudden and extremely intense bursts of anxiety) and the onset of agoraphobia. Estimates of the progression from panic to agoraphobia range from a low of 85 per cent of the cases (Aronson & Logue, 1987) to 100 per cent (Franklin, 1987; Kleiner & Marshall, 1987).

Since the focus in this chapter is on agoraphobia and panic, a current definition of each will provide the platform for a critical examination of the clinical and theoretical disagreements about the conceptualisation and treatment of each. Starting with agoraphobia, if one were to construct a list of the situations that elicit anxiety, it would be a very long one, and would include travelling in trains, planes, buses and cars (especially if others are driving), being forced to wait in any of a variety of situations such as supermarket queues, hairdressers, bridge traffic, sitting through long meals in restaurants, or in the homes of others. In specific detail, the list of concerns and environments which elicit anxiety is seemingly endless. Some writers (Glick, 1967) have a preference for separating each condition by adding the word 'phobia' to the various situations (for example, hairdresser phobia, bridge phobia, shopping phobia). This practice can lead to an unacceptable proliferation of phobias distinguished only by locale. Factor-analytic studies of agoraphobic fears indicate a small number of common themes underlying all of these seemingly disparate concerns. The research (see Mathews, Gelder & Johnston, 1981) concludes that the list of anxiety environments and situations can be tied to two distinct themes: phobic anxiety triggered by a separation by some crucial distance (which will differ from one individual to the next) from what is perceived by the agoraphobic as a 'safe place'; the second theme which can be abstracted from the large variety of anxiety-evoking situations is travelling without a 'significant other'. In the most intense varieties of agoraphobia, the agoraphobic person may press for constant companionship even while at home.

Of these two separation concerns, the ones associated with anxiety during travel and the consequent reduction in free, untroubled mobility have, without question, received the most attention from clinical writers on the subject. A perusal of the behavioural therapy literature reveals that until recently agoraphobia was treated as more or less synonymous with travel phobia. If the agoraphobic has a strong dependency on an attachment figure, the latter would doubtless take issue with this as a narrow, restrictive definition. The constant appeals to the attachment figure for company and reassurance can be very burdensome. So, were one to ask these significant others to nominate the central problem they may well indicate the excessive reliance and dependence upon them. To get the perspective of the agoraphobic, we asked 53 agoraphobics with concurrent panic attacks to rate all of the stresses in terms of the quality and quantity of the anxiety which they evoke. Forty-one of the respondents listed neither travelling nor separation anxiety as the most dreaded event — that place was given, unhesitatingly, to panic attacks.

Panic attacks

Panic reactions are sudden and severe attacks of anxiety which are accompanied by a diverse set of physiological reactions: over-breathing or hyperventilation, tachycardia (racing heart) and excessive physical tension. The psychological symptoms that accompany this 'autonomic firestorm', as one agoraphobic patient described it (Clarke & Wardman, 1985), are 'simply terrifying'. In general terms, during panic upheavals there is cognitive disorganisation, dizziness, fear of loss of support ('jelly legs') and, most importantly, belief that collapse, insanity and even death are imminent. Many of these panic reactions appear to come without apparent cause — from 'out of the blue'. While the duration can vary from a few moments to half an hour, clients report that it is their lack of ability to predict and control panic reactions which is especially terrifying.

In addition to these debilitating attacks, and the two anxiety themes of travel and isolation, there are likely to be a host of related problems. Chief among these is the 'fear of fear' (Goldstein & Chambless, 1978), which is believed by some (for example, Foa & Kozak, 1991) to be an important, indeed the major, source of agoraphobic avoidance. Foa and Kozak argue that the true source of avoidance is the dread of suffering an (unexpected) panic attack in a strange locale where help or assistance may not be readily available.

Another component of the syndrome is depression, which increases with the degree of agoraphobic avoidance (Klosko et al., 1986.) Finally, agoraphobics may show excessive reliance on alcohol and tranquillisers, used in most instances to cope with anxiety reactions (see Miller & Reise, 1991).

The information given above summarises the descriptive knowledge of agoraphobia and panic. The data provide a starting point for understanding the disorders, but do not answer a number of critical questions concerning the way in which the components of the two interact, the processes underlying them nor the role of panic in agoraphobic avoidance. The answers to each of these questions has serious implications for clinical treatment.

The main aims of the chapter are to examine the problems of agoraphobia and panic. The close association between agoraphobia and panic disorders has long been noted. The point of controversy, however, is the nature of the link between them. Until the mid-1980s (American Psychiatric Association, *Diagnostic and Statistical Manual of Mental Disorders,* third edition, 1980 (DSM-III)) agoraphobia and panic were considered as two separate disorders. Recently, it has been argued that agoraphobia is merely a component of panic condition. A corollary of this view is that the treatment of agoraphobia amounts to the treatment of panic. A further assumption is that, quite simply, there is no phobia in agoraphobia. A rival view, presented through the following case study of an agoraphobic woman, is based on the proposition that agoraphobia is a complex disorder in which two different forms of anxiety — phobic and panic — interact to produce and maintain the syndrome.

Case study of panic disorder and agoraphobia

The case to be examined in detail in this chapter is of Juliana B who was aged 37 when she made contact with the Psychology Clinic at the University of New South Wales. Juliana was born in Holland; she is married with two teenage children, and lives in a western suburb of Sydney. Sixteen years ago she moved to Australia from Athens with her Greek husband George. Juliana and George met in Amsterdam where George had found employment as a 'guest worker'. Because of the uncertainty of his security of tenure they left Holland to travel to Australia via Athens. Juliana had great misgivings about leaving her widowed mother and the security and familiarity of her home and the routines of daily life. She voiced her fears to George, who reassured her that once they were settled in Sydney her mother could come to visit and, if she wished, could give up her home in Amsterdam and live with them in Australia. Juliana relented and shortly thereafter Mr and Mrs B emigrated to Australia. On the ship voyage, Juliana experienced periods of chronic anxiety. She had always been mildly insecure when parted from her mother for extensive periods, but the persistence of these reactions was new to her. She interpreted her anxiety as a response to the irrevocable separation from home and her mother because the anxiety was at its most disturbing when she reflected on the great changes in her life and her longing to see her mother. By the time the ship arrived in Perth, Juliana was constantly anxious and deeply unhappy. The themes of her anxiety were the well-being of her mother, the unknown challenges awaiting her and George in Sydney, and general fears of being unable to cope in a strange land.

Soon after arriving in Sydney she and her husband purchased a house with their combined savings. They were able to do this because George worked at two jobs and Juliana obtained employment in a real estate office. Matters took a turn for the worse 18 months later when Juliana discovered that she was pregnant. Neither Juliana nor her husband wanted a child at that time, but their religious convictions put the option of abortion out of the question. The prospect of paying off the house on her husband's income alone and other financial pressures forced Juliana to take a weekend job at a newsagent in a nearby suburb. The demands of running a house and working two jobs added to the already existing distress she was experiencing from morning sickness early in her pregnancy. Just at that time her mother informed her that she was planning a trip to Australia. Given the circumstances, Juliana was delighted at the news that her mother was coming for a three-month visit. Unfortunately the visit helped to re-establish the dependence on her mother which had been a feature of their relationship since she was a young girl. The trip was not a success largely because Juliana's mother missed her home and friends in Holland. On the day prior to her mother's departure, when Juliana was in a generally anxious mood, she experienced her first full-blown panic attack. On the day in question she was on her way to work when she felt an intense and unexpected anxiety reaction. It occurred when she was disembarking from the bus just around the corner from her office. Immediately her thoughts turned from her general worries and concerns about her mother's departure to a sharply focused awareness of the tightness in her chest and the rapid beating of her heart. She attempted to take her pulse and stopped after 15 seconds when she counted 30 heart beats. Her breathing became extremely laboured and, as she recalls, very rapid, so much so that a passer-by in the street stopped to ask her if she were having an asthma attack. Juliana could not guess at the cause of those physical and emotional changes that exploded so violently and without warning. It seemed to her that what had happened was catastrophically bad and possibly foretold death or impending madness. That evening at home her husband was sympathetic but assured her the anxiety was really nothing but a 'bit of nerves'. Despite this attempt at reassurance, she made an appointment with her general practitioner. After listening to her fears of a heart attack, he examined her and reassured her that she was well. She nevertheless pressed him for a referral to a specialist in cardiovascular medicine. She received a clean bill of health from the specialist and her fears were calmed after she remained vigilant to changes in her physiological reactions. Matters went on in this way until the delivery of the child a few months later. Juliana had a difficult labour and delivery and though the health of mother and child were excellent she did go through a period of serious post-partum depression. Upon returning home the depression eased but for the next six months she remained anxious and apprehensive about having another panic attack and also about the well-being of her mother in Amsterdam.

Sometime towards the end of the first year after the birth Juliana received news that her mother had suffered a mild heart attack. On hearing the news, Juliana was struck with a series of panics which extended over the following week. These caused her to seek further medical advice and yet again the tests revealed no cardiovascular dysfunctions. By this time new problems had begun to appear. She found travelling away from the house so frightening and exhausting that she soon gave up attempts to venture more than 100 metres or so in either direction from the house. When accompanied by her husband she discovered that the range was extended considerably and that going 500 metres to the end of the street was possible without too much discomfort. It puzzled her that the presence of others — friends, acquaintances, neighbours — did not ease her fears as much as did her husband's presence, even though he was often openly critical of her for her 'silly worries'. In her car she could go much further (for example, to nearby shopping centres) as long as she was driving and in control. Under these conditions the perimeter of safety extended to a few kilometres in any direction from around the house.

From that time onwards Juliana began to display the full range of symptoms and signs of agoraphobia and panic. With some day-to-day variation her mobility was sharply restricted. She also became more dependent on her husband to the point where she would become anxious if he were to be away from home or out of telephone contact. Panic frequency varied from two to four per week with most of these striking her while she was out of the house. Despite the increase in the number of attacks, Juliana showed no habituation to the impact of panic. The attacks always surprised her and left her badly shaken; she also experienced grave doubts about her health and sanity during and just after the attacks. Depression too, was a daily feature of her life. There was variation in the levels of depression according to how well she perceived herself to be functioning, but even on 'good' days her mood was dysphoric.

During the following year she took a friend's advice and agreed to see a psychiatrist. Her husband supported her in this decision and drove her to and from the therapy sessions but took no part in them nor did the therapist request him to do so. The content of the therapy was psychodynamic but without some of the trappings of the classical Freudian arrangements. Juliana sat face-to-face with the analyst and was never asked to lie on a couch. The therapist also took a more active role in the interaction and offered suggestions for behaviour change as well as interpretations of her free associations and dreams. Juliana recalls the therapist as friendly and considerate and their relationship as mainly a good one. However, whenever she pressed him for information about the causes of her travelling anxiety and her panic attacks, he remained non-committal. When questioned about the forces maintaining the problems, he offered the suggestion that the source of her tensions was a fear of her sexual urges getting out of control in public and moreover that, by 'holding onto her symptoms', she was in fact exerting control over her husband. These interpretations worried her greatly and led to her discontinuing therapy after 10 sessions.

A year later, with no change in any of her problems, Juliana sought the help of another clinician. He told her that the main problem was depression, gave her a biochemical explanation of her disorder and placed her on a schedule of antidepressant medication. She tried this for a week but was so intolerant of the side effects that she discontinued the medication and her visits to that doctor. Shortly afterwards she obtained a prescription for a minor tranquilliser from a local GP and continued to use it daily.

Discussion

As stated at the opening of this chapter anxiety disorders are prevalent and disabling. Juliana's problems were numerous, including panic disorder (PD), agoraphobic avoidance (PDA), recurrent unipolar depression, generalised anxiety disorder (GAD) and general demoralisation. Of the nine categories of anxiety disorder listed in the *Diagnostic and Statistical Manual of Mental Disorders*, third edition, revised (DSM-III-R) (American Psychiatric Association, 1987), PD is given special prominence. The signs and symptoms of panic include heart palpitation, respiratory distress, dilation of blood vessels which causes sweating, loss of fine motor control, a dread of collapse or insanity or death (Holt & Andrews, 1989) and a sense of being powerless to control these reactions.

Recent research suggests that panic attacks may not be as rare as the low prevalence rates suggested. Norton, Dorward and Cox (1986) estimated the prevalence in a population of university students and found that 35 per cent had experienced one or more panic attacks within the last year and 25 per cent within the preceding three weeks. These do seem very high figures and had the authors used a clinical interview method rather than the paper and pencil assessments the figures may have been lower. There is no question that Juliana met the frequency and severity criteria as outlined in the DSM-III-R criteria for PD.

Juliana also qualified for a GAD diagnosis, the essential features of which are maladaptive, unreasonable or excessive anxiety about two or more life circumstances. In her case these worries were centred on the health of her mother (which, given her complete recovery, was excessive), her sons, who were in fact never seriously ill, and being abandoned by her husband, which was never a prospect at any stage in her marriage. Juliana had the motor tensions, worried preoccupation, and the feeling of being on edge and other autonomic over-reactions that characterise GAD. She also had the depressive symptoms that are commonly present in GAD. Depression also features in PD and agoraphobic avoidance and thus tying it to any one of those three was not possible. It was not until significant inroads were made into the agoraphobic fears and avoidance that the depression lifted (see below).

Turning to the agoraphobia component, Juliana's reactions showed an excellent fit to the clinical profile as outlined in DSM-III-R. She was restricted in her mobility, felt better when travelling with a trusted companion, and if she had to endure travelling beyond safety areas or alone, she did so under the pressure of strong avoidance inclinations. Juliana displayed the full array of agoraphobic fears (standing in a queue, travelling by bus, train or plane or, in general, whenever she believed that she could not reach safety with speed and dignity).

Juliana occasionally used alcohol and tranquillisers to excess, a problem which is by no means uncommon and can be found in one-third or more of those diagnosed as social phobics or agoraphobics (see Clarke & Saunders, 1988). It follows that the clinician should always have a high index of suspicion for the presence of these problems whether or not the patient makes explicit mention of them. Recent research (Norton et al., 1989) has distinguished between individuals who experience panic or agoraphobia first and then turn to alcohol to reduce anxiety as opposed to those whose drinking predated these disorders. It has been suggested those in the latter group have a greater proportion of alcohol disorders in their family of origin. The authors conclude that the different groups 'may require different treatment programs' (page 171) to reduce excessive alcohol intake. Fortunately, Juliana had no physiological dependence to or withdrawal reactions from either substance when alcohol or tranquillisers were unavailable. There was a suggestion of a psychological dependence on Valium, in her desire to take them with her while travelling even after she stopped using them altogether.

Treatment: conceptual issues

Theories of the aetiology and nature of agoraphobic and panic disorder influence the treatment that will be considered. Apart from psychoanalytic therapies pharmacological approaches have the longest history in the treatment of both. Of the great variety employed, the two most widely used pharmacotherapies are minor tranquillisers and antidepressant medications. The former lower muscle tension and have a central mood-altering effect. Onset is rapid with the effects noticed within 30 to 60 minutes. Psychologically their availability can be a source of relief even if not actually consumed, as indicated in Juliana's desire to have them within reach at all times. Antidepressants have a mixed record. There is some disagreement over their mode of action, with some arguing for direct anti-panic effects (Zitrin, 1981) and others insisting that they are of value mainly, or only, in those who experience significant levels of depression (Marks, 1987). On a more practical note, agoraphobics often complain of unpleasant side effects (Zitrin, 1981) and many discontinue as did Juliana, rather than put up with the side effects. Moreover, even when agoraphobic panickers can be persuaded to persist with the medication regimen the record shows that, upon discontinuation, after months of successful use relapse rates can approach 80 per cent (Sheehan, 1982).

The literature on the psychological treatment of panic anxiety is too small to permit any but the most tentative conclusions. There is, however, a measure of agreement that hyperventiliation and catastrophic interpretations of the physiological changes associated with it play an important role (Rapee & Murrell, 1988). The focus, therefore, has been on breathing control and cognitive restructuring therapies. Juliana benefited somewhat from both when used separately, but substantial improvement did not eventuate until the two were combined. This involved the introduction of a desensitisation-like procedure, which involved the deliberate escalation of the intensity of panicky reactions via faster and faster rates of breathing. Once these reactions were triggered, Juliana was coached in the use of adaptive cognitive strategies to reinterpret the significance of the reactions. Whether through controlled exposure to the physical sensations of panic, the challenge to catastrophic cognitions under these conditions (the evocation of and challenge to 'hot cognitions'), or both, Juliana did not overcome her panic disorder until the two — hyperventilation and cognitive restructuring — were brought together in this component of the treatment package.

More is known about the value of exposure for phobias — in the cognitive behavioural literature on agoraphobia it has become an indispensable tool in therapy. There is a broad consensus and an abundance of evidence that systematic exposure to phobic environments is a critical element in treatment. The data from scores of well-controlled experiments can be distilled into three recommendations: (1) to get the person to enter the phobic areas; (2) under the right conditions; and (3) to remain there until there is a drop in anxiety (Marshall, Gauthier & Gordon, 1979; Williams, Turner & Peer, 1985). The main differences among the varieties of exposure therapy concern the role of anxiety evocation and control during exposure. It seems critical that during exposure some degree of anxiety is aroused (Lang, 1977; Foa & Kozak, 1991), which could possibly explain why agoraphobics respond better to flooding forms of exposure where anxiety is accentuated than to systematic desensitisation where anxiety is kept to the lowest possible level. Some clinicians who favour flooding go so far as to claim that teaching patients methods of anxiety control is of no value whatsoever. Indeed, Marks (1987) suggested that during exposure agoraphobic patients might want to bring a book to read or knitting while waiting for the extinction of fear. This view seems to cast the patient into the role of the passive recipient and automatic habituator to environment stressors during exposure. In direct contrast, Williams, Turner and Peer (1985) and Williams and Zane (1989) have demonstrated therapist-assisted exposure to be superior to exposure alone. The clear advantage of guided treatment over standard stimulus exposure lead the authors to interpret their results as a 'call for recognising the role of the therapist in phobia treatment. The exposure concept that now heavily influences phobia treatment accords the therapist's role little beyond encouraging the agoraphobic to go and place herself in the presence of the phobic stimuli for a prolonged duration. The present findings show that active therapist assistance contributes significantly to outcomes' (Williams & Zane, 1989, page 244).

Finally, the role of expectancies deserves mention. Juliana's therapist spent considerable time in giving information dispelling misconceptions about agoraphobia and its treatment and attempting to generate positive expectancies for change. A powerful example of the role of expectancy and justification for this strategem was reported by Southworth and Kirsch (1988). Agoraphobics were given the same number of hours of exposure but those in the low-expectancy group were told the exposure was designed for assessment purposes only. The high-expectancy group were told that exposures constituted a powerful intervention. Post-test analysis showed the high-expectancy ('therapy') group significantly improved in comparison to the low-expectancy group (Kazdin & Wilcoxin, 1975). These results and others like them (see Clarke, 1991 for a review) call for a reappraisal of the processes of change in exposure and suggest a critical role for cognitive changes, as well as through extinction or habituation.

Treatment: applications and techniques

Initially Juliana stated her wishes in very general terms ('to feel better', 'be less anxious'). After discussion, she and the therapist refined the global statements into precise goals and specific interventions for particular problems. The idea of the short-term time-limited therapy appealed to her, as did the pragmatic, technique-focused approach to psychotherapy.

As a first step, the therapist gave an overview of what phobias are, the similarities and differences between monosymptomatic phobias and agoraphobia, and the special problem of panic. Because Juliana listed panic as the most pressing of her concerns apart from her wishes to be able to travel freely, panic, by mutual agreement, was selected as the first target for treatment. To start, the therapist asked her to keep a panic diary listing the time, place and duration of the attacks, plus a brief description of what she had been doing, thinking and feeling just prior to and following the attacks. Juliana was at first reluctant to comply believing as she did that these attacks were visited upon her from 'out of the blue'. With further requests in which the task was described as a kind of detective work, experimental and exploratory in nature, she cooperated fully in the exercise. To her surprise the diary did reveal clear patterns. Most of the panic attacks occurred when she was outside of the home, and the majority of those on days when she had slept poorly. Fewer than 10 per cent of the attacks took place in the home, and most of these were linked to excessive drinking, for example, after she had taken alcohol the night before to assuage her anxieties about an imminent and particularly worrying task. She was reluctant to speak openly about her drinking for fear of being labelled an alcoholic. It was explained to her that there was a qualitative and quantitative difference between physiologically dependent drinkers ('addicts') and the much larger number of non-dependent problem drinkers who use alcohol, as it were, as a kind of liquid tranquilliser. Juliana's score on the Severity of Alcohol Dependence questionnaire was a low 6 out of a possible 60. The low dependence score was consistent with her claim that she used alcohol as a means of anxiety control. However, as has been noted elsewhere (Clarke & Saunders, 1988), the days following excessive consumption of alcohol are typically marked by periods of sensitisation, the exacerbation of insecurities, more and more severe panics and great difficulties in travelling. When a perusal of the panic diary revealed the truth of these connections, Juliana stopped taking alcohol immediately.

Three related interventions were begun in the treatment program for panic. The first was informational. Juliana believed that one day she might 'go crazy' when panicking. To counter this belief the therapist read to Juliana excerpts of schizophrenic speech and thought descriptions of the disorder (from Neale & Oltmans, 1980). With great relief she acknowledged that never in her worst periods had her behaviour or thoughts held the slightest resemblance to the 'word salad' and impenetrable logic of a schizophrenic patient.

The second strand of treatment focused on the immediate connection between overbreathing or hyperventilation and feelings of impending panic. Juliana was unaware and unconvinced of this connection until, at the request of the therapist, she engaged in a five-minute period of hyperventilation. This produced the parasthesias ('tingling' in the extremities), fears of losing consciousness and vivid memories of previous panics. Once convinced of the major contribution to panic of overbreathing, it was pointed out that while hyperventilation could very quickly produce panic-like symptoms, continuous overbreathing (deep sighs, yawning) was a more likely, though less dramatic, contribution to panic. To cope with imminent or actual panic Juliana was advised to purchase a watch with a sweep hand and to ensure that the number of breathing cycles never exceeded 12 per minute (Rapee, 1985).

Lastly, the role of cognitions, internal sensations and belief in panic was outlined. The counselling, reduced to its essentials, was founded on the claim that physical arousal by itself did not constitute panic. Attention to sensations arising from physiological changes plus catastrophic interpretations of these completed the picture. Physiology plus cognition plus overbreathing were labelled as the 'terrible trio', and panic reaction depended upon all three occurring. Juliana was resistant to this explanation and her idea of 'causeless' panic persisted for a number of sessions. However, motivated by her desperate fear of panic, she practised the exercises. The cognitive corrections proved especially troublesome, because in the midst of her turmoil she either forgot them or got them hopelessly muddled. Cognitive disorganisation in panic is the rule rather than the exception in agoraphobic panickers (Clarke & Wardman, 1985) and Juliana's reactions were typical of the population. In order to lessen the reliance upon memory at such times a number of basic facts about panic were printed on a white index card which she carried in her purse and placed on her bed table at night.

This psychoeducational program and the associated practice won her confidence and she followed the suggestions given to her. Within four sessions some progress was noted but it was modest, with the reduction from an average of four panics per week to half that number. Beyond this, however, there was little change and a new 'panic exposure' component was added. This was based on the work of Lang (1977) and Foa and Kozak (1991) which maintains that in order to access the structure of fear memories it is necessary to evoke all of the dimensions of the fear complex including those linked to the physiological changes aroused in anxiety reactions.

To start, Juliana was asked to relax and sit with her eyes closed and then to increase her rate of breathing up to the point where she first became aware of the thoughts and feelings of approaching panic. Focusing first on the maladaptive thoughts was less effective for Juliana in triggering physiological arousal because she reported that the content of the thoughts was 'intellectual' and not affective in impact. Increasing the rate of breathing was preferable, beginning as it did with the generation of affectively laden thoughts ('hot cognitions'). When she signalled their presence by raising her left index finger, the therapist intervened forcibly to: (a) have her exert control over her breathing to the prearranged level; and (b) to take out her index cards and read them aloud. Later she was asked to read them subvocally and, finally, to memorise the contents and dispense with the cards. When she could reliably bring her anxiety levels to 20 out of 100 on the fear thermometer, the hyperventilation rates were escalated and prolonged. She was urged to produce even more catastrophic thoughts during these periods. This desensitisation-like procedure reduced the frequency of panics to an average of one per month. Interestingly, the cognitive restructuring techniques (see below) did not supplant the catastrophic interpretations. Afterwards, when she experienced one of her rare panics, in the first instant or two she would be captured by the familiar catastrophic cognitions until the use of corrective breathing and adaptive counter panic cognitions limited their intensity and duration to a brief moment or two.

This finding raises the possibility that 'cognitive restructuring' may be more accurately conceived as 'cognitive competition' training: maladaptive catastrophic interpretations were not supplanted/restructured in a literal sense of the word. Instead, her reports, typical of so many, were that she now began to engage in a dialogue of conflict in which she would alternate between negative cognitions and corrective counter reactions. With practice the relative strengths of the two altered in favour of the latter.

The next stage in the general plan was to put into place a combined exposure therapy and cognitive restructuring program directed at her avoidance reactions and her negative interpretations of travelling and of being alone. The fundamental premise common to all the varieties of cognitive-behavioural therapy (CBT) is that it is often the meaning that we attach to the feared situations of our lives and not the objective events themselves which lie behind so much of our unhappiness. In its conventional form, the argument states that the sentences we say to ourselves are the proximal causes of anxiety, anger or depression depending on the content of these interpretations and utterances. There was indeed some validity to these claims in Juliana's case.Without prompting, she volunteered a number of her habitual monologues ('I think I am going to faint' in response to light-headedness caused by overbreathing; 'If I have to leave the shopping queue and all of my goods in the basket and run out of here, people will think that I am crazy'). The aim of the therapy was to modify the unpleasant affect by altering the pattern of thinking that is believed to be responsible for that stress. Juliana accepted the logic of the CBT, but had little success in identifying anxiety-related thoughts — apart, that is, from the dramatic and terrifying cognitions which occurred during panic and which overshadowed all other thoughts. In Juliana's case, however, it was her unshakable conviction that being in a phobic situation itself lead directly to the anxiety without any conscious mediation of maladaptive beliefs and self-statements. When the therapist put the question to her 'But what were you thinking just before you began to be frightened?' her reply was 'Nothing that I can remember'. Homework assignments unearthed no internal sentences or 'automatic thoughts'. The clinical point to be made here is that maladaptive cognitions may be the cause of psychological misery and behavioural problems. Some of these cognitions are in full awareness and take the form of imagery and internal sentences. Others appear to operate outside of or below the level of awareness. Insisting to the client that they *must* have been entertaining negative thoughts can, in compliant individuals, produce 'causal' cognitions supplied to please the therapist's demand for such material.

As noted, in many instances Juliana's experience was that the fear came first and the fear-laden thoughts afterwards. In these instances the negative self-statements would then come to awareness and she could counter these with adaptive inner speech ('its OK, I can go a little further'; 'there is nothing to fear and my distress is just of the flight/fight system working and it will pass shortly'). These cognitions seemed to act as an inhibitory break on the phobic reactions. It is worth noting in this regard that in the first weeks of exposure therapy, Juliana's estimation of the likelihood of panic just prior to departure was in the vicinity of 50 per cent, which at that time represented a significant overestimation. However, the estimations of the anxiety she was likely to experience outside of the zone of safety in the area around her house and immediate neighbourhood were in proportion to the distance travelled, likely delays at her destination, and the availability of support from her companion (therapist or husband). In her words, distant places were feared not because panic might ensue, but because such places were a long distance from home base and safety and the further the distance the greater the predicted and experienced anxiety. Likewise, when the therapist accompanied her on these trips it was his proximity that reassured her. Once more, fear of panic and being without assistance did not, in the great majority of cases, cause Juliana to worry about being separated from her therapist. Again and again it emerged from her report that she feared places far from home, because the places *were* far from home, or because the therapist was too far away.

Prior to initiating the exposure component of the treatment program, Juliana and her therapist agreed that exposure alone had accomplished little in the past. She had managed, when absolutely necessary, to carry through the journeys required of her, (for example, to do the shopping, to visit a sick relative or husband, to get her child to the emergency ward of a distant hospital) but these efforts took a tremendous toll and left her no better able next time to cope with travel or separation. When the idea of a non-pharmacologic anxiety control strategy was proposed, she was sceptical at first. However, she agreed and she was reinforced by the therapist's reminders that the tranquillisers gave only temporary relief and that she complained of being tense and anxious at home with others. One of the reasons for Juliana's lack of enthusiasm was the failure to benefit from relaxation therapy tapes she had used a few years earlier. She used the tapes only once or twice, the usual fate for tape-only relaxation therapy (Borkovec & Sides, 1979). The inefficacy of the tapes further biased her against non-medical interventions for the control of tension and anxiety. Once she relented, she was asked which of the many standard relaxation techniques did she feel was best suited for her. It was explained that some techniques work on the principal of establishing a calming mental imagery with the assumption that this will bring about physical relaxation. Others begin with physical relaxation, sometimes called deep muscle-relaxation training, relying on mental calm to follow.

Juliana expressed a preference for the mental exercises first with deep-muscle relaxation to be used perhaps at some later time. She was drawn to the suggestion of mental control over tension because of her unrewarding efforts with relaxation tapes. Her therapist pointed out that she had practised with these too seldom to make a difference but she persisted in her preference for imagery-based relaxation. With the assistance of the therapist she suggested a number of relaxation scenes. The effects of this training were immediate and positive. Juliana's respiration rate declined from 14–15 cycles per second to an average of 6–8 within five minutes, while her pulse rate dropped from 75–80 per minute to 60–63 within ten minutes. By the time the 20-minute session had finished, her self-report rating on the tension scale was zero and 20 on the anxiety scale, down from 80 and 90 respectively. From the speed and depth of her response, it was apparent that Juliana had great skills at mental imagery and appeared deeply hypnotised, though no formal hypnotic induction was attempted because of her fears of hypnosis. However, after three weeks' daily practice, when the exposure trials began (see below) and she became anxious, she was unable to make effective use of the techniques. The most that she could manage was to call to mind brief fragments of the calming imagery and her sense of anxiety control was minimal and sporadic. This forced a change of strategy and deep-muscle relaxation was begun in line with the techniques and conceptualisation developed by Ost (1987) — applied relaxation training (ART). The client sits in a comfortable position with eyes closed and is asked to produce and release tension in different muscle groups around the body. Typically, maximal degrees of tension levels are requested for up to 10 seconds and then instruction is given for either gradual reduction or an all-at-one release to level zero. An important issue to be addressed in relaxation therapy is the purpose to be achieved — ostensibly to become relaxed while performing the technique. Juliana's therapist endorsed this goal but pointed out a second and more important one, which is to become aware of muscle tension in its earliest stages and to apply the counter-tension procedures at that point before it progresses to less manageable levels. He also informed her of the findings from the experimental literature that 'unshielded' exposure to stressful or anxiety-provoking environments does not in itself automatically bestow gains in the form of anxiety reduction — a fact that Juliana had long since discovered for herself. Coping techniques, relaxation among them, can accelerate the benefits of exposure therapy and limit the risks of sensitisation (Williams & Zane, 1989). Since Juliana had a poor to nonexistent awareness of the early signs of tension her therapist advised that training begin at the levels typically experienced and/or when she did tend to become aware of tension distress. The program, therefore, was designed to maximise transfer of training. The rules across all categories of skill training are that transfer of training is always greatest when training and test environments and conditions are as similar as possible. Consequently, since Juliana never reported acute tension level in the 90–100 range but rather more often chronic tension levels ranging from 40 to 70 on the tension scale, the focus of training to begin with was in the region of intermediate tension levels.

The use of intermediate levels for full and immediate versus gradual release of tension proved to be satisfactory, however stage two of the ART program was not effective — nor has it been for most of the agoraphobics seen in our clinic. The aim in stage two of ART is to omit the tension-induction component, with the only request being that the patient breathe calmly and relax each muscle group starting from the top of the head and moving down to the tip of the toes. Juliana complained that the releasing phase, without at least some tension induction, was so difficult that attempts to do this were counter-productive and lead to increases in tension. The therapist therefore made an adjustment to the ART procedure, which was to generate low perceptible levels of tension and then to relax these. With these changes to ART, Juliana mastered the technique within six sessions. In the final stages of ART cue-control relaxation was added (Ost, 1987). This involved having Juliana say the word 'tense' as she increased muscle tension, always when inhaling, and say the word 'relax' when releasing tension as she exhaled. This helped to give her cognitive control and awareness of muscle tension. Within a few sessions she found that when she began to get physically tense she would actually hear the word 'tense' in her mind. This acted as a 'bell ringer' and a reminder to begin the inhibitory work of muscle tension-relaxation. In the final stages of ART, she was taught differential relaxation, in which she was asked to distinguish the muscle tension levels required for the proficient completion of a routine activity such as writing a letter or driving a car, and the concurrent production of excessive tensions in other parts of the body not required. By this time Juliana had achieved control over panic and perfected the relaxation techniques. This set the stage for the final phase, exposure therapy.

Strictly speaking, exposure was not entirely new to Juliana. Although she was described as 'housebound' she did get out on almost a daily basis. In addition to her desperate forays to the nearby shopping mall she had, on her own, unwittingly been practising exposure on an informal basis (for example, driving daily, brief walks with her sons or her young niece who came to visit with Juliana whenever her sister-in-law needed child-minding assistance for the day).

The principles of exposure therapy were presented along with answers to the question that agoraphobics invariably ask: 'If getting out is the means by which phobias are eliminated, why in all this time haven't I "cured" myself?' The therapist's answer was that in fact she had done so, to some degree. Had she never gone out the evidence, from those who are truly housebound, is that her agoraphobia would be considerably worse in all respects. The therapist also pointed out that there were a number of crucial differences between the 'then', prior to therapy, and the 'now', on the threshold of exposure therapy:

1. In the past any travelling/separation anxiety was interpreted as threatening and dangerous; now she could challenge counter-productive interpretations with cognitive coping techniques.
2. In place of her former reliance upon sheer 'willpower' and a 'do-or-die' attitude, she now was equipped with tension and anxiety management skills to counter escape-avoidance reactions.
3. Her travel efforts, such as they were, had been haphazard in response to the demands of the moment instead of the 'step-at-a-time' of exposure therapy.
4. She had never remained outside, and alone, for a period long enough for her anxiety to decline while in the shopping mall or wherever. Thus, she 'suffered' a reduction in anxiety while fleeing the phobic situation which thereby strengthened the association between escape and anxiety relief.
5. Her attributions for 'success' on a given venture had been along the lines of 'Thank God I was lucky enough to survive this time' instead of to the systematic execution of a specific plan based on the acquisition of effective coping techniques.

After 'rationale therapy' (Kirsch, 1990) a hierarchy of feared tasks was constructed around the two themes of travel distance and degree of therapist support (or of her husband who also heard the rationale for exposure therapy and eagerly agreed to accompany her on daily sessions whenever possible). In each session there were two systematic manipulations. The first was of distance from home and the second the degree of separation from the support companion. Distance alone was actually not as important as proximity to home and perceived ease of access to escape routes. Thus, going from her car to the shopping mall was rated 40 on a 'fear thermometer (0-100)' if the task for the day was to enter an uncrowded shop where she could choose an item, pay quickly and leave. A crowded shop, though closer to the car, could get a rating of 70–80. Or, later, when she went to cinemas, sitting on the aisle in the middle of the theatre was rated as less difficult than sitting in the middle of a crowded row nearer to the exit. Second, in all of these situations, ratings were lower when accompanied. The general strategy, then, was for each session to extend the distance, reduce escape accessibility, and reduce personal contact with the other. Before leaving the house the therapist would remind Juliana of the fundamental principles and specific techniques of cognitive corrections and breathing control. Immediately before departing Juliana was asked to estimate the likelihood of panic, and on a graph of the 'fear thermometer' the amount of anxiety anticipated at five-minute intervals. While on the trip, she would indicate on the same graph the actual anxiety experienced.

For the first three weeks estimated levels always exceeded the actual 'fear thermometer' ratings, but by smaller amounts each week. By the fourth week Juliana was no longer 'overshooting' in her pre-trip estimates. Panic probabilities remained essentially unchanged at 30 per cent. Across this period, anxiety ratings declined as did her pulse rate, but neither significantly. What was especially puzzling was the failure to show transfer of the within-session changes on the same or similar tasks. The answer to the problem was traced to the timing and the amount of tranquilliser used. A few minutes before leaving she would take a substantial amount. The action of the drugs functioned to isolate her pharmacologically from the full range of anxiety experiences. While this left her in relative comfort during the trip it gave her only a restricted opportunity to experience and master higher intensities of anxiety (Lang, 1977; Foa & Kozak, 1991). More specifically, the use of high doses of tranquilliser inclined her to attribute her successes to the drug. When the problem was explained to her she agreed, reluctantly at first, to limit her intake to one 5 mg tablet taken no sooner than 20 minutes before leaving for an exposure trial. Following this change she reported a reduction in her motivation to continue with exposure therapy. Interestingly, the effect of reducing her intake of tranquillisers was greater on 'anticipatory' than it was on 'impact' anxiety as reflected in a return to overestimations of expected, as compared to experienced, anxiety. Previous improvements in the range of her behaviour were maintained and within a further two weeks she began to show more 'matching' and less 'overshooting'. Progress was steady with only the occasional setback. By week 15 Juliana was ready to discontinue weekly therapy for monthly 'booster' visits. Shortly afterwards she had a relapse when she had to take antibiotics after infecting her finger. This immediately intensified her separation and travel anxieties, panic attacks doubled, and depression, as measured by the Beck Depression Inventory, climbed from a low-to-moderate score of seven to a much higher one of 18. We have observed this pattern before, but there is no obvious psychological or physiological explanation to account for the adverse effects of antibiotics. Fortunately when the antibiotics washed out of the system the gains achieved earlier in treatment were re-established.

Today, Juliana is virtually free of her agoraphobia. She can travel by car or on foot, and has never again scored highly on a depression inventory. She has a panic attack once every few months usually when she is fatigued or allows her intake of alcohol to exceed two drinks per day. When the panics occur she is prone to the catastrophic thoughts but she reports that by breathing control and cognitive techniques she can calm herself quickly. The one limitation which remains, although mild, is a continued dependence upon her husband. She is able to be alone and at ease at home and to travel unaided, but she still prefers to have her husband nearby. With this limitation in mind, the significant drop in fear levels and panic frequency and the total discontinuation of Valium, and depression scores well within the normal range testify to the clinical value of these gains. At present she is receiving booster sessions once every three months and counselling on how to deal with setbacks and lapses. Her marital adjustment, as measured by a marriage adjustment scale which was low but within the normal range at the start of therapy, at the conclusion revealed much higher levels of satisfaction and no more than the usual levels of marital dysfunction.

Aetiological considerations

In this case study, the two most salient and disturbing problems in the clinical picture were panic disorder and agoraphobic avoidance. Until recently, they were considered two distinct but overlapping problems each with its own aetiology and mechanisms, and each susceptible to quite different modes of treatment. For example, in the *Diagnostic and Statistical Manual of Mental Disorders,* third edition (DSM-III) (American Psychiatric Association, 1980), PD was defined in much the same way as it is today (with some minor exceptions, one being that in DSM-III-R four attacks are required within four weeks for the diagnosis of a PD whereas in the earlier edition it was three attacks within a three-week period) and agoraphobia was included under the separate category of phobia. Then, the criterion definition for a phobic was 'the persistent irrational fear ... (which) the person recognises is excessive or unreasonable' (DSM-III-R, 1987, pages 243–4). Quite clearly the critical criterion in the definition of phobia is unaltered. What has changed in DSM-III-R and the soon-to-be-published DSM-IV is the loss of status of agoraphobia as a problem category in its own right. It is now grouped with PD as a subvariety of that disorder. In other words, agoraphobia is to be seen as a more severe version of PD. Within this new perspective, agoraphobic avoidance is no more than a precautionary reluctance by PD individuals to place themselves in a position where they might panic: 'Agoraphobia: Fear of being in places or situations from which escape might be difficult (or embarrassing) or in which help is not available in the event of a panic attack ... As a result of this fear, the person either restricts travel or needs a companion when away from home' (DSM-III-R, pages 238-9).

In effect DSM-III-R has, by this change in definition and conceptualisation, taken the phobia out of agoraphobia. In this new perspective, once panic strikes the person does not recognise that his or her fear is 'excessive and unreasonable'.

There is a certain appeal in this new formulation. 'Occam's razor' and the Law of Parsimony require scientists to use no more than the necessary number of concepts to capture a range of phenomena. Empirically it is established that panic attacks always precede agoraphobia. (As we have seen, estimates of the quantitative linkage and progression range from 85 per cent to 100 per cent of cases.) By contrast, there are very few findings that agoraphobic avoidance precedes panic reactions (Clum & Knowles, 1991). Whether these findings allow us to conclude that 'if agoraphobia always or usually follows the development of panic attacks then it is a more severe variant of panic disorder' (Clum & Knowles, page 297) is open to question.

Starting with the aetiology of PD it, like agoraphobia, has a sudden onset, usually in the mid-twenties, but unlike agoraphobia it is equally common in males and females. There is evidence for a genetic risk factor in PD (Torgersen, 1983) but the exact processes by which this predisposition is activated are not known. Panic reactions can be triggered by a wide range of provoking agents including overbreathing, infusions of sodium lactate-concentrated inhalations of carbon dioxide, and caffeine challenges (Clarke, 1991). Panics have also been linked to periods of stressful life events (de Loof et al., 1989). They are known to be affected by cognitive misinterpretations of what are objectively non-threatening physiological changes (Rapee, Mattick & Murrell, 1986) and there is evidence from the present case study and other reports (Rapee, 1985) that cognitive-behavioural treatments show promise in the alleviation of PD.

Whatever the mechanisms (and a diathesis-stress model (Meehl, 1962) may well be the most fruitful approach to the study of panic), the question remains: Why do some people with panic later become agoraphobic avoiders, while others do not? We can look to the particulars of Juliana's case for suggestions, if not answers, to this vexed and vexing question.

A number of proposals have been advanced to answer the question of what, apart from the symptoms themselves, distinguishes PD from agoraphobic avoidance. An obvious candidate is the severity of the panic. Do avoiders experience more severe panic attacks? The answer is that the two groups do not differ on this variable (Fleming & Faulk, 1989; Adler et al., 1989), nor does the number of symptoms distinguish the two groups (Rapee & Murrell, 1988). One study cited in support of the relationship between panic severity and avoidance was conducted by Noyes et al. (1987). This report carried the provocative title which expresses precisely the question addressed in this chapter: 'Is agoraphobia a variant of panic disorder or a separate illness?' Noyes et al. concluded in favour of the former. In their study a significant number of PDA patients reported more symptoms than PD (alone) patients. But the symptoms referred to were those problems which interfered with everyday activities. The difficulty with this line of reasoning is that it tends towards circularity, in that patients were more likely to report interference of daily activities involving travelling (for example, shopping). Other variables that have failed to distinguish PD patients from those with agoraphobia are age of onset (Thyer et al., 1985), frequency of attacks (Mavissakalian, 1988), duration (Noyes et al., 1987), location of first attack (Rapee & Murrell, 1988) or scores on the widely-used Anxiety Sensitivity Index (ASI) (Reiss et al., 1986). On the other side, it has been reported that outcome expectancies were more negative in avoiders than in those with PD alone. Noyes et al. (1987) looked at fears of dying or going crazy which did distinguish statistically between those who did and those who did not avoid following panic. Nevertheless, of those with no avoidance, 65 per cent did report catastrophic cognitions compared with 84 per cent with limited avoidance and 93 per cent of those with extensive avoidance. These data portray an association between catastrophic thinking and avoidance. However, it should be noted that two out of every three PD patients without avoidance had the same number and severity of catastrophic cognitions, and between eight and nine out of every 10 with limited avoidance did so as well.

The forgoing review leaves little doubt as to the connection between panic and the onset of agoraphobia. At the same time, it gives no warrant for contentions that 'If agoraphobia always … follows the development of panic attacks then it (agoraphobia) is (simply) a more severe variant of panic disorder' (Clum & Knowles, 1991, page 297). Sequence is not causality nor does it enlighten us as to the processes of the two disorders and their interaction. Few would argue that the expectations of panics and fear of fear contribute to agoraphobic avoidance. In keeping with the 'fear of fear' theory of avoidance, avoidance was more pervasive when expectancies of panic were higher, regardless of the validity of these estimates. What is not easily reconciled with the DSM-III-R position and those of its supporters is the high correlation between Juliana's ratings of fear of travelling and distance from home or trusted companion whether panic expectancies were high or low.

Early in therapy Juliana's anxiety responses were a composite of panic and phobic fears with overlap in their psychophysiological expression. Caution is thus required lest the distinction between phobic and panic anxiety be pressed too far. Nevertheless, a study of her self-reports suggests that the differences between the two is more than just an inquiry into terminology. In answer to the question given during the exposure exercise 'How reasonable is the anxiety you are experiencing now?', the mean score for the first 16 occasions was seven out of ten (zero indicated 'completely unreasonable' and ten 'completely reasonable'). Over the last 16 measurement occasions when panic estimates and frequencies were significantly lower, the mean score was 2.7 on this scale. She made it clear that as she was confident that panic was very unlikely it was 'silly' to be fearful while in a cinema or walking by herself. Juliana likened these 'unjustified' reactions to her vigorous resistance in the past to being left at home alone. She recalled a number of episodes when she refused her husband's request to take both boys away for a weekend trip. She would insist on having at least one present even when both were under the age of five. She had no difficulty in appreciating the illogic of her request. 'It was just so silly' she remarked to her therapist. 'Had I gone into a panic attack, what help could a child be? I knew that but still I had to have someone in the family with me.' Also consistent with DSM-III-R criterion of a phobic response, and by her own estimate, too, was the sharp and immediate increase in anxiety when she walked around the corner and out of sight of her house. This example is especially telling because she could walk nearly twice the distance from home in the other direction because it was within visual access. The final strand of evidence that the travel and separation distress has a phobic quality to it are their positive responses to exposure therapy in Juliana's case, and as reported in the experimental literature (Foa & Kozak, 1991). Despite the forgoing, in the present case it is not possible to assert that exposure was the therapy of choice or that it alone had an impact on the phobias. A range of interventions from expectation manipulations, cognitive restructuring and rational self-talk together with ART was combined with exposure so that the effects of any one cannot be disentangled from the others. Moreover, it is safe to suppose that CBT did make an important contribution to therapy. Early assessments of her cognitive activities during exposure revealed that Juliana did engage in negative self-talk associated with what Beck would term a negative 'set' or 'schema' (Beck, Emery & Goldberg, 1985). Following the introduction of CBT Juliana came to recognise the role of cognitive distortions and 'catastrophising' in the exacerbation of her travel, separation and, especially, panic reactions. Finally, there is convincing evidence that CBT, when added to exposure, significantly diminishes phobic anxiety (Clarke, 1991). Moreover, it should be recognised that exposure is a procedure and not a statement of the mechanisms or processes of change, and these remain to be elucidated. However, the relative inefficacy of CBT alone for phobias (Bandura, 1977; Ellis, 1977), compared with the apparent superiority of CBT for non-phobic social-performance anxieties (Emmelkamp, 1979) and the acknowledged power of exposure therapy for phobias is consistent with the details from the present case and suggest the presence of a phobic disorder in PDA clients.

If agoraphobia is seen as a separate disorder and not as a variant of panic disorder, how does it originate and what are the core processes in its development? The two most influential theories of phobias have come from psychoanalytic and learning theories. There are a variety of psychoanalytic theories and no one explanation of Juliana's anxieties would be forthcoming from all. Most, though, would view her difficulties with travel and separation as surface manisfestations of repressed urges and conflicts.The presenting anxieties would be seen as symptoms and not as the real, underlying disorder, which would be interpreted as a conflict between forbidden psychosexual urges and ego defenses against their undisguised presentation. Freud (1959) taught that the agoraphobic's desire to stay near home and to be with others is a form of (unconsciously arranged) protection against powerful impulses towards promiscuous behaviour — as indeed Juliana's first therapist concluded. It could be argued further that these impulses originated because of Juliana's strong hostilities towards her mother, who was a rival with her for her father's affections. Or perhaps Juliana was searching for the father whose divorce from her mother took him out of Juliana's life at too early an age. By any of these accounts direct attempts to modify the symptoms, as in CBT and exposure therapy, without due consideration of the underlying repressed conflicts should lead to symptom substitution. Against this prediction was the lack of any evidence for the appearance of the presenting problems. If anything, there was improvement in untreated areas (for example, her depression) as well as significant diminutions in panic, separation and travel anxiety.

Until the coming of the 'cognitive revolution' of the last decade the major opposition to psychodynamic theory came from learning theory. The learning or conditioning models have all descended by one path or another from the Pavlovian theory of classical conditioning. The paradigmatic case is that of 'Little Albert', the 11-month-old boy made fearful of a tame rat whose introduction was paired with a loud, aversive noise (Watson & Rayner, 1920).

More recently the conditioning-associative model has been expanded to include acquisition of phobias via direct observation or the symbolic pairing of the phobic-conditioned stimulus with a traumatic unconditioned stimulus. The learning models were designed to explain the origins of circumscribed phobias with the tacit assumption that the differences amongst phobias are those of content only. This assumption fails to account for the differences in age of onset, sex distributions and associated symptomatology that distinguish so-called 'simple' from 'complex' or 'clinical' phobias (Emmelkamp, 1979; Marks, 1987). It is not clear what any of the learning-associative models would say about the separation phobias of agoraphobia. If one views panic as analagous to an aversive internal unconditioned stimulus then one might expect the particular locale of its occurrence, and others like it, to become by association conditioned aversive stimuli. There was in fact some evidence for this in Juliana's strong avoidance tendencies towards places which had been associated with especially severe panics. But what is not explained by any of the learning theories was the presence of strong fears where panics have never occurred. As to the modelling accounts, when she was a young girl Juliana remembers being aware of her mother's apprehensions about either her or Juliana going out alone. Her mother's worries did not diminish, even when Juliana was well into her teenage years. If these recollections are correct her mother may well have had a subclinical form of agoraphobia.

Despite its plausibility the conditioning-associative model in all of its forms has been subjected to a number of serious criticisms. One is, that when asked, many adult phobics recall any traumatic events which brought the phobia into being (Clarke & Jackson, 1983). Another is they fail to accord any special significance to the evolutionary significance of phobic events as do the European ethologists. Bowlby (1975, page 171) sums up the views of the ethological position in his remarks that:

> 'In the past there have been theorists who have postulated that ... all stimuli derive their fear-arousing properties from becoming associated with pain. Not only is the theory false, but a moment's thought shows it to be hardly plausible. As a natural clue to potential danger, the experience of physical pain is in a special category. The clues to which attention has so far been directed are distal clues perceived by the distance receptors ... By giving warnings while potential danger is still more or less remote, these clues enable an animal or man to take precautions in good time. By contrast ... to await events until pain is experienced may well be to wait too long. Physical pain has the status of last ditch.'

Bowlby is saying, with Lorenz (1969) and Tinbergen (1951), that to the eyes of the intellectual city dweller (and the psychotherapist), phobic reactions 'may seem irrational and childish, and may even be attributed to pathological fancy (but) to the eye of the biologist, a deeper wisdom is apparent. Examination shows, indeed, that, so far from being irrational or foolhardy, to rely initially on the naturally occurring clues to danger and safety is to rely on a system that has been both sensible and efficient over millions of years' (Bowlby, 1975, page 168). Why are we not all phobically anxious to these cues? If it is supposed that phobias are a form of survival instinct why do they not emerge at birth and persist across a lifetime? In considering the question, Clarke and Jackson (1983) offered a reply distilled from the writing of Hebb (1946) and Bowlby (1975) and the ethologists. They state that some phobias are apparent at birth but most do not make their appearance until months or years later. It is no answer to cite 'maturational processes', but in our ignorance about the specific mechanisms, all that can be said is that given the time required for the acquisition of the normal background experiences, most members of the species will show these reactions on first encounter (Hebb, 1946). Regarding the elimination or alleviation of phobic anxieties, this poses no problem so long as we are careful not to accept the invalid dichotomy of 'innate' and 'learned' reactions.

Environmental manipulations can potentiate or subdue phobic reactions. The latter, of course, is the clinical goal. In the previous sentence we chose the word 'subdue' instead of 'extinguish' or 'extirpate' or any other word implying the total and final elimination following their 'extinction'. This reservation is in line with the core notions in Seligman's conditioning theory (1970) as well as the 'instinct' position of Bowlby and the European ethologists. Phobic anxiety is 'most clearly apparent during childhood and old age, sometimes disguised or discounted during adult life [but] these biases nevertheless remain with us. From the cradle to the grave they are an intrinsic part of human nature' (Bowlby, 1975, page 168).

One well-documented example of the ontogeny of fear in children without the requirement of prior aversive training is the universal separation distress (from familiar places and caretakers) displayed in humans, apes and monkeys once they achieve the powers of self-locomotion (Bowlby, 1975). From the evolutionary-adaptive perspective these reactions make good sense. When infants become mobile, yet are too weak to cope with the dangers they may encounter or are without the experience and cognitive development to elaborate realistic estimates of threat, they are at great risk. The tendency for separation-attachment reactions is supposed to function to instil caution in the face of a situation (for example, being alone in an unknown locale) where 'learning by experience' can lead to injury or death. What, though, does this tell us about agoraphobia? As noted, it has an onset time in the early twenties long after separation reactions have abated even in those who develop agoraphobia. There is, as yet, no evidence of a 'pre-agoraphobic personality' in the late adolescent years just prior to the onset of panic which progresses to full-blown agoraphobia. What has been suggested is that childhood separation traumas (for example, death of a parent, threats of abandonment) constitute a diathesis or underlying vulnerability that is dishabituated by panic attacks (Clarke & Wardman, 1985; Bowlby, 1975). This hypothesis was examined by Thyer, Himle and Fischer (1988) who found no difference in the frequencies of separation trauma between avoiders and non-avoiders. Their methodology was criticised by Friedman and Paradis (1991) for adopting a too restrictive definition of separation. By including separation stressors other than death (for example, extended hospitalisation of a significant caretaker) they were able to find support for the separation anxiety hypothesis.

Though framed in a different terminology from that employed by the ethologists, Donald Klein (1981) has proposed an account of agoraphobia which can be recast into an adaptive evolutionary framework. Klein's contention is that agoraphobics are especially sensitive to separation anxiety. Separation threats in adulthood (somehow) lead to panic reactions which in turn sensitise these unfortunate individuals to become incapacitated by anticipatory fears (of further panics and separation).

A third perspective, Rachman's (1984) safety-signal hypothesis, similarly emphasises the agoraphobic's desire for safety. This safety can be accomplished by keeping ready access to a safety-figure or place (for example, one's home or automobile). As in Klein's account, the aim of the agoraphobic is to do whatever is necessary to preserve at least a minimum sense of safety. The greater the spatial or temporal separation from perceived safety signals the greater the amount of agoraphobic distress.

If Juliana's memories of an over-protective mother were not coloured by experiences since the start of her panics and agoraphobia, they fit well to the sensitisation-separation phobia hypothesised in the models of Klein, Friedman and others. The major limitation is that there is too little predictive power in any of these models. Second, there are many children who suffer grievous losses in childhood without becoming panickers or avoiders. It may be the case that these and a physiological vulnerability together set the individual on a course for agoraphobia after the onset of panic attacks. It is not necessary to assume that the diathesis must be exclusively of a physiochemical nature. Beck, Emery and Goldberg (1985) have demonstrated that agoraphobics are prone to cognitive distortions maintained by overactive danger schema. The existence of a complex diathesis-stress disorder gains support from findings that cognitive restructuring therapies alone have not proved as effective as exposure therapy with agoraphobia but the two together appear to be superior to either alone (Clarke, 1991).

To conclude this section on aetiology, and the chapter, the argument expressed in the two major positions, that agoraphobia is simply a severe form of PD, and its opposite, that the two are distinct forms of psychopathology, remains to be settled. One fact is clear: the role of panic in agoraphobia is of undoubted importance, and this understanding constitutes a major advance from earlier times when agoraphobia was considered as separate from panic. The place of panic can be considered from three perspectives in the aetiology, maintenance and treatment of agoraphobia. As to aetiology, the evidence is unequivocal: panic is highly correlated with the development of agoraphobia and associated avoidance tendencies (though it should be noted that not all people with panic disorders become agoraphobic; put another way, without panic there is little chance of the development of agoraphobia, but some panickers never develop agoraphobia). Once experienced, the fear of panic is a powerful motivation for avoidance. And, ideally, the treatment of panic should be an integral part of the earliest stage of the intervention program. (However, there are reports of successful outcomes where panic concerns are not the focus of treatment (see Marshall, Gauthier & Gordon, 1979).) These findings give support to the argument for the subordination of agoraphobia in theory and in therapy to the understanding of the causes and treatment of panic. However, the seeming non-rational nature of the attachment reactions reported by Juliana of the kind long noted in the clinical literature (for example, Marks, 1969) and the similarity of the exposure treatments and their efficacy for other phobias and agoraphobia, question the DSM-III-R (American Psychiatric Association, 1987) and similar positions which render agoraphobia as a cognitive disorder. The position advanced in this chapter is that it is not helpful to ask whether agoraphobia is a phobia or a cognitive disorder (for example, expectancies of panic anticipated, a fear of fear). Rather it should be asked: in what way do cognitive processes operate in panic disorders and in agoraphobia? The question is still debated. Nevertheless, from the experimental evidence cited earlier and from the details of Juliana's case history, it appears premature at this stage to dismiss the phobia from agoraphobia.

James T. Quinn
Liverpool Hospital

12 Multiple personality disorder

Compared with the other disorders discussed in this book, multiple personality disorder (MPD) is relatively rare. The cases that have been identified number in the thousands rather than the millions as for schizophrenia (Chodoff, 1987). Despite this, MPD has captured public and professional attention. Books, films and television shows have all been made about this astonishing condition. There seems to be something fascinating and captivating about MPD.

Until recently, it has been difficult to study MPD because too few subjects were available. This seems to be changing, however (see Coons, Bowman & Milstein, 1988; Putnam et al., 1986, for example). We are now beginning to accumulate a reasonable body of knowledge about this most enigmatic of disorders. Yet, just about every aspect of MPD remains controversial (Fahy, 1988). This chapter begins with a detailed case study of a woman with MPD. This is followed by a discussion of some of MPD's cardinal features and describes some treatment options. The final section reviews recent controversies about the origin, nature and treatment of this peculiar condition.

Case study

John Barraclough, the Dean of Health Sciences in a large metropolitan university, was facing a distasteful task. He was about to interview Jackie, a senior academic who was creating a problem for one of the departments in his faculty. Jackie, a senior lecturer in social work, had joined the university seven years before and had been promoted from tutor to senior lecturer within that period. During that time, she performed well, published in respected journals, and became a popular teacher among students. However, in the last year or so, John had been hearing disturbing rumours in academic circles about Jackie's drinking and, more recently, there had been complaints from students that she had not turned up for lectures. She was a member of the faculty liaison committee which John chaired and on three occasions she had not turned up for meetings, even though she was secretary of the committee. John had made some discreet inquiries among the staff of her department and discovered that there had been a number of unexplained absences lasting a few days to a week when Jackie simply disappeared.

The problem was made more delicate because Jackie's husband was also an academic. He was professor of anthropology and a senior academic politician within the university. He had caused some raised eyebrows recently by conducting a fairly public affair with a young, attractive Ph.D. student. John was aware that Jackie had been having a lesbian relationship with a senior lecturer in nursing, also in John's faculty. There had been two unpleasant scenes between Jackie and her husband on campus to the embarrassment of other university staff.

Despite his background in clinical psychology, John was unsure how he should deal with this problem. After appropriate preliminaries, he indicated to Jackie that there had been student and staff complaints about her absences and asked for an explanation. Jackie apologised for the absences but offered no real explanation, stating that she had been working very hard and had recently undertaken extra duties teaching a course on human sexuality to nursing students. She was also deeply involved, with other colleagues, in a research project into the sexual abuse experienced by some students in the faculty. Jackie explained that young female students who remembered unpleasant childhood experiences as a response to filling out the questionnaires in the sex abuse survey were coming to the student counselling service for assistance. Because of her social work background, the student counselling service had co-opted her to counsel some of the more difficult cases. This only added to Jackie's extensive responsibilities.

John was sympathetic and accepted that Jackie was overworking. He suspected that her drinking, which had not been raised in the interview, could be a response to this excessive emotional and work pressure as well as the real explanation for her unexplained absences. However, he indicated to Jackie that the university was unhappy and could not tolerate her unexpected and unexplained absences forever. He promised that at the end of the present semester he would review her workload with her department head and he also suggested that she agree to see the head of the student counselling service for what he described as 'stress management'. John did not raise Jackie's marital problems or her alcohol abuse, but he hoped that these would be dealt with as part of that referral. Jackie agreed to accept a referral for counselling.

Dr Stephen Roche, the head of the student counselling service, arranged an appointment for Jackie. When Jackie arrived for her interview, Dr Roche settled her down with more than the usual care. He was tentative about conducting a clinical interview with Jackie, who was both a staff member and a member of his research team. He asked Jackie if she was comfortable in seeing him professionally and when she said she was, he proceeded to take a psycho-social history.

Dr Roche discovered that Jackie was the daughter of a couple who had lived in a suburb close to the university at the time of Jackie's birth, but who had moved to the country when Jackie was 7 years old because her father, a clergyman, had been transferred to a rural parish. The family had returned to the area when Jackie was 15 years old. She had been a good school student, had easily obtained entry into a teaching course and, some years later, left teaching to train as a social worker. On qualifying as a social worker she had worked for three years in a large hospital where she had shown great promise and co-authored a number of papers with physicians and surgeons in the hospital. This led to a career as a tutor in her present department where she had demonstrated superior academic ability and had been promoted to senior lecturer. Jackie had been remarkably free from emotional problems throughout her life, although she had never been a good mixer. She had played few games at school, but she had a deep interest in music and played the violin competently. Overall, she appeared to Dr Roche to be a serious, rather rigid and somewhat tense individual.

Jackie reported that she had a warm and fulfilling relationship with her father who was rather domineering, outgoing and a popular clergyman. She described her mother as kind, quiet and serious, rather like herself. Jackie disclosed later in the interview that she was the youngest of three adopted children. Jackie's family had been comfortably well-off throughout her life. She had left home when she was 17 years old to study as a teacher and had kept up regular contact with both her parents until her father's death.

She admitted that she had been distressed and upset by her father's death. Since then, she had maintained only limited contact with her family and had lost contact with her brother and sister. She admitted that the decision to leave teaching and study social work might have been related to disillusionment and sadness following her father's death.

Jackie met and married her husband, Ralph, after she joined the staff of the university. He was 20 years her senior and she was his second wife. They have one child, a 5-year-old daughter, Margaret. Dr Roche inquired about Jackie's marital relationship and her psychosexual development. Jackie said that she had had very few sexual encounters prior to marriage. She described herself as not very interested in sex but admitted that at times during the marriage her sexual interest had been quite high. She and Ralph had drifted apart following the birth of their daughter; they now fought intermittently. Jackie admitted that they both were drinking too much and that both had partners outside the marriage. She described her homosexual relationship, which had existed for a period of two years, as very important and satisfying. She had a high level of sexual interest in this relationship.

Jackie admitted that she had been drinking more heavily in the previous 18 months and ascribed this to the marital problems and the excessive workload. She also said that she had gaps of memory during her drinking and had only the haziest recall of what had happened during those periods when she had been absent from home or work for two or more days.

Dr Roche decided that he should make a more formal assessment of Jackie's problems and formulate a detailed treatment plan. He explained this proposal to Jackie. They agreed that whatever else emerged as a result of the more complete assessment, Jackie would seek a detoxification and alcohol rehabilitation program combined with marital therapy and stress management training in the long vacation. Jackie agreed to attend the counselling service for a formal assessment.

First assessment

The student counselling service was proud of its computerised assessment system. In addition to a self-administered structured interview which generates DSM-III-R diagnoses (*Diagnostic and Statistical Manual of Mental Disorders*, third edition, revised) (American Psychiatric Association, 1987), the system also administers a battery of psychological tests and a symptom checklist. Dr Roche received a report of Jackie's computerised assessment a few days after testing.

The report was not especially alarming. Jackie's responses to the structured interview questions indicated that she satisfied the DSM-III-R criteria for Alcohol Abuse and Dependence. These included blackouts, vomiting blood, physical fights, 'DTs' (hallucinations and fever) and two weeks in which she drank seven or more drinks every day. Jackie stated that she first got drunk at the age of 11, first had problems with drinking when she was 35 and that she was 37 years of age when the problems had last occurred. The assessment indicated that Jackie was presently anxious and that she hoped that one outcome of treatment would be a reduction in anxiety. She also indicated a desire to control her drinking.

Other than anxiety and drinking, Jackie felt that she had no other particular problems, and the remaining tests seemed to agree. Jackie's scores on a symptom checklist were all either at or below the mean for general outpatients. Her score on the Beck Depression Inventory (Beck et al., 1961) indicated a minimal level of depression. On the State-Trait Anxiety Inventory (Spielberger, Gorsuch & Lushene, 1970), a measure of a person's 'state' of anxiety at the time of testing as well as the person's typical, 'trait', anxiety level, Jackie's state anxiety fell in the bottom 20 per cent of females of her age and her trait anxiety score fell in the bottom quarter. Her score on the Rathus Assertiveness Inventory (Rathus, 1973), a measure of social assertiveness, showed that she was rather assertive. There was no sign of other disorders.

Dr Roche was a little surprised by Jackie's apparent emotional stability given her past and present problems with alcohol. He arranged to see Jackie again in two week's time. At this meeting he planned to review the results of her assessment.

First clues

Dr Roche was absent from his department for three days. On his return, just as he was about to commence a staff meeting, he received an urgent phone call from John Barraclough. John was concerned because Jackie had disappeared. She had not attended her lectures and she had missed an important meeting. When John rang her home, her husband, Ralph, told him that she was not at home. To John's surprise Ralph told him that, throughout their marriage, Jackie had disappeared for a day or two at a time. Ralph was not convinced that this was entirely due to alcohol and believed that she had some secret relationship. Despite many rows and bitter recriminations, Jackie had never given him a convincing explanation of these absences.

Dr Roche was puzzled and concerned to learn that Jackie's absences were nothing new but he put these worries aside and commenced the staff meeting. He immediately discovered that the first item on the agenda also concerned Jackie. She had been involved in a major crisis at the counselling centre.

One of the young women involved in the sexual abuse project had arrived at the centre in an agitated state. She had suddenly remembered her father's sexual abuse. The details were particularly distressing because they involved physical torture and her father making her available to his drinking friends for sexual purposes. The abuse had involved oral, anal and vaginal intercourse. The girl had completely forgotten these experiences until her involvement in the abuse project even though the abuse had occurred on a very frequent basis between the ages of 9 and 17. Jackie had spent a number of hours with this girl during which time the girl's agitation appeared to decrease. When the girl appeared more settled, Jackie had suggested that they have a cup of coffee. She left the girl alone and, on her return, Jackie discovered her on the floor bleeding profusely from a deep cut in her left forearm. Jackie handled the situation magnificently and called for assistance from the university's medical officer. Jackie accompanied the girl in the ambulance to the hospital but, shortly after the girl had been admitted, Jackie disappeared.

Two days later, Dr Roche received a phone call from a hospital in a neighbouring town. That morning an unknown woman in a red dress had been admitted. She was suffering from an overdose of minor tranquillisers. The only form of identification she held was Dr Roche's professional card. Dr Roche set out for the hospital immediately. Once there, he was able to identify the still unconscious woman as Jackie. Dr Roche met the hospital psychiatrist, Dr Jones, who agreed to admit Jackie to the hospital's psychiatric unit for assessment and to keep in contact with Dr Roche. The following week, Dr Roche received a report which indicated that Jackie had settled down very quickly in hospital and that no psychiatric condition had been diagnosed. The hospital had made contact with Jackie's G.P., Dr Thompson, who had undertaken to contact Dr Roche.

Dr Thompson came to see Dr Roche a few days later. He told him that Jackie had been consulting him for a considerable period of time, complaining of depression, anxiety, tension, panic attacks and migraine. As the family G.P., he had known Jackie since her childhood. He had lost touch with her when she left the family to begin teaching but she had started to see him again when she returned to the area to take up her position at the university.

According to Dr Thompson, Jackie had been a pretty child, very close to her father and his favourite child. Although he was a clergyman, her father had private means and was quite wealthy. Her mother was a rather vague and colourless individual. Dr Thompson considered that her family life had been reasonably happy. At the time of her father's death, following a short illness, Jackie (who was then around 22 years old) developed severe migraines and panic attacks. She had episodes of 'blindness' and a number of seizures. She saw a neurologist who diagnosed 'migraines'. At the time, Jackie also suffered from an intermittent skin disease which Dr Thompson was unable to diagnose; this eventually disappeared without the intervention of a specialist.

Dr Thompson attended Jackie during her pregnancy which had been marred by severe vomiting throughout. She had great difficulty conceiving, which Dr Thompson believed was due to a previous history of pelvic inflammatory disease of unknown origin. She had also complained of episodes of cystitis. Jackie was remarkably brave and had shown no distress through what was a painful labour. Eventually, the baby was delivered by forceps and on recovering from the anaesthetic Jackie had appeared vague and confused. She did not appear to understand that she had delivered a baby. This confusion cleared up rapidly.

Dr Thompson was aware that Jackie found her workload difficult to manage and he knew that she had problems in her marriage. Recently, he had been treating her for what he regarded as stress-related symptoms, including panic attacks and sleeplessness, with minor tranquillisers and light sedation. He had previously tried various medications for her depression with no useful result. Curiously, Dr Thompson was unaware of her alcohol abuse.

Dr Roche was now very puzzled and worried. The facts were just not adding up. He was concerned that Jackie had not told him many of the things that Dr Thompson was now telling him. He decided he would have another interview with Jackie. However, before an appointment could be scheduled, Jackie contacted Dr Roche in a state of considerable distress asking to see him urgently. He agreed to see her later that day. On her arrival, it was clear that Jackie was depressed and extremely anxious. Dr Roche inquired why she was feeling this way and she replied that she had always felt like this. When he asked whether anything had precipitated her present depression she replied that her depression had become worse following a frightening dream. Jackie said that, in her dream, she had seen a small child in a large bed; a dark figure was leaning over the child who was crying. Jackie could not identify the figure because the dream was misty and unclear.

Suddenly, while describing the dream, Jackie had a clear-cut hyperventilation panic attack (see chapter 11 for a description of such attacks). When the panic attack subsided, Dr Roche asked whether anything unusual had happened the previous day. Jackie replied that she had been counselling a student who had recounted an episode of incest. While eliciting this history she experienced a panic attack which she described as similar to the one that had just occurred.

Dr Roche raised the issue of her recent disappearance and admission to hospital. Jackie said that she remembered having a panic attack after the suicidal student had been admitted to hospital, but she had no memory of what transpired during her disappearance. She believed that she had been drinking because she was told that her breath had the odour of alcohol when she was admitted to hospital, but Jackie claimed that she did not remember drinking. Once again, Dr Roche found himself puzzled; he could not reconcile Jackie's story with what he had learned from other sources. He was convinced that Jackie had a major alcohol problem and was having blackouts but he was now suspicious that, despite her apparently happy childhood, Jackie's reaction to stories of sexual abuse may be the result of her own abuse as a child. He asked gently whether anything of a traumatic nature occurred during her childhood. Jackie replied, 'There are large parts of my childhood that I do not remember. I only remember things clearly from around the time of my fifteenth birthday'. Dr Roche felt that Jackie's case was now taking a very different turn. There was a suggestion, at least, that at some stage in her childhood Jackie had been a victim of some sort of trauma. Dr Roche asked her to undergo a new assessment and Jackie agreed.

Second assessment

This time Jackie presented a very different picture. In contrast to the earlier assessment in which her only self-described problems were anxiety and drinking, Jackie revealed a variety of additional problems. First there were fears. Jackie indicated that she would like to feel less anxious in enclosed places and that she wanted to overcome her fear of darkness. Jackie also seemed to be obsessive. She said that she wanted to stop thinking the same depressing, suicidal and guilt-provoking thoughts over and over. She worried about her health (she wanted to reduce her use of painkillers for headaches). She was also concerned about work, especially her social awkwardness. She said that she took criticism badly, was uneasy in groups and would like to be more comfortable talking to others. She wanted to stop swearing at other people when they made her angry. More ominously, Jackie feared giving in to her desire to hurt other people or to be hurt by them.

The computerised interview indicated that Jackie satisfied many of the DSM-III-R criteria for a 'major depressive episode'. These included weight loss, 'slower' thoughts, attempted suicide, trouble concentrating, trouble sleeping and worthless, sinful, guilty feelings. In addition to depression, the interview also indicated that Jackie had many simple phobias, agoraphobia and panic attacks. But this was not all. Jackie also had many of the signs of a somatoform disorder including nausea, amnesia, vomiting, chest pains, constipation, shortness of breath and other non-specific complaints.

The computer-administered psychological tests confirmed that Jackie was experiencing considerable distress. She was depressed, anxious and had paranoid ideas. Unlike her previous assessment, this time her Beck Depression Inventory score reflected a serious state of depression and the State-Trait Anxiety Inventory placed her at the top end of both state and trait anxiety. Also in direct contrast to her earlier assessment, her score on the Rathus Assertiveness Inventory indicated an exceedingly low level of assertiveness. On a test of 'dissociative experiences', Jackie scored in the high range, suggesting for the first time that she may be suffering from a dissociative disorder.

Personalities revealed

This assessment was obviously very different from the first. At their next session, Dr Roche said to Jackie, 'I have just reviewed your recent assessment and I am puzzled because it is quite different from your previous one. We have discussed your drinking problem and your disappearances. The history I have obtained from your general practitioner suggests that you have had a lot of emotional problems and some physical ones as well, yet the first time that I saw you, you did not appear distressed. I am concerned that you are apparently having panic attacks when you have been dealing with clients who have been sexually abused and I am beginning to wonder whether you might have had some trauma in your own childhood that you don't remember'.

These words produced a dramatic change in Jackie. She sat upright, folded her arms, looked much more aggressive and said in a loud and hostile voice 'It is time that I talked to you. That pathetic wimp knows nothing about what that bastard did to us. She was too weak to stop that shit of a father raping her'. Dr Roche was startled by this sudden change and said 'What are you talking about, Jackie?'.

She replied, 'I have always been opposed to her wasting her time seeing a clown like you. You cannot even tell the difference between us'. They proceeded to have the following extraordinary conversation:

'Are you telling me that you are in some way different from Jackie?'

'You have only to use your eyes. I am obviously different. Can't you see the difference?'

'Do you have a different name?'

'It's none of your business. You don't need to know.'

'If we are to talk together I need to call you something.'

'Oh, very well, you can call me Stephanie. I suppose it will stop you confusing me with that pathetic bitch. Don't you understand I'm not even the same age as her.'

'What age are you?'

'I'm an adult.'

'But what age are you?'

'I'm 15 but you must treat me as an adult, I look after her, somebody has to.'

'What do you know about what your father did to you when you were a child, Stephanie?'

'That bastard is not my father and I have never been a child. I came around when she was 15.'

'What do you do?'

'I look after her, like I told you. She's pathetic. All that crying and carrying on. I was the one that had sex with that sanctimonious bastard. I didn't care, I didn't feel it. I used to make him give us money. Do you know that he even used to pray with her afterwards. I used to go into his room when he was dying and he used to ask me for sex and I used to laugh at him and tell him he was a useless old pervert.'

'Are you sexually active now?'

'Piss off, you're just a dirty old pervert too. I'm not going to talk about my sex life with you. I'm going.'

Suddenly her body posture and facial expression changed and Jackie was sobbing in front of him. Dr Roche asked, 'Do you know what has just happened?'

'You have been talking to her.'

'Do you know her name?'

'No, but I can hear her voice talking to me, she says I'm pathetic.'

Dr Roche now knew that he was dealing with a major dissociative disorder, a case of multiple personality. The strange inconsistencies in the history, the amnesia for childhood, the disappearances which he had been so ready to view as alcohol amnesias, the substance abuse all began to make sense. The odd illnesses after her father's death, the blindness and the seizures, the strange indifference to pain during pregnancy, the failure to recognise that she had a baby and her intense reactions to histories of incest, even the dream about the child, were all symptoms of multiple personality disorder (MPD).

Two days later, Dr Roche was contacted by the local police station who had been given his name by a woman they had just arrested for soliciting and suspicion of drug dealing. She would not give the police her name. She had been observed acting in a most provocative manner and openly soliciting clients in one of the main streets of town. She was wearing a short red dress with black boots and a white belt and when arrested was discovered to have in her possession a quantity of heroin. They also found a key with an address on it and they had gone to that address. They found a tidy flat with one bedroom filled with mirrors and a gaudy decor suggesting that it was used for sexual purposes. They also found business cards from an escort agency with the name 'Freya' printed on them. Another room was decorated in red colours with white and black drapes. There was a heavy cloying smell of candle smoke and several crosses of different sizes on a small table which was covered in a purple linen cloth.

Dr Roche found Jackie in a cell, cradling a child's colouring book and pencils to her chest. Jackie had become upset in police custody; one of the policewomen had bought a colouring book for her own child and Jackie had pleaded to be given the book and the pencils. She had remained in the cell quietly colouring the book and behaving in a way the police described as childish.

Dr. Roche entered the cell and greeted her.

'Hello, Jackie.'

A child-like voice replied, 'Hello, who are you'.

'Don't you know who I am? I'm Dr Stephen Roche. I'm a psychologist. I have been treating you.'

'Oh, I see, Jackie has told us that you are a doctor who is looking after us. Will I get into trouble? Have I done something wrong? Stephanie told me I was not to talk with you. Will I get into trouble? She will be cross with me.'

Dr Roche realised he was talking to a child personality and asked, 'What is your name?'

'My name is Jaqueline.'

'What age are you?'

'I'm 6.'

Dr. Roche rang Jackie's husband who arrived at the police station, posted bail for Jackie and took her home.

Dr. Roche saw Jackie the next day when she arrived at his office with a bandage on her left wrist. Jackie appeared very agitated. She said, 'I want to kill myself. I have disgraced myself and my family. Ralph is furious with me. What will happen to my job? I have been arrested for prostitution and for possessing drugs. I want to die! I'm no good. I have always been bad. They tell me I'm bad'.

'Who tells you you're bad?', Dr Roche asked.

'The voices in my head.'

'Whose voices do you hear?'

'I don't know all of them.'

'How many are there?'

'I'm not sure, I think there are five'.

'Are there any differences between the voices?'

'One is a deep male voice. I think there is an old woman's voice. There is a child's voice but I'm not sure about the others.'

'Do they have names?'

'I think the child is called Jaqueline. She cries a lot. I can hear her crying now.'

'Do you know any other names?'

'There is one called Stephanie. I don't know the names of the others.'

'How long have you heard these voices?'

'As long as I can remember. Before I did social work I thought everybody heard voices, I thought it was normal.'

'Why did you not tell me about these voices?'

'The voices have always warned me not to tell people about them. Anyway, I thought if I told you about the voices, you would think I was mad.'

'I don't think you are mad, but I think you may have what we call a dissociative disorder. I think you may have a multiple personality disorder.'

'Do you mean I have schizophrenia?'

'No, this is not schizophrenia, it's a dissociative disorder. Can I ask you about that bandage on your arm?'

'When I woke this morning, there was a cut on my arm and there was blood all over the bed. It has happened before.'

'Look, I think we should try to find out what happened to your arm. If I can get you to relax deeply I may be able to help you find out how your arm got cut.'

'Are you going to hypnotise me?'

'No, that's not necessary. I am simply going to ask you to take several deep breaths and count slowly from one to ten. Each time you breathe out I want you to say the word "relax" to yourself.'

When Jackie had completed the relaxation exercise, Dr Roche asked 'Do you feel relaxed, Jackie?'.

Jackie replied in a distant voice, 'Yes'.

'Now, I want you just to let things happen. Does anybody know about the cutting of the arm?'

Suddenly a calm, unemotional voice replied, 'What do you want to know?'.

'Who are you?', Dr Roche asked.

'I don't have a name', was the answer.

'What do you do?'

'I see and hear all that is happening. I don't do anything.'

'Can you tell me about the cutting of the arm?'

'Yes. The child's arm was cut because she talked to you.'

'Who cut the child's arm?'

'You are not allowed to know.'

'Do you know Stephanie?'

'Yes, she looks after Jackie and the child.'

'Did Stephanie cut the arm?'

'No, you are not allowed to know the name of the person who cut the arm.'

'Can you help me any more?'

'No.'

'May I talk to you again.'

'If you wish.'

'Thank you. Jackie, can you hear me?'

'Yes.'

'Now we can stop being relaxed. We'll count from ten to one.'

Although he had not set out to hypnotise her, Dr Roche had put Jackie in something similar to a hypnotic state. The ease with which this occurred took him a bit by surprise. It was at this point that Dr Roche became understandably concerned that he had neither the experience nor the time to treat a complex case of MPD. He referred Jackie to a colleague, Dr Jacobs, a specialist in dissociative disorders.

Treatment

In the past, the goal of treatment was to support the most 'competent' personality (Thigpen & Cleckley, 1957). This approach is rarely successful, however. Therapy often elicits many more personalities. This was certainly the case for Jackie. Dr Jacob's treatment revealed the following personalities:

1. A so-called 'host personality', Jackie, who was depressed and had panic attacks and nightmares. The nightmares became more specific during therapy. They consisted of scenes of child abuse perpetrated by her father and other men.
2. A 'child personality', Jaqueline.
3. A 'protector personality', Stephanie, who looked after Jackie and Jaqueline.
4. A 'promiscuous substance abuser', Freya. Freya was the prostitute who knew about drug use and who held regular seances in the flat which the police discovered when 'Jackie' was arrested.
5. A 'no-name personality' called 'the observer'. This was the serene, helpful alternate personality who told Dr Roche about the arm-cutting incident.
6. A 'persecutor', a witch-like figure who was one of the voices heard by Jackie and who was responsible for the arm-cutting. This personality believes that she can harm the body by cutting it or arranging overdoses because she is separate from Jackie and the others and will survive the death of the body.
7. A 'cross-gender male personality', Brad, who is tough and acts as Freya's pimp and who also knows where to get drugs.
8. An 'administrator personality'. This alternate personality does not get anxious or depressed, is highly sociable and can give lectures and tutorials as well as chair committees. This personality specialises in coping with the work situation.

Today, the preferred treatment involves trying to integrate the disparate personalities into a single whole or at least an untroubled coalition (Putnam, 1989; Ross, 1989; Kluft, 1987). The therapist begins by establishing trust and safety within therapy and then progresses to a very gradual process of getting to know the relationships between the parts and a cautious exploration of the dissociated traumatic memories. An attempt to favour one personality over another is misguided and trying to suppress an unattractive or angry part is fruitless and dangerous. Sometimes, videotapes are used to 'introduce' a part to another, or different parts may be enouraged to begin conversations with each other.

Hypnosis is used by many therapists but is not essential. The use of hypnosis to recover or abreact memories requires great caution and skill. Contrary to common expectation, hypnosis is most useful in controlling access to traumatic material rather than its aggressive exploration or abreaction.

When there is sufficient trust and cooperation between the therapist and the parts and between the parts themselves, the dissociated emotions are dealth with by a process essentially similar to the graded exposure or abreactive techniques used in post-traumatic stress disorder (PTSD). This process is prolonged, it is always fraught with difficulty and is punctuated by crises involving suicide attempts, aggression, self-mutilation and episodes of dramatic dissociation. At the end of this process an attempt at integration is often successful.

Jackie has a no-name personality called 'the observer' — such personalities can be very useful and may guide and advise the therapist during therapy, especially where dangerous material is being dealth with. While the ultimate aim of therapy is integration, this cannot be achieved until all traumatic emotions have been processed by some form of exposure technique.

Coping and stress management skills are also taught to provide the patient with alternative ways of coping with stress so that dissociation will no longer be the preferred mode of coping.

Dr Jacobs undertook therapy with Jackie. He explained that treatment could last some considerable months or even years but that he thought the outcome would eventually be favourable. He requested that Dr Roche approach the university authorities and seek a reduction in Jackie's workload and asked that allowance be made for her absences from work during therapy. Therapy is currently underway.

Main features of MPD

At one time, multiple personality was considered to be a form of hysteria. The reason for this is the frequency of somatoform disorders (especially conversion hysteria) among MPD patients. Jackie's palpitations, chest pains, dizziness, blurred vision, amnesia, paralysis and muscle weakness are fairly typical.

With experience, however, clinicians realised that the problems of MPD patients go well beyond those of hysteria. As already noted, the DSM-III-R categorises MPD as a dissociative disorder, a disorder in which there is 'a sudden temporary alteration in the normally integrative functions of consciousness, identity or motor behavior' (page 253). The diagnostic criteria are:

A. The existence within a person of two or more distinct personalities or personality states (each with its own relatively enduring pattern of perceiving, relating to, and thinking about the environment and self).

B. At least two of these personalities or personality states recurrently take full control of the person's behavior (page 272).

According to the DSM-III-R, the transition between these personalities or personality states is often abrupt. Prior to the DSM-III-R, there was also a third criterion, 'an inability to recall important personal information that is too extensive to be explained by ordinary forgetfulness'. It is proposed to reinstate this criterion in the DSM-IV because it is so common among MPD patients (American Psychiatric Association, 1991). Amnesia for parts of one's personal history is central to the disorder. Whole sections of an individual's life can be lost. Few people, other than those with MPD, forget who they are or what they have done.

Additional symptoms and signs have been also identified (Kluft, 1987). For example, patients may report 'lapses', times when they were unaware of what was transpiring. They report being told of things that they have said or done but which they cannot remember. Patients refer to themselves by different names, use the word 'we' to describe themselves, are easily hypnotised and often report finding letters in their handwriting that they do not recall writing. A history of severe headaches, blackouts and seizures is also common in the histories of people diagnosed as suffering from MPD.

Signs in Jackie's case

Jackie's case history shows how MPD may first appear in a covert way. In Jackie's case, alcohol abuse and amnesia initially masked the MPD. Overt symptoms only emerged in response to stress. As the case developed, the first suggestion of an alternate personality occurred, the red dress. Next, the 'hidden' history known to the G.P. and not disclosed by Jackie to Dr Roche, was revealed. There were, in addition, dramatic differences between the initial history, the first assessment, the history known to the G.P. and the second assessment. These differences were the result of memory gaps that occurred to different degrees within Jackie's various personalities. This is a common occurrence in MPD. As Putnam (1989) has rightly pointed out, when a clinician takes a history and finds loose ends that cannot be tied together or when there are marked inconsistencies in a history, MPD should be considered.

Ultimately, Jackie was found to have had all of the common MPD signs. Using the Dissociative Disorders Interview Schedule (Ross, 1989), Dr Jacobs found Jackie a fairly typical example of an MPD patient. She had a history of severe headaches as well as a number of somatoform symptoms. Her history of substance abuse was also fairly typical. Jackie, like many people with MPD, had a history of major depression.

Dr Jacobs found that Jackie had heard voices arguing in her head as well as voices commenting on her actions. She had felt that her feelings, thoughts and actions were being controlled by someone or something outside her. None of these experiences happened while she was under the influence of either drugs or alcohol and they were not part of a major depressive episode. These symptoms are common among patients suffering from MPD although they also occur frequently in schizophrenia. Indeed, MPD patients may frequently be mis-diagnosed as schizophrenic (Rosenbaum, 1980).

Although Jackie had never walked in her sleep, she had trance-like episodes during which she stared off into space, lost awareness of what was going on around her and lost track of time. Jackie stated that these episodes had occurred more than 50 times. Such trance-like episodes are frequent in multiple personality and other dissociative disorders.

Jackie told Dr Jacobs of being physically and sexually abused as a child. The abuse started when she was 3 years old and was carried out by her father and other males. Jackie reported she was subjected to more than 50 separate incidents of sexual abuse until the abuse stopped when she reached the age of 15. The sexual abuse involved genital touching, other types of fondling, intercourse with a male, being forced to perform oral sex on a male and oral sex carried out on her by a male, anal sex with a male and enforced sex with animals. Physical and sexual abuse is common in the reported histories of people with MPD (Coons & Milstein, 1986). In fact, because MPD patients have often endured sexual and physical abuse, it is possible that at least some of their symptoms may be the result of PTSD; a delayed reaction to intense stress. Dr Jacobs, for example, found that Jackie scored high on several measures designed to measure PTSD.

Jackie reported noticing personal possessions missing (or finding new possessions) without knowing where things went or where they came from. She found papers in her handwriting that she did not recall writing. Jackie said that apparent strangers often talked to her as if they knew her and that people told her that she had done or said things that she could not recall doing or saying. She had 'blank' spells, periods of missing time that she could not remember. She had found herself in an unfamiliar place, not sure how she had got there. She had memories that came back to her all of a sudden, in a flood, and she experienced long periods when she felt unreal, as if in a dream, or as if she was not really there. These are all typical signs of MPD.

Jackie said that there were large parts of her childhood which she could not remember and said that she spoke about herself using the words 'we' and 'us'. On many occasions she felt that there was another person or persons inside her.

Over the course of her life, Jackie had often been impulsive and unpredictable. She had trouble controlling her spending, gambling, substance use, eating, and her sexual appetites. She had also engaged in physically self-damaging acts, especially when depressed or bored. These problems, which are typical of patients with borderline personality disorders, are common in MPD.

Jackie reported that she was unsure of the number of different personalities within her but felt that the personality or part of her that was dominant at any particular time controlled her behaviour and also reported that two or more different personalities had been in control of her body on at least three separate occasions. Some type of amnesia or combination of types of amnesia existed among the different personalities. She agreed that each individual personality was complex and had behaviours and social relationships that were not shared by the other personalities.

Jackie is an example of what is known as a high-functioning MPD. Her system of alternative personalities, while quite complex, did not interfere unduly with her successful professional career. Her story is not actually a single case history but one based on several Australian cases. The melding is deliberate and intended to protect patient confidentiality. Although all cases are different, Jackie is fairly typical.

Conclusions and controversies

Prevalence

Multiple personality disorder is not a new phenomenon; it is likely that many of the cases of 'demonic possession' reported over the years may actually have been cases of MPD (Putnam, 1989). Although once considered exceedingly rare, the number of cases being reported seems to be increasing (Bliss, 1980). Some writers have claimed that MPD is more common than most researchers believe (Bliss, 1986; Greaves, 1980). They argue that the condition has frequently been confused with schizophrenia and the hysterical neuroses. These claims have been challenged, however (Chodoff, 1987). Until careful studies of the incidence and prevalence of MPD are conducted, we must leave the issue of frequency of MPD undecided.

Dissimulation

The possibility that people might pretend to have alternative personalities has arisen mainly in the legal arena. The most infamous example was the case of Kenneth Bianchi, California's 'Hillside Strangler'. Clinicians who hypnotised Bianchi discovered a submerged personality called Steve who claimed responsibility for the murders.

An expert psychiatrist, Martin Orne, called in by the prosecution claimed that Bianchi was only feigning (Orne, Dinges & Orne, 1984). According to Orne, the hypnotists inadvertently provided Bianchi with cues as to what they expected. By asking to talk to other personalities and by indicating that one personality may not recall the words of the other, they let Bianchi know how they expected MPD patients to behave, and he acted accordingly. Bianchi was convicted so the jury must have agreed with Orne.

Most patients, of course, are not on trial for murder. They do not have such a strong reason for malingering. Nevertheless, they may still be inadvertently influenced by therapists. Sarbin and Coe (1979) argue that the therapist acts as a kind of stage director guiding a suggestible but highly inventive and imaginative patient in the production of MPD. This argument was proposed quite early in the history of MPD. It is known as the iatrogenic argument and was one reason for a decline in interest in MPD in the early part of this century.

It is, of course, possible that therapists unintentionally provide patients with cues as to how to behave and then reward them with attention and concern. Certainly, some therapists appear to treat many more MPD cases than others (see, for example, Allison, 1984; Bliss, 1980). It is at least possible that these therapists may subtly encourage patients to display MPD symptoms.

Such a possibility was explored in a laboratory experiment by Spanos, Weekes and Bertrand (1985). University students were asked to play the role of an accused murderer being examined by a psychiatrist. They were told to use whatever cues they could to behave appropriately. The students were hypnotised and some were then interviewed using questions taken from transcripts of Kenneth Bianchi's interviews. These students produced behaviour similar to Bianchi's. They adopted new names and feigned amnesia.

Although this study showed that some of the phenomena of multiple personality can be faked and that the hypnotic interview is not necessarily the most objective way to demonstrate that someone has MPD, it would be an exaggeration to conclude that such studies prove that MPD does not exist. Many of the phenomena associated with MPD occur completely outside hypnosis. Jackie, for example, revealed her alternate personality through her behaviour (her disappearances, her prostitution) and in the course of a conversation with Dr Roche. These revelations preceded any attempt to hypnotise her. In some cases, alternate personalities have been found to have different heart rates, different blood pressures and even different EEG patterns. These physiological indices are exceedingly difficult to fake (Lester, 1977).

While it seems reasonable to warn psychologists to be careful when doing hypnotic interviews, in order to ensure that they do not inadvertently bias the results, the research conducted so far does not lead to the conclusion that all MPD cases are either feigning or responding to subtle cues produced by clinicians. The numerous examples of MPD phenomena that are unrelated to hypnosis suggest that the MPD diagnosis does not rely solely on hypnotic manifestations. The similarity in presentation across MPD patients is far greater than that found in many other mental disorders, for example, schizophrenia.

Aetiology

Perhaps the most important common finding in the histories of MPD patients is sexual and physical abuse (Coons & Milstein, 1986). This has led to the hypothesis that there may be a link between MPD and PTSD. Central to the concept of PTSD is the idea that it is the result of exceptional trauma. The DSM-III-R refers to PTSD occurring when 'The person has experienced an event that is outside the range of usual human experience and that would be markedly distressing to almost anyone'. The trauma reported by MPD patients is typically horrific, or as Putnam (1989) puts it, Gothic. Some critics of the MPD concept have questioned the reliability of the reports of abuse, especially when they are so horrific as to appear unlikely. Such denials are not new. Freud himself, having initially believed the women who told him they had been abused, subsequently claimed that they must have fantasised this abuse. To avoid making premature judgements either way, we need to do further research into the relationship between early trauma and MPD.

In his aetiological theory which was based on an analysis of 14 cases, Bliss (1986) does not insist on a history of physical and sexual abuse but he certainly assumes that some major problem occurs in the lives of MPD patients when they are between 4 and 6 years old. The first alternate personality is created to protect the child from direct involvement with the problem. The child is usually a female and highly vulnerable to the development of MPD because of a special susceptibility to self-hypnosis (the ability to put one's self into hypnotic states). The child finds that creating an alternate personality does protect her from the emotional problem, so, in the future, problems are dealt with by creating additional personalities. Although there is need for more research, Bliss's self-hypnosis theory seems to fit with the clinical evidence presently available.

There is no doubt that MPD patients in clinical settings are very disturbed individuals. The condition is now being diagnosed in many countries with increasing frequency and there is a growing opportunity for the systematic study of a reasonably large series of cases. As suggested above, one promising approach is the examination of the relationship between dissociative phenomena and PTSD especially if this is combined with rigorous objective studies using sophisticated psychophysiological and psychometric techniques. Studies of other dissociative disorders and their relationship to carefully established childhood abuse will not only add to our knowledge in this area but will also serve to resolve some of the controversies surrounding MPD.

References

Adams, P. L. (1985). The obsessive child: A therapy update. *American Journal of Psychotherapy, 39*, 301–13.

Adler, C., Craske, M. Kirshenbaum, S. & Barlour, D. H. (1989). 'Fear of panic': An investigation of its role in panic occurrence, phobia avoidance, and treatment outcome. *Behaviour Research and Therapy, 27*, 391–96.

Agras, N., Sylvester, D. & Oliveau, D. (1969). The epidemiology of common fears and phobiae. *Comprehensive Psychiatry, 10*, 151–56.

Alexander, J. F. & Parsons, B. V. (1982). *Functional family therapy.* Monterey, Calif.: Brooks/Cole.

Alexopoulos, G. (1989). Biological abnormalities in late-life depression. *Journal of Geriatric Psychiatry, 22*, 25–34.

Allen, R. (1984). Treatment resistant depression and electroconvulsive treatment: One approach. *American Journal of Social Psychiatry, 4*, 44–46.

Allison, R. B. (1984). Difficulties diagnosing the multiple personality syndrome in a death penalty case. *International Journal of Clinical and Experimental Hypnosis, 32*, 102–17.

Allsopp, M. & Verduyn, C. (1989). A follow-up of adolescents with obsessive compulsive disorder. *British Journal of Psychiatry, 154*, 829–34.

Allsopp, M. & Verduyn, C. (1990). Adolescents with obsessive compulsive disorder. *Journal of Adolescence, 13(2)*, 157–69.

American Heart Foundation. (1987). Conference on behavioral medicine and cardiovascular disease. *Circulation* (supplement 1).

American Psychiatric Association (1952). *Diagnostic and statistical manual of mental disorders* (1st ed.). Washington, D.C.: American Psychiatric Association.

American Psychiatric Association (1968). *Diagnostic and statistical manual of mental disorders* (2nd ed.). Washington, D.C.: American Psychiatric Association.

American Psychiatric Association (1980). *Diagnostic and statistical manual of mental disorders* (3rd ed.). Washington, D.C.: American Psychiatric Association.

American Psychiatric Association (1987). *Diagnostic and statistical manual of mental disorders* (3rd ed. rev.). Washington, D.C.: American Psychiatric Association.

American Psychiatric Association (1991). DSM-IV Options Book: Work in Progress. Washington, D.C. American Psychiatric Association.

Andersen, B. L. (1981). A comparison of systematic desensitisation and directed masturbation in the treatment of primary orgasmic dysfunction in females. *Journal of Consulting and Clinical Psychology, 49*, 568–70.

Anderson, A. E., Morse, C. & Santmyer, K. (1985). Inpatient treatment for anorexia nervosa. In D. M. Garner & P. E. Garfinkel (eds), *Handbook of psychotherapy for anorexia nervosa and bulimia.* New York: Guilford Press.

Anderson, B. J. & Wolf, F. M. (1986). Chronic physical illness and sexual behaviour: Psychological issues. *Journal of Consulting and Clinical Psychology, 54*, 168–75.

Andreasen, N. C. (1982). Negative symptoms in schizophrenia. *Archives of General Psychiatry, 39*, 784–88.

Andreasen, N. C. (1989). *Brain imaging: Applications in psychiatry.* Washington: American Psychiatric Press.

Andreasen, N. C. (1990). *Modern problems of pharmacopsychiatry: Positive and negative symptoms and syndromes*. Basel, Switzerland: S. Karger.

Andreasen, N. C. & Flaum, M. (1991). Schizophrenia: The characteristic symptoms. *Schizophrenia Bulletin, 17*, 27–49.

Andreasen, N., Grove, W., Endicott, J., Coryell, W., Scheftner, W., Hirschfeld, R. & Keller, M. (1988). The phenomenology of depression. *Psychiatry and Psychobiology, 3*, 1–10.

Andrews, J. (1966). Psychotherapy of phobias. *Psychological Bulletin, 66*, 455–80.

Anscombe, R. (1987). The disorder of consciousness in schizophrenia. Schizophrenia Bulletin, 13, 241–260.

Antonuccio, D., Akins, W., Chatham, P., Monagin, J., Tearnan, B. & Ziegler, B. (1984). An exploratory study: The psychoeducational group treatment of drug-refractory unipolar depression. *Journal of Behaviour Therapy and Experimental Psychiatry, 15*, 309–13.

Apter, A., Bernhout, E. & Lyano, S. (1984). Severe obsessive compulsive disorder in adolescence: A report of eight cases. *Journal of Adolescence, 7(4)*, 349–58.

Aronson, T. & Logue, C. (1987). On the longitudinal course of panic disorder: Developmental history and predictors of phobic complications. *Comprehensive Psychiatry, 28*, 344–55.

Asperger, H. (1944). Die 'Autistischen Psychopathen' in Kindesalter. *Archiv fur Psychiatrie und Nervenkrankheiten, 117*, 76–136.

Baillie, A. J., Mattick, R. P. & Hall, W. (1991). *Review of smoking cessation literature: A meta-analysis*. (Submitted for publication.)

Baker, C. D. & De Silva, P. (1988). The relationship between male sexual dysfunction and belief in Zilbergald's Myths: An empirical investigation. *Sexual and Marital Therapy, 3*, 229–39.

Ban, T. (1987). Prolegomenon to the clinical prerequisite: Psychopharmacology and the classification of mental disorders. *Progress in Neuro-Psychopharmacology and Biological Psychiatry, 11*, 527–80.

Bandura, A. (1977). Self-efficacy: Toward a unifying theory of behavior change. *Psychological Review, 84*, 191–215.

Bandura, A. & Walters, R. (1963). *Social learning and personality development.* New York: Holt, Rinehart & Winston.

Barbach, L. (1980). *Women discover orgasm.* Free Press: New York.

Barkley, R. A. (1987). The assessment of attention deficit hyperactivity disorder. *Behavioural Assessment, 9*, 207–33.

Barlow, D. H. (1986). Causes of sexual dysfunction: The role of anxiety and cognitive interference. *Journal of Consulting and Clinical Psychology, 54*, 104–48.

Barlow, D. H., Hayes, S. C. & Nelson, R. O. (1984). *The scientist-practitioner: Research and accountability in clinical and educational settings*. New York: Pergamon Press.

Barnes, T. R. & Liddle, P. (1990). Evidence for the validity of negative symptoms. In N. C. Andreasen (ed.), *Modern problems of pharmacopsychiatry: Positive and negative symptoms and syndromes*. Basel, Switzerland: S. Karger, pp. 43–72.

Baron-Cohen, S. (1988). Social and pragmatic deficits in autism: Cognitive or affective? *Journal of Autism and Development Disorders, 18(3)*, 379–402.

Bartak, L. & Rutter, M. (1976). Differences between mentally retarded and normally intelligent autistic children. *Journal of Autism and Childhood Schizophrenia, 6*, 109–20.

Bates, A., Burns, D. & Moorey, S. (1989). Medical illness and the acceptance of suffering. *International Journal of Psychiatry in Medicine, 19*, 269–80.

Bebbington, P. & Kuipers, L. (1988). Social influences on schizophrenia. In P. Bebbington & P. McGuffin (eds), *Schizophrenia: The major issues*. London: Heinemann, pp. 201–25.

Beck, A. (1963). Thinking and depression: I. Idiosyncratic content and cognitive distortions. *Archives of General Psychiatry, 9*, 324–33.

Beck, A. (1964). Thinking and depression: II. Theory and therapy. *Archives of General Psychiatry, 10*, 561–71.

Beck, A. (1983). Cognitive therapy of depression: New perspectives. In P. Clayton & J. Barrett (eds), *Treatment of depression: Old controversies and new approaches.* New York: Raven Press, pp. 265–84.

Beck, A. (1987). Cognitive models of depression. *Journal of Cognitive Psychotherapy, 1*, 5–37.

Beck, A., Emery, G. & Goldberg, L. (1985). *Anxiety disorders and phobias: A cognitive perspective*. New York: Basic Books.

Beck, A., Epstein, N., Brown, G. & Steer, R. (1988). An inventory for measuring clinical anxiety: Psychometric properties. *Journal of Consulting and Clinical Psychology, 56*, 893–97.

Beck, A., Epstein, N. & Harrison, R. (1983). Cognitions, attitudes and personality dimensions in depression. *British Journal of Cognitive Psychotherapy, 1*, 1–16.

Beck, A., Rush, A., Shaw, B. & Emery G., (1979). *Cognitive therapy of depression*. New York: Guilford Press.

Beck, A., Ward, C., Mendelson, M., Mock, J. & Erbaugh, J. (1961). An inventory for measuring depression. *Archives of General Psychiatry, 41*, 53–63.

Beck, A. T., Ward, C., Mendelson, M., Mock, J. & Erbaugh, J. (1962). Reliability of psychiatric diagnoses: A study of consistency of clinical judgement and ratings. *American Journal of Psychiatry, 119*, 351–57.

Beck, A., Weissman, A., Lester, D. & Trexler, L. (1974). The measurement of pessimism: The Hopelessness Scale. *Journal of Consulting and Clinical Psychology, 54*, 861–65.

Beech, H. R. & Vaughan, M. (1978). *Behavioural treatment of obsessional States*. Chichester: John Wiley & Sons.

Bemporad, J. (1979). Adult recollections of a formerly autistic child. *Journal of Autism and Developmental Disorders, 9(2)*, 179–97.

Bentler, P. M. (1967). Heterosexual behaviour assessment: I. Males. *Behaviour Research and Therapy, 5*, 21–25.

Bentler, P. M. (1968). Heterosexual behaviour assessment: II. Females. *Behaviour Research and Therapy, 6*, 27–30.

Berrios, G. E. (1985). Positive and negative symptoms and Jackson: A conceptual history. *Archives of General Psychiatry, 42*, 95–97.

Berrios, G. & Quemada, J. (1990). Depressive illness in multiple sclerosis: Clinical and theoretical aspects of the association. *British Journal of Psychiatry, 156*, 10–16.

Berrios, G. & Samuel, C. (1987). Affective disorder in the neurological patient. *Journal of Nervous and Mental Disease, 175*, 173–76.

Beumont, P. J. V., Al-Alami, M. & Touyz, S. W. (1988). Relevance of a standard measurement of undernutrition to the diagnosis of anorexia nervosa: Use of Quetelet's body mass index. *International Journal of Eating Disorders, 3*, 399–406.

Birchwood, M. & Cochrane, R. (1988). Families coping with schizophrenia: Coping styles, their origins and correlates. *Psychological Medicine, 20*, 857–65.

Birrell, P. C. (1989). Improving behavioural interventions against CHD: The importance of stress management and of multi-focussed programmes. In P. F. Lovibond & P. H. Wilson (eds), *Clinical and abnormal psychology.* Amsterdam: North Holland.

Birrell, P. C. & Lovibond, S. H. (1988). Stress and acute cardiovascular events. *Medical Journal of Australia, 149*, 510.

Bleuler, E. (1911). *Dementia praecox, or the group of schizophrenias.* (Trans. J. Zinkin.) New York: International University Press, 1950.

Bliss, E. L. (1980). Multiple personalities: A report of 14 cases with implications for schizophrenia and hysteria. *Archives of General Psychiatry, 37*, 1388–97.

Bliss, E. L. (1986). *Multiple personality, allied disorders and hypnosis.* Oxford: Oxford University Press.

Bolton, D., Collins S. & Steinberg, D. (1983). The treatment of obsessive compulsive disorder in adolescence: A report of fifteen cases. *British Journal of Psychiatry, 142*, 456–64.

Bolton, D. & Turner, T. (1984). Obsessive compulsive neurosis with conduct disorder in adolescence: A report of two cases. *Journal of Child Psychology and Psychiatry, 25(1)*, 133–39.

Borkovec, T. & Sides, J. (1979). Critical procedural variables related to the physiological effects of progressive relaxation: A review. *Behaviour Research and Therapy, 17*, 119–25.

Borland, B. L. & Heckman, H. K. (1976). Hyperactive boys and their brothers: A 25-year follow-up study. *Archives of General Psychiatry, 33*, 669-75.

Bowlby, J. (1975). *Attachment and loss*, (vol. 2). Middlesex, England: Penguin Books.

Boyd, J. & Crump, T. (1991). Westphal is agoraphobia. *Journal of Anxiety Disorders*, 5, 77–86.

Broadbent, D. E. (1958). *Perception and communication.* London: Pergamon Press.

Brockington, J. F., Kendell, R. E. & Leff, J. P. (1978). Definitions of schizophrenia: Concordance and prediction of outcome. *Psychological Medicine*, *8*, 387–98.

Brown, G. W. & Rutter, M. L. (1966). The measurement of family activities and relationships. *Human Relationships*, *19*, 241–63.

Brown, R. A. & Sollod, R. (1988). Ethical and professional issues in sex therapy. In R. A. Brown & J. R. Field (eds), *Treatment of sexual problems in individual and couples therapy*. New York: PMA.

Bruch, H. (1973). *Eating disorders: Obesity, anorexia nervosa and the person within*. New York: Basic Books.

Burd, L., Kerbeshian, J. & Cook, J. (1988). Tourette disorder in North Dakota. *Neuroscience and Biobehavioural Reviews*, *12(3–4)*, 223–28.

Burns, A. (1990). Editorial: Disorders of affect in Alzheimer's disease. *International Journal of Geriatric Psychiatry*, *5*, 63–66.

Caine, E. D., McBride, M. C., Chiverton, P., Bamford, K. A., Rediess, S. & Shiao, J. (1988). Tourette's syndrome in Monroe County school children. *Neurology*, *38(3)*, 472–75.

Callaway, E. & Naghdi, S. (1982). An information processing model for schizophrenia. *Archives of General Psychiatry*, *39*, 339–47.

Cantwell, D. P. (1976). Genetic studies of hyperactive children. In R. R. Fieve, D. Rosenthal & H. Brill (eds), *Genetic research in psychiatry*. Baltimore: John Hopkins University Press.

Carney, M., Roth, M. & Garside, R. (1965). The diagnosis of depressive syndromes and the prediction of ECT response. *British Journal of Psychiatry*, *111*, 659–74.

Carpenter, W. T. & Strauss, J. S. (1974). Cross-cultural evaluation of Schneider's first-rank symptoms of schizophrenia: A report from the international pilot study of schizophrenia. *American Journal of Psychiatry*, *131*, 682–87.

Carpenter, W. T., Strauss, J. S. & Bartko, J. J. (1974). Flexible system for the diagnosis of schizophrenia: A report from the WHO Pilot Study of Schizophrenia. *Science*, *182*, 1275–78.

Casper, R. C. (1987). Psychotherapy in anorexia nervosa. In P. J. V. Beumont, G. D. Burrows & R. C. Casper (eds), *Handbook of eating disorders: Part 1. Anorexia and bulimia nervosa*. Amsterdam, Elsevier, pp. 255–69.

Chalmers, J. & Cowen, P. (1990). Drug treatment of tricyclic-resistant depression. *International Review of Psychiatry*, *2*, 239–48.

Chapman, L. J. & Chapman, J. P. (1973). *Disordered thought in schizophrenia*. New York: Appleton-Century Crofts.

Charney, D., Price, L. & Heninger, G. (1986). Desipramine-yohimbine combination treatment of refractory depression. *Archives of General Psychiatry*, *43*, 1155–61.

Chiarello, C. (1980). A house divided? Cognitive functioning with callosal agenesis. *Brain and Language*, *11*, 128–58.

Chodoff, P. (1987). More on the multiple personality disorder. *American Journal of Psychiatry*, *144*, 124.

Clark, D. A. & Bolton, D. (1985). An investigation of two self-report measures of obsessional phenomena in obsessive compulsive adolescents. *Journal of Child Psychology and Psychiatry*, *26(3)*, 429–37.

Clarke, J. C. (1991). Managing mood: Depression and anxiety. In B. Hesketh & A. Adams (eds.), *Psychological perspectives on occupational health*. Sydney: Harcourt Brace Jovanovich.

Clarke, J. C. & Jackson, J. A. (1983). *Hypnosis and behavior therapy: The treatment of anxiety and phobias*. New York: Springer.

Clarke, J. C & Saunders, J. B. (1988). *Alcoholism and problem drinking: Theories and treatment*. Sydney: Pergamon.

Clarke, J. C. & Wardman, W. (1985). *Agoraphobia: A clinical and personal account*. Sydney: Pergamon.

Clum, G. & Knowles, S. (1991). Why do some people with panic disorders become avoidant? A review. *Clinical Psychology Review, 11*, 293–313.

Collins, D. & Lapsley, H. (1991). *Estimating the economic costs of drug abuse in Australia*. Canberra: Australian Government Publishing Service.

Conners, C. K. (1973). Rating scales for use in drug studies with children. *Psychopharmacology Bulletin. Special Issue*, 28–54.

Cooke, R. (1990). T3 augmentation of a tricylic antidepressant in a patient receiving T4 maintenance therapy. *American Journal of Psychiatry, 147*, 255.

Coons, P. M., Bowman, E. S. & Milstein, V. (1988). Multiple personality disorder: A clinical investigation of 50 cases. *Journal of Nervous and Mental Disease, 176*, 519–27.

Coons, P. M. & Milstein, V. (1986). Psychosexual disturbance in multiple personality: Characteristics, aetiology and treatment. *Journal of Clinical Psychiatry, 47(3)*, 106–10.

Cooper, J. (1970). The Leyton obsessional inventory. *Psychological Medicine, 1*, 48–64.

Cooper, J. E., Kendell, R. E., Gurland, B. J., Sharp, E. L., Copeland, J. R. M. & Simon, R. (1972). *Psychiatric diagnoses in New York and London: A comparative study of mental hospital admissions.* London: Oxford University Press.

Corsini, R. J. & Wedding, D. (eds) (1989). *Current psychotherapies*. Itasca, Ill.: Peacock Publishers Inc.

Creamer, M. (1987). Cognitive interventions in the treatment of obsessive-compulsive disorders. *Behaviour Change, 4(1)*, 20–27.

Crow, M. (1980). The molecular pathology of schizophrenia: More than one disease process. *British Medical Journal, 280*, 66–68.

Curtiss, S. (1985). The development of human cerebral lateralisation. In D. F. Benson & E. Zaidel (eds), *The dual brain, hemispheric specialisation in humans; UCLA 26*. New York: The Guilford Press, pp. 97–116.

Dadds, M. R. (1987). Families and the origins of child behavior problems. *Family Process, 26*, 341–57.

Dadds, M. R. (1989). Child behaviour therapy and family context: Research and clinical practice with maritally distressed families. *Child and Family Behavior Therapy, 11*, 27–44.

Dadds, M. R. & Powell, M. B. (1991). The relationship of interparental conflict and global marital adjustment to aggression, anxiety and immaturity in aggressive and nonclinic children. *Journal of Abnormal Child Psychology, 19*, 553–68.

David, O. J. (1974). Association between lower level lead concentrations and hyperactivity in children. *Environmental Health Perspectives*, *7*, 17–25.

Davis, G., Armstrong, H., Donovan, D. & Temkin, N. (1984). Cognitive-behavioral treatment of depressed affect among epileptics: Preliminary findings. *Journal of Clinical Psychology*, *40*, 930–35.

Davison, G. C. & Neale, J. M. (1990). *Abnormal psychology*, (5th ed.). New York: John Wiley & Sons.

Day, R. (1986). Social stress and schizophrenia: From the concept of recent life events to the notion of toxic environments. In G. D. Burrows & T. R. Norman (eds), *Handbook of studies of schizophrenia*. Amsterdam: Elsevier, pp. 71–82.

De Loof, C., Zandbergan, J., Lonsbergen, H., Pols, H. & Grieze, E. (1989). The role of life events in onset of panic disorder. *Behaviour Research and Therapy*, *27*, 461–63.

De Myer, M. K., Hingten, J. & Jackson, R. (1981). Infantile autism reviewed: A decade of research. *Schizophrenia Bulletin*, *7*, 388–451.

Deicken, R. (1987). Combined alprazolam and phenelzine treatment of refractory depression with panic attacks. *Biological Psychiatry*, *22*, 762–66.

Dembroski, T. M., MacDougall, J. M., Williams, R. B., Haney, T. L. & Blumenthal, J. A. (1985). Components of Type A, hostility and anger-in: Relationship to angiographic findings. *Psychosomatic Medicine*, *47*, 219-33.

Derogatis, L. R., Fagan, P. J., Schmitdt, C. W., Wise, T. N. & Gilden, K. S. (1986). Psychological subtypes of anorgasmia: A marker variable approach. *Journal of Sex and Marital Therapy*, *12(3)*, 197–210.

Derogatis, L. R. & Meyer, J. K. (1979). A psychological profile of the sexual dysfunctions. *Archives of Sexual Behaviour*, *8*, 210–23.

Desmarais, P. & Lallee, Y. (1988). Severe obsessive-compulsive syndrome in a 10-year-old: A 3-year follow-up. *Canadian Journal of Psychiatry*, *33*, 405–8.

Dessauer, M., Goetze, U. & Tolle, R. (1985). Periodic sleep deprivation in drug-refractory depression. *Neuropsychobiology*, *13*, 111–16.

Devenyi, P. & Saunders, S. J. (1986). *Physicians' handbook for medical management of alcohol and drug-related problems*. Toronto: Addiction Research Foundation of Ontario.

Deykin, E. Y. & MacMahon, B. (1979). Incidence of seizures among children with autistic symptoms. *American Journal of Psychiatry*, *136 (10)*, 1310–12.

DiClemente, C. C., Prochaska, J. O., Fairhurst, S., Velicer, W., Velasquez, M. & Rossi, J. (1991). The process of smoking cessation: An analysis of precontemplation, contemplation and determination stages of change. *Journal of Consulting and Clinical Psychology*, *59*, 295–304.

Dobinson, I. & Poletti, P. (1989). *Buying and selling heroin: A study of heroin user/dealers*. Sydney: New South Wales Attorney General's Department.

Dobson, K. (1989). A meta-analysis of the efficacy of cognitive therapy for depression. *Journal of Consulting and Clinical Psychology*, *57*, 414–19.

Donchin, E. (1979). Event-related potentials: A tool in the study of human information-processing. In H. Bergleiter (ed.), *Evoked brain potentials and behavior*. New York: Plenum Press, pp. 13–88.

Douglas, V. I. (1988). Cognitive deficits in children with attention deficit disorder and hyperactivity. In L. M. Bloomingdale & J. Sergeant (eds), *Attention deficit disorder: Criteria, cognition and intervention*. Oxford: Pergamon.

Douglas, V. I. & Peters, K. G. (1979). Toward a clearer definition of the attention deficit of hyperactive children. In G. A. Hale & M. Lewis (eds), *Attention and cognitive development*. New York: Pergamon.

Duggan, C., Lee, A. & Murray, R. (1991). Do different subtypes of hospitalized depressives have different long-term outcomes? *Archives of General Psychiatry, 48*, 308–12.

Duncan, C. C., Morihisa, J. M., Fawcett, R. W. & Kirch, D. G. (1987). P300 in schizophrenia: State or trait marker. *Psychopharmacology Bulletin, 23*, 497–501.

Dyck, M. & Stewart, B. (1991). Cognitive vulnerability to depression. *Journal of Cognitive Psychotherapy, 5*, 115–29.

Eaves, G. & Rush, A. (1984). Cognitive patterns in symptomatic and remitted unipolar major depression. *Journal of Abnormal Psychology, 93*, 31–40.

Edwards, G. (1987). *The treatment of drinking problems: A guide for the helping professions*. London: Blackwell Scientific Publications.

Edwards, G., Arif, A., & Hodgson, R. (1981). Nomenclature and classification of drug and alcohol-related problems: A WHO memorandum. *Bulletin of the World Health Organization, 59*, 225–42.

Elkin, I., Shea, T., Watkins, J., Imber, S., Sotsky, S., Collins, J., Glass, D., Pilkonis, P., Leber, W., Docherty, J., Fiester, S. & Parloff, M. (1989). National Institute of Mental Health treatment of depression collaborative research program: General effectiveness of treatments. *Archives of General Psychiatry, 46*, 971–82.

Elkins, R., Rapoport, J. L. & Lipsky, A. (1980). Obsessive-compulsive disorder of childhood and adolescence: A neurobiological viewpoint. *Journal of the American Academy of Child Psychiatry, 19*, 511–24.

Ellis, A. (1977). A note on the treatment of agoraphobics with cognitive modification versus prolonged exposure *in vito*. *Behaviour Research and Therapy, 17*, 162–64.

Emmelkamp, P. (1979). Clinical phobias. In M. Hersen, R. M. Eisler & P. Miller (eds), *Progress in Behaviour Modification*, vol. 8. New York: Academic Press.

Emmelkamp, P. M., Van-Linden-Van-den-Heuvell, C., Ruphan, M. & Sanderman, R. (1989). Home-based treatment of obsessive-compulsive patients. *Behaviour Research and Therapy, 27(1)*, 89–93.

Endicott, J., Nee, J., Fleiss, J. L., Cohen, J., Williams, J. B. & Simon, R. (1982). Diagnostic criteria for schizophrenia. *Archives of General Psychiatry, 39*, 884–89.

Englehardt, D. N., Rosen, H., Feldman, J., Englehardt, J. A. Z. & Cohen, P. (1982). A 15-year follow-up of 646 schizophrenic outpatients. *Schizophrenia Bulletin, 8*, 493–503.

Erdreich, M. (1988). Selective pharmacology and psychotherapy in compulsive eating disorders. *Dynamische-Psychiatrie, 21(5)*, 448–55.

Ersner-Hershfield, R. & Kopel, S. (1979). Group treatment of preorgasmic women: Evaluation of partner involvement and spacing of sessions. *Journal of Consulting and Clinical Psychology, 47*, 750–59.

Extein, I. & Gold, M. (1988). Thyroid hormone potentiation of tricyclics. *Psychosomatics, 29*, 166–74.

Fahy, T. A. (1988). The diagnosis of MPD: A critical review. *British Journal of Psychiatry, 153*, 597–606.

Farmer, A. & McGuffin, P. (1989). The classification of the depressions: Contemporary confusion revisited. *British Journal of Psychiatry, 155*, 437–43.

Fennell, M. & Teasdale, J. (1982). Cognitive therapy with chronic, drug-refractory depressed outpatients: A note of caution. *Cognitive Therapy and Research, 6*, 455–59.

Fine, S. (1973). Family therapy and a behavioral approach to obsessive compulsive neurosis. *Archives of General Psychiatry, 28*, 695-97.

Flament, M. F., Koby, E., Rapoport, J. L., Berg, C. J., Zahn, T., Cox, C., Denckla, M. & Lenane, M. (1990). Childhood obsessive-compulsive disorder: A prospective follow-up study. *Journal of Child Psychology and Psychiatry, 31(3)*, 363–80.

Flament, M. F., Rapoport, M. D., Berg, C. J., Sceery, W., Kilts, C. & Mellstrom, L. M. (1985). Clomipramine treatment of childhood obsessive-compulsive disorder: A double-blind control study. *Archives of General Psychiatry, 42(10)*, 977–83.

Flament, M.F., Whitaker, A., Rapoport, J.L., Davies, M. (1988). Obsessive compulsive disorder in adolescence : An epidemiological study. *Journal of the American Academy of Child and Adolescent Psychology, 127 (6)*, 764–71.

Flaum, M. & Andreasen, N. C. (1991). Diagnostic criteria for schizophrenia and related disorders: Options for DSM-IV. *Schizophrenia Bulletin, 17*, 133–42.

Fleming, B. & Faulk, A. (1989). Discriminating factors in panic disorder with and without agoraphobia. *Journal of Anxiety Disorders, 3*, 209–19.

Flor-Henry, P., Yeudall, L. T., Koles, Z. J. & Howarth, B. G. (1979). Neuropsychological and power spectral EEG investigations of the obsessive-compulsive syndrome. *Biological Psychiatry, 14*, 119–30.

Foa, E. B., Grayson, J. B., Steketee, G., Doppelt, H. G., Turner, R. M. & Latimer, P. L. (1983). Success and failure in the behavioral treatment of obsessive-compulsives. *Journal of Consulting and Clinical Psychology, 15*, 287-97.

Foa, E. & Kozak, M. (1991). Emotional processing: Theory research and clinical implications for anxiety disorders. In J. Safran & L. Greenberg (eds), *Emotion, psychotherapy, and change*. New York: Guilford Press.

Forster, E. & Holthausen, V. S. (1979). Obsessive compulsive disorder in adolescence. *Zeitschrift fur Kinder und Judenpsychiatrie, 7*, 5–18.

Francis, G. (1988). Childhood obsessive compulsive disorder: Extinction of compulsive reassurance seeking. *Journal of Anxiety Disorders, 2*, 361–66.

Franklin, J. (1987). The changing nature of agoraphobic fears. *British Journal of Psychology, 26*, 127–33.

Freidman, J. M., Weiler, S. J., Lo Piccolo, J. & Hogan, D. R. (1982). Sexual dysfunctions and their treatment: Current status. In A. S. Bellack, M. Hersen & A. E. Kazdin (eds), *International handbook of behaviour modification and therapy.* New York: Plenum.

Freud, S. (1959). Analysis of a phobia in a five-year-old boy. In S. Freud, *Collected Papers*, vol. 1. New York: Basic Books.

Freund, K. & Blanchard, R. (1981). Assessment of sexual dysfunction and deviation. In M. Hersen & A. S. Bellack (eds), *Behavioural assessment: A practical handbook.* Pergamon Press: New York.

Friedman, A., Cowitz, B., Cohen, H. & Granick, S. (1963). Syndromes and themes of psychotic depression. *Archives of General Psychiatry, 9*, 504–9.

Friedman, D., Cornblatt, B., Vaughan, H. G. & Erlenmeyer-Kinsky, L. (1988). Auditory event-related potentials in children at risk for schizophrenia: The complete initial sample. *Psychiatry Research, 26*, 203–21.

Friedman, D., Vaughan, H. G. & Erlenmeyer-Kimling, L. (1982). Cognitive brain potentials in children at risk for schizophrenia: Preliminary findings. *Schizophrenia Bulletin, 8*, 514–31.

Friedman, S. & Paradis, C. (1991). African-Americans and panic disorder. *Journal of Anxiety Disorders, 5*, 35–41.

Frith, C. D. (1979). Consciousness, information processing and schizophrenia. *Journal of Psychiatry, 134*, 225–35.

Frith, C. D. (1987). The positive and negative symptoms of schizophrenia reflect impairments in the perception and initiation of action. *Psychological Medicine, 17*, 631–48.

Frith, U. (1989). *Autism: Explaining the enigma.* Oxford: Basil Blackwell.

Frith, U. (1991). *Autism and Asperger syndrome.* Cambridge: Cambridge University Press.

Gajzago, C. & Prior, M. (1974). Two cases of 'recovery' in Kanner syndrome. *Archives of General Psychiatry, 31*, 264–68.

Garner, D. M. (1985). Iatrogenesis in anorexia nervosa and bulimia nervosa. *International Journal of Eating Disorders, 4*, 4701–26.

Garner, D. M. & Bemis, K. M. (1985). Cognitive therapy for anorexia nervosa. In D. M. Garner & P. E. Garfinkel (eds), *Handbook of psychotherapy for anorexia nervosa and bulimia.* New York: Guilford Press.

Garner, D. M. & Garfinkel, P.E. (1979). The Eating Attitudes Test: An index of the symptoms of anorexia nervosa. *Psychological Medicine, 9*, 273–79.

Garner, D. M. & Olmsted, M. A. (1984). Eating disorder inventory manual. New York: Psychological Assessment Resources, Inc.

Geffen, G. M., Forrester, G. M., Jones, D. L. & Simpson, D. A. (1992). Auditory verbal learning and memory in cases of callosal agenesis. In M. Lassonde & M. A. Jeeves (eds), *Callosal agenesis: The natural split-brain.* New York: Plenum Press (in press).

Geffen, G. M., Moar, K. J., O'Hanlon, A. P., Clark, C. R. & Geffen, L. B. (1990). Performance measures of 16- to 86-year-old males and females on the Auditory Verbal Learning Test. *The Clinical Neuropsychologist*, *4*, 45–63.

Gerstley, L. J., Alterman, A. I., McLellan, A. T. & Woody, G. E. (1990). Antisocial personality disorder in patients with substance abuse disorders: A problematic diagnosis? *American Journal of Psychiatry*, *147*, 173–78.

Gewirz, G., Malaspina, D., Hatterer, J., Feureisen, S., Klein, D. & Gorman, J. (1988). Occult thyroid dysfunction in patients with refractory depression. *American Journal of Psychiatry*, *145*, 1012–14.

Gibson, E. & Walk, R. (1960). The visual cliff. *Scientific American*, *202*, 2–9.

Gillan. P. W. (1977). Stimulation therapy for sexual dysfunction. In E. R. Wheeler (ed.), *Progress in sexology*. New York: Plenum.

Gillberg, C. (1989). Asperger syndrome in 23 Swedish children: A clinical study. *Developmental Medicine and Child Neurology*, *31*, 520–31.

Gillberg, C. (1990). Autism and pervasive development disorders. *Journal of Child Psychology and Psychiatry*, *31(1)*, 99–199.

Gillberg, C., Carlstrom, G. & Rasmussen, P. (1983). Hyperkinetic disorders in seven-year-old children with perceptual, motor and attentional deficits. *Journal of Child Psychology & Psychiatry*, *24*, 233–46.

Gillberg, C. & Gillberg, C. (1989). Asperger syndrome — Some epidemiological considerations: A research note. *Journal of Child Psychology and Psychiatry*, *30(4)*, 631–38.

Gillberg, C., Steffenburg, S. & Jakobssen, G. (1987). Neurological findings in 20 relatively gifted children with Kanner-type autism on Asperger syndrome. *Developmental Medicine and Child Neurology*, *29*, 641–49.

Glick, B. (1967). *Archives of General Psychiatry*, *17*, 577–83.

Goldstein, A. & Chambless, D. (1978). A reanalysis of agoraphobia. *Behavior Therapy*, *9*, 45–59.

Goldstein, J. M. & Tsuang, M. T. (1988). The process of subtyping schizophrenia: Strategies in search of homogeneity. In M. T. Tsuang & J. C. Simpson (eds), *Handbook of schizophrenia vol. 3: Nosology, epidemiology and genetics of schizophrenia*. Amsterdam: Elsevier, pp. 63–84.

Goodman, A. G., Rall, T. W., Nies, A. S. & Taylor, P. (1990). *Goodman and Gilman's the pharmacological basis of therapeutics* (8th ed.). New York: Pergamon Press.

Greaves, G. B. (1980). Multiple personality: 165 years after Mary Reynolds. *Journal of Nervous and Mental Disease*, *168*, 577–96.

Gubman, G. D., Tessler, R. C. & Willis, G. (1987). Living with the mentally ill: Factors affecting household complaints. *Schizophrenia Bulletin*, *13*, 727–36.

Haaga, D., Dyck, M. & Ernst, D. (1991). Empirical status of cognitive theory of depression. *Psychological Bulletin*, *109*, 215–36.

Halgren, E. (1990). Insights from evoked potentials into the neuropsychological mechanisms of reading. In A. B. Schiebel & A. F. Wechsler (eds), *Neurobiology of higher cognitive function*. New York: Guilford Press.

Hanna, G. L., McCracken, J. T. & Cantwell, D. P. (1991). Prolactin in childhood obsessive-compulsive disorder: Clinical correlates and response to clomipramine. *Journal of the American Academy of Child Psychiatry, 30*, 173–78.

Happe, F. (1991). The autobiographical writings of three Asperger syndrome adults: Problems of interpretation and implications for theory. In U. Frith (ed.), *Autism and Asperger syndrome*. Cambridge: Cambridge University Press, pp. 207–42.

Harbison, J. M., Graham, P. J., Quinn, J. T., McAllister, H. & Woodward, R. (1974). A questionnaire measure of sexual interest. *Archives of Sexual Behaviour, 3*, 357–66.

Harburg, E. & Hauenstein, L. (1980). Parity and blood pressure among four race-stress groups of females in Detroit. *American Journal of Epidemiology, III*, 356–66.

Harpin, R., Liberman, R., Marks, I., Stern, R. & Bohannon, W. (1982). Cognitive-behavior therapy for chronically depressed patients: A controlled pilot study. *Journal of Nervous and Mental Disease, 170*, 295–301.

Hawton. K. (1985). *Sex therapy: A practical guide*. Oxford: Oxford University Press.

Hawton, K., Salkovskis, P. M., Kirk, J. & Clark D. M. (eds) (1989). *Cognitive behaviour therapy for psychiatric problems: A practical guide*. Oxford: Oxford Medical Publications.

Heather, N. (1989). Disulfiram treatment for alcoholism: Deserves re-examination. *British Medical Journal, 299*, 471–72.

Heather, N., Tebbutt, J., Mattick, R. P. & Zamir, R. (1991). Development of a scale for measuring impaired control over alcohol consumption. *Journal of Studies on Alcohol*. (Submitted for publication.)

Heatherton, T. F., Kozlowski, L. T., Frecker, R. C. & Fagerstrom, K.O. (1991). The Fagerstrom test for nicotine dependence: A revision of the Fagerstrom tolerance questionnaire. *British Journal of Addiction, 86*, 1119–27.

Hebb, D. O. (1946). On the nature of fear. *Psychological Review, 53*, 259–76.

Heiman, J., Lo Piccolo, L. & Lo Piccolo, J. (1976). *Becoming orgasmic: A sexual growth programme for women*. N.J.: Prentice-Hall.

Hemsley, D. R. (1975). A two-stage model of attention in schizophrenia research. *British Journal of Social and Clinical Psychology, 14*, 81–89.

Herink, R. (1975). *Systems of psychotherapy.* San Luis Obispo, California: San Luis Obispo Press.

Hermelin, B. (1976). Coding and the sense modalities. In L. Wing (ed.), *Early childhood autism* (2nd ed.). Oxford: Pergamon Press, pp. 135–68.

Hetherington, E. M., Cox, M. & Cox, C. R. (1982). Effects of divorce on parents and children. In M. Lamb (ed.), *Nontraditional families*. Hillsdale, N.J.: Erbaum.

Hetherington, E. M. & Martin, B. (1986). Family factors and psychopathology in children. In H. C. Quay & J. S. Werry (eds), *Psychopathological disorders of childhood* (3rd ed.). New York: John Wiley & Sons.

Hillyard, S. A., Picton, T. W. & Regan, D. M. (1978). Sensation, perception and attention: Analysis using ERPs. In E. Callaway, P. Tveting & S. Coslow (eds), *Event-related brain potentials in man*. N.Y.: Academic Press.

Hodgeman, C. H. (1983). Current issues in adolescent psychiatry. *Hospital and Community Psychiatry, 34(6)*, 514–21.

Hodgson, R. J. & Rachman, S. (1977). Obsessional-compulsive complaints. *Behaviour Research and Therapy, 15*, 389-95.

Hoffmann, W. & Prior, M. (1982). Neuropsychological dimensions of autism in children: A test of the hemispheric dysfunction hypothesis. *Journal of Clinical Neuropsychology, 4(1)*, 27–42.

Hogarty, G., Anderson, A. M. & Reiss, D. J. (1987). Family psychoeducation, social skills training and medication in schizophrenia: The long and short of it. *Psychopharmacological Bulletin, 23*, 12–13.

Hogarty, G., Schooler, N. R., Ulrich, R. F., Mussare, F., Ferro, P. & Herron, E. (1979). Fluphenazine and social therapy in the aftercare of schizophrenic patients. *Archives of General Psychiatry, 36*, 1283–94.

Hollingshead, A. B. & Redlich, F. C. (1958). *Social class and mental illness: A Community Study.* New York: John Wiley & Sons.

Hollingsworth, C. E., Tanquay, P. E., Grossman, L. & Pabst, P. (1980). Long term outcome of obsessive-compulsive disorder in childhood. *Journal of the American Academy of Child Psychiatry, 19*, 134–44.

Hollon, S., Kendall, P. & Lumry, A. (1986). Specificity of depressotypic cognitions in clinical depression. *Journal of Abnormal Psychology, 95*, 52–59.

Holt, P. & Andrews, G. (1989). Provocation of panic. *Behaviour Research and Therapy, 27*, 253–61.

Honjo, S., Hirano, C., Murase, S. et al. (1989). Obsessive compulsive symptoms in childhood and adolescence. *Acta-Psychiatrica-Scandinavica, 80(1)*, 83–91.

Hoon, E. F., Hoon, P. W. & Wincze, J. P. (1976). An inventory for the measurement of female sexual arousability. *The SAI Archives of Sexual Behaviour, 5,* 291–301.

Howlin, P. & Rutter, M. (1987). *Treatment of autistic children*. New York: John Wiley & Sons.

Hoy, E., Weiss, G., Minde, K. & Cohen, N. (1978). The hyperactive child at adolescence: Cognitive, emotional and social functioning. *Journal of Abnormal Child Psychology, 6*, 311–24.

Huessy, H. & Cohen, A. (1976). Hyperkinetic behaviors and learning disabilities followed over seven years. *Pediatrics, 57*, 4–10.

Hullett, F. & Bidder, T. (1983). Phenelzine plus triiodothyronine combination in a case of refractory depression. *Journal of Nervous and Mental Disease, 171*, 318–20.

Hunkeler, W., Mohler, H., Pieri, L., Polc, P., Bonnetti, E. P., Cumin, R., Schaffner, R. & Haefely, W. (1981). Selective antagonists of benzodiazepines. *Nature, 290*, 514–16.

Jacobson, E. (1929). *Progressive relaxation*. Chicago: University of Chicago Press.

Janet, P. (1903). *Les obsessions et la psychathenie*. Paris: Ballieve.

Jaspers, K. (1913). *General psychopathology.* (Trans.) Manchester: Manchester University Press, 1963.

Jeeves, M. A. (1990). Agenesis of the corpus callosum. In F. Boller & J. Grafman (eds), *Handbook of neuropsychology,* vol. 4. Amsterdam: Elsevier Science, pp. 99–114.

Jeeves, M. A. & Silver, P. H. (1988). Interhemispheric transfer of spatial tactile information in callosal agenesis and partial commissurotomy. *Cortex*, *24*, 601–4.

Jehu, D. (1979). *Sexual dysfunction: A behavioural approach to causation, assessment and treatment*. London: John Wiley & Sons.

Jenike, M. A. (1983). Obsessive-compulsive disorder. *Comprehensive Psychiatry, 24*, 99–115.

Johnson, D. A. W. (1988). Drug treatment of schizophrenia. In P. Bebbington & P. McGuffin (eds), *Schizophrenia: The major issues*. London: Heinemann, pp. 158–71.

Johnson, D. A. W., Pasterski, G., Ludlow, J. M., Street, K. & Taylor, R. D. W. (1983). The discontinuation of maintenance neuroleptic therapy in chronic schizophrenic patients: Drug and social consequences. *Acta Psychiatrica Scandinavica*, *67*, 339–52.

Johnstone, E. C., Crow, T. J., Frith, C. D., Husband, J. & Kreel, L. (1976). Cerebral ventricle size and cognitive impairment in chronic schizophrenia. *Lancet*, *ii*. 924–26.

Josiassen, R. C., Shagass, C., Roemer, R. A. & Straumanis, J. J. (1985). Attention-related effects on somatosensory evoked potentials in college students at high risk for psychopathology. *Journal of Abnormal Psychology, 94*, 507–18.

Judd, L. (1965). Obsessive compulsive neurosis in children. *Archives of General Psychiatry, 12*, 136–44.

Kameyama, T., Niwa, S.I., Hiramatsu, K.I., Saitoh, S., Fukuda, M., Nakagome, K. & Itoh, K. (1987). Event-related potential correlates of psychotropic drug effects on attentional and hemispheric dysfunction in schizophrenia. In R. Takahashi, P. Flor-Henry, J. Gruzelier & S. Niwa (eds), *Cerebral dynamics, laterality and psychopathology*. Amsterdam: Elsevier, pp. 221–30.

Kanner, L. (1943). Autistic disturbance of affective contact. *Nervous Children*, *2*, 217–50.

Kantor, D., McNevin, S., Leichner, P., Harper, D. & Krenn, M. (1986). The benefit of lithium carbonate adjunct in refractory depression: Fact or fiction? *Canadian Journal of Psychiatry, 31*, 416–18.

Kaplan, H. S. (1974). *The new sex therapy: Active treatment of sexual dysfunction*. New York: Brunner/Mazel.

Kaplan, H. S. (1983). *The evaluation of sexual disorders: Psychological and medical aspects*. New York: Brunner/Mazel.

Kaplan, M. D. & Sadock, B. J. (eds) (1988). *Synopsis of psychiatry —behavioural sciences clinical psychiatry.* Baltimore, Md.: Williams and Wilkins.

Kazdin, A. (1987). Treatment of antisocial behaviour in children: Current status and future directions. *Psychological Bulletin*, *102*, 187–203.

Kazdin, A. (1988). *Child psychotherapy.* New York: Pergamon Press.

Kazdin, A. & Wilcoxin, L. (1975). Systematic desensitization and non-specific treatment effects: A methodological evaluation. *Psychological Bulletin*, *83*, 729–58.

Kearney, C. A. & Silverman, W. K. (1990). Treatment of an adolescent with obsessive compulsive disorder by alternating response prevention and cognitive therapy: An empirical analysis. *Journal of Behaviour Therapy and Experimental Psychiatry, 21(1)*, 39–47.

Kendell, R. (1976). The classification of depressions: A review of contemporary confusion. *British Journal of Psychiatry, 129*, 15–28.

Kendell, R. E. (1975). *The role of diagnosis in psychiatry.* Oxford: Blackwell Scientific Publications.

Kennedy, S. & Joffe, R. (1989). Pharmacological management of refractory depression. *Canadian Journal of Psychiatry, 34*, 451–56.

Khanna, S., Kaliaperumal, V. G. & Channabasavanna, S. M. (1986). Reactive factors in obsessive compulsive neurosis. *Indian Journal of Psychological Medicine, 9(2)*, 68–73.

Kiloh, L. & Garside, R. (1963). The independence of neurotic depression and endogenous depression. *British Journal of Psychiatry, 109*, 451–63.

Kirsch, I. (1990). *Changing expectations: A key to effective psychotherapy.* Pacific Grove, Calif.: Brooks/Cole.

Klein, D. F. (1981). Anxiety reconceptualized. In D. F. Klein & J. Rabkin (eds), *Anxiety: New research and changing concepts*. New York: Raven Press.

Kleiner, L. & Marshall, W. (1987). The role of interpersonal problems in the development of agoraphobia with panic attacks. *Journal of Anxiety Disorders, 1*, 313–24.

Klerman, G. & Cole, J. (1965). Clinical pharmacology of imipramine and related antidepressant compounds. *Pharmacology Review, 17*, 101–41.

Klerman, G. (1985). The scientific status of neurotic depression. *Psychopathology, 18*, 167–73.

Klosko, J., Shadick, R., Heimberg, R. & Barlow, D. (1986). *The attributional style of patients diagnosed with agoraphobia with panic versus patients diagnosed with panic disorder.* Paper presented at the annual meeting of the Association for the Advancement of Behavior Therapy. Chicago, November.

Klulft, R. P. (ed.) (1987). *Childhood antecedents of multiple personality.* Washington, D.C.: American Psychiatric Press.

Koenigsberger, H. W. & Handley, R. (1986). Expressed emotion: From predictive index to clinical construct. *American Journal of Psychiatry, 143*, 1361–73.

Kolakowska, T., Williams, A. O., Ardeen, M., Reveley, M., Jambor, K., Gelder, M. & Mandelbrote, B. (1985). Schizophrenia with good and poor outcome: Early clinical features, response to neuroleptics and signs of organic dysfunction. *British Journal of Psychiatry, 146*, 229–39.

Kovacs, M. & Beck, A. T. (1977). An empirical clinical approach toward a definition of child depression. In J. G. Schulterbrandt & A. Raskin (eds), *Depression in children: Diagnosis, treatment and conceptual models.* New York: Raven Press, pp. 1–25.

Kraepelin, E. (1896). *Demential praecox and paraphrenia.* (Trans. M. Barclay.) Edinburgh: Livingstone, 1919.

Kramlinger, K. & Post, R. (1989). The addition of lithium to carbamazepine. *Archives of General Psychiatry, 46*, 794–800.

Krasnov, V. & Kohanenko, E. (1989). Izmeneniya gormalnih pokazatele v terapevtichesko dinamike depressi raslichno nozologii. *Zhurna l Neuropatologii i Psikiatrii, 89*, 101–5.

Kulish, N. (1988). Precocious ego development and obsessive compulsive neurosis. *Journal of The American Academy of Psychoanalysis, 16(2)*, 167–87.

Kuriansky, J. B., Deming, W. E. & Gurland, B. J. (1974). On trends in the diagnosis of schizophrenia. *American Journal of Psychiatry, 126*, 1213.

Lang, P. (1977). Imagery in therapy: An information-processing analysis of fear. *Behavior Therapy, 8*, 862–86.

Langer, G., Neumark, J., Koinig, G., Graf, M. & Schonbeck, G. (1985). Rapid psychotherapeutic effects of anaesthesia with isoflurane (ES narcotherapy) in treatment-refractory depressed patients. *Neuropsychobiology, 14*, 118–20.

Larcombe, N. & Wilson, P. (1984). An evaluation of cognitive-behaviour therapy for depression in patients with multiple sclerosis. *British Journal of Psychiatry, 145*, 366–71.

Last, C. G. & Strauss, C. C. (1989). Obsessive compulsive disorder in childhood. *Journal of Anxiety Disorders, 3(4)*, 295–302.

Leff, J. P., Kuipers, L., Berkowitz, R., Eberlein-Fries, R. & Sturgeon, D. (1982). A controlled trial of social intervention in schizophrenic families. *British Journal of Psychiatry, 141*, 121–34.

Leff, J. P. & Vaughn, C. E. (1985). *Expressed emotion in families*. New York: Guilford Press.

Leonard, H. L., Swedo, S. E., Rapoport, J. L., Koby, E. V., Lenane, M., Cheslow, D. & Hamburger, S. D. (1989). Treatment of obsessive compulsive disorder with clomipramine and desipramine in children and adolescents. *Archives of General Psychiatry, 46(12)*, 1088–92.

Lester, D. (1977). Multiple personality: A review. *Psychology, 14*, 54–9.

Lewis, S. W., Murray, R. M. & Owen, M. (1988). Obstetric complications in schizophrenia: Methodology and mechanisms. In S. C. Schulz & T. Tamminga (eds), *Proceedings of the First International Congress of Schizophrenia*. New York: Oxford University Press.

Lidz, T., Cornelison, A. R., Fleck, S. & Terry, D. (1957). The intrafamilial environment of the schizophrenic patient. *Psychiatry, 20*, 329–42.

Liebowitz, M. R., Hollander, E., Fairbanks, J. & Campeas, R. (1990). Fluoxetine for adolescents with obsessive compulsive disorder. *American Journal of Psychiatry, 14(3)*, 370–71.

Linet, L. (1989). Treatment of a refractory depression with a combination of fluoxetine and d-amphetamine. *American Journal of Psychiatry, 146*, 803–4.

Lipsedge, M. S. & Prothero, W. (1987). Clonidine and clomipramine in obsessive compulsive disorder. *American Journal of Psychiatry, 144(7)*, 965–66.

Lo Piccolo, L. & Heiman, J. R. (1978). Sexual assessment and history interview. In J. Lo Piccolo & L. Lo Piccolo (eds), *Handbook of sex therapy*. New York: Plenum Press.

Lobitz, W. C. & Lobitz, G. K. (1978). Clinical assessment in the treatment of sexual dysfunctions. In J. Lo Piccolo & L. Lo Piccolo (eds), *Handbook of sex therapy.* Plenum Press: New York.

Loeber, R. (1982). The stability of antisocial and delinquent child behaviour: A review. *Child Development*, *53*, 1431–46.

Loeber, R. (1991). Antisocial behavior: More enduring than changeable? *American Academy of Child and Adolescent Psychiatry*, *30*, 393–97.

Looke, H. & Wallace, K. (1959). Short marital-adjustment and prediction tests: Their reliability and validity. *Marriage and Family Living*, *21*, 251–55.

Lorenz, K. (1969). Innate basis of learning. In K. Pribram (ed.), *On the biology of learning*. New York: Harcourt Brace Jovanovich.

Lovaas, O. I. (1987). Behavioural treatment and normal educational and intellectual functioning in young autistic children. *Journal of Consulting and Clinical Psychology*, *55*, 3–9.

Lovibond, S. H., Birrell, P. C. & Langeluddecke, P. (1986). Changing coronary heart disease risk-factor status: The effects of three behavioral programs. *Journal of Behavioral Medicine*, *9*, 415–37.

Lustman, P., Kulkarni, S. & Amado, H. (1983). Treatment of depression accompanying panhypopituitarism. *Psychosomatics*, *24*, 7–75.

Luxenberg, J. S., Swedo, S.E., Flament, M.F. & Friedland, R.P. (1988). Neuroanatomical abnormalities in obsessive compulsive disorder detected with quantitative X-ray computed tomography. *American Journal of Psychiatry*, *145(9)*, 1089–93.

Mackay, A. V. P. & Crow, T. J. (1980). Positive and negative symptoms and the role of dopamine. *British Journal of Psychiatry*, *137*, 379–86.

MacMillan, J. F., Gold, A., Crow, T. J., Johnson, A. L. & Johnson, E. C. (1986). Expressed emotion and relapse in first episodes of schizophrenia. *British Journal of Psychiatry*, *151*, 741–44.

Madanes, C. (1980). Protection, paradox and pretending. *Family Process*, *19*, 73–85.

Mai, F. (1989). Depression in physical illnesses. *Psychiatric Journal of the University of Ottawa*, *14*, 354–55.

Malmo, R. (1975). *On emotions, needs, and our archaic brain*. New York: Holt, Rinehart, Winston.

Marks, I. (1969). *Fears and phobias*. London: Academic Press.

Marks, I. (1972). Flooding (implosion) and allied treatments. In W. Agras (ed.), *Behaviour modification: Principles and clinical applications*. Boston: Little, Brown.

Marks, I. (1987). *Fears, phobias and rituals*. New York: Oxford University Press.

Marks, R. C. & Luchins, D. J. (1990). Relationship between brain imaging findings in schizophrenia and psychopathology: A review of the literature relating to positive and negative symptoms. In N. C. Andreasen (ed.), *Modern problems of pharmacopsychiatry: Positive and negative symptoms and syndromes*. Basel, Switzerland: S. Karger, pp. 89–123.

Marlatt, G. A. & George, W. H. (1984). Relapse prevention: Introduction and overview of the model. *British Journal of Addiction, 79*, 261–73.

Marlatt, G. A. & Gordon, J. R. (1985). *Relapse prevention.* New York: Guilford Press.

Marshall, W., Gauthier, J. & Gordon, A. (1979). The current status of flooding therapy. In M. Herson, R. Eisler & Miller (eds), *Progress in behaviour modification*, vol. 7. New York: Academic Press.

Maslow, A. H. (1968). *Toward a psychology of being.* New York: van Nostrand-Reinhold.

Masters, W. H. & Johnson, V. E. (1970). *Human sexual inadequacy.* Boston: Little, Brown and Co.

Mathews, A., Gelder, M. & Johnston, D. W. (1981). *Agoraphobia: Nature and treatment.* London: Guilford Press.

Mattick, R. P. & Baillie, A. (1992). *An outline for approaches to smoking cessation: Quality assurance project.* Canberra: Australian Government Publishing Service.

Mattick, R. P. & Hall, W. (1992). *A treatment outline for approaches to opiate/polydrug dependence.* Canberra: Australian Government Publishing Service. In press.

Mattick, R. P. & Jarvis, T. (1992). *An outline for the management of alcohol dependence and abuse.* Canberra: Australian Government Publishing Service (in press).

Mattick, R. P. & Newman, C. (1991). Social phobia and avoidant personality disorder. *International Review of Psychiatry, 3*, 163–73.

Mattick, R. P. & Peters, L. (1988). Treatment of severe social phobia: Effects of guided exposure with and without cognitive restructuring. *Journal of Consulting and Clinical Psychology, 56*, 251–60.

Mattick, R. P., Peters, L. & Clarke, J. C. (1989). Exposure and cognitive restructuring for social phobia: A controlled study. *Behavior Therapy, 20*, 3–23.

Mattick, R. P. & Ward, J. (1992). Drug and alcohol treatment research, policy and practice: An Australian perspective. *Journal of Drug Issues* (in press).

MavissaKalian, M. (1988). The relationship between panic, phobic, and anticipatory anxiety in agoraphobia. *Behaviour Research and Therapy, 26*, 235–40.

Mayeux, R. (1990). Parkinson's disease: A review of cognitive and psychiatric disorders. *Neuropsychiatry, Neuropsychology, and Behavioral Neurology, 3*, 3–14.

McConaghy, N. (1960). Modes of abstract thinking and psychosis. *American Journal of Psychiatry, 117*, 106–10.

McConaghy, N., Catts, S. V., Michic, P. T., Fox, A. M., Ward, P. B. & Shellcy, A.M. (in revision). *P300 indexes thought disorder in schizophrenics but allusive thinking in normals.*

McCord, W. & McCord, J. (1969). *Origins of crime.* Montclair, N.J.: Patterson Smith.

McGhie, A. & Chapman, J. (1961). Disorders of attention and perception in early schizophrenia. *British Journal of Medical Psychology, 34*, 103–17.

McMullen, S. & Rosen, R. C. (1979). Self-administered masturbation training in the treatment of primary orgasmic dysfunction. *Journal of Consulting and Clinical Psychology, 47*, 912–18.

McPherson, A. H., Ward, P. B., Michie, P. T., Catts, S. V., Mitchell, P., McConaghy, N., Andrews, S. & Shelley, A. M. (1991). An event-related potential (ERP) analysis of attention in acute and remitted psychotic patients with schizophrenic symptoms. *Biological Psychiatry, 29*, 224S.

Mednick, S. A. (1958). A learning theory approach to research in schizophrenia. *Psychological Bulletin, 55*, 316–27.

Meehl, P. (1962). Schotaxia, schiotypy, schizophrenia. *American Psychologist, 17*, 827–38.

Mehta, M. (1990). A comparative study of family-based and patient-based behavioural management in obsessive compulsive disorder. *British Journal of Psychiatry, 157*, 133–35.

Meichenbaum, D. H. & Genest, M. (1980). Cognitive behavior modification. In F. H. Kanfer & A. P. Goldstein (eds), *Helping people change: A textbook of methods*. New York: Pergamon Press.

Meyer, A. (1917). The aims and meaning of psychiatric diagnosis. *American Journal of Insanity, 74*, 163–68.

Miller, G. A., Simons, R. F. & Lang, P. J. (1984). Electro-cortical measures of information processing deficit in anhedonia. *Annals of the New York Academy of Sciences, 425*, 498–602.

Miller, I., Bishop, S., Norman, W. & Keitner, G. (1985). Cognitive-behavioural therapy and pharmacotherapy with chronic, drug-refractory depressed inpatients: A note of optimism. *Behavioural Psychotherapy, 13*, 320–27.

Miller, N. & Reise, R. (1991). Drug and alcohol dependence and psychiatric populations: The need for diagnosis, intervention, and training. *Comprehensive Psychiatry, 32*, 268–76.

Miller, W. (1975). Psychological deficit in depression. *Psychological Bulletin, 82*, 238–60.

Miller, W. R. (1983). Motivational interviewing with problem drinkers. *Behavioural Psychotherapy, 11*, 147–72.

Miller, W. R. (1987). Behavioral alcohol treatment research advances: Barriers to utilization. *Advances in Behavior Research and Therapy, 9*, 145–64.

Miller, W. R. & Rollnick, S. (1991). *Motivational interviewing: Preparing people to change addictive behaviours*. New York: Guilford.

Miller, W. R., Sovereign, R. G. & Krege, B. (1988). Motivational interviewing with problem drinkers: II. The drinker's check-up as a preventive intervention. *Behavioural Psychotherapy, 16*, 251–68.

Mitchell, P. F., Andrews, S., Fox, A. M., Catts, S. V., Ward, P. B. & McConaghy, N. (1991). Active and passive attention in schizophrenia: An ERP study of information processing in a linguistic task. *Biological Psychology, 32*, 101–24.

Monti, P. M., Abrams, D. B., Kadden, R. M. & Cooney, N. L. (1989). *Treating alcohol dependence: A coping skills training guide*. New York: Guilford.

Murphy, S. M., Kilpatrick, D. G., Amick-McMullan, A., Veronen, L. J. et al. (1988). Current psychological functioning of child sexual assault survivors: A community study. *Journal of Interpersonal Violence, 3(1)*, 55–61.

Murray, R. M., Lewis, S. W., Owen, M. & Foerster, A. (1988). The neurodevelopmental origins of dementia praecox. In P. Bebbington & P. McGuffin (eds), *Schizophrenia: The major issues*. London: Heinemann, pp. 90–108.

Nathan, P. E. (1991). Substance use disorders in the DSM-IV. *Journal of Abnormal Psychology, 100*, 356–61.

Nathan, S. G. (1986). The epidemiology of the DSM-III psychosexual dysfunctions. *Journal of Sex and Marital Therapy. 12*, 267–81.

Neale, J. & Oltmans, T. (1980). *Schizophrenia*. New York: John Wiley & Sons.

Neisser, U. (1976). *Cognition and reality: Principles and implications of cognitive psychology*. San Francisco, Calif.: Freeman.

Nierenberg, A. & Amsterdam, J. (1990). Treatment-resistant depression: Definition and treatment approaches. *Journal of Clinical Psychiatry, 51(6)*, Supplement, 39–47.

Njiokiktjien, C. (1991). Absence of the corpus callosum: Clinicopathological correlations. In G. Ramaekers & C. Njiokiktjien (eds), *The child's corpus callosum: Pediatric Behavioural Neurology*, vol. 3. Amsterdam: Suyi Publications, pp. 235–50.

Norman, T., Sartor, D. & McIntyre, I. (1988). Clinical and experimental studies on the potentiation of antidepressant drugs by thyroid hormones. *Medical Sciences Research, 16*, 545-50.

Norman, W., Miller, I. & Keitner, G. (1987). Relationship between dysfunctional cognitions and depressive subtypes. *Canadian Journal of Psychiatry, 32*, 194–98.

Norman, W., Miller, I. & Klee, S. (1983). Assessment of cognitive distortion in a clinically depressed population. *Cognitive Therapy and Research, 7*, 133–40.

Norton, G., Dorward, J. & Cox, B. (1986). Factors associated with panic attacks in nonclinical subjects. *Behaviour Therapy, 17*, 239–52.

Norton, G., Malan, J., Cairns, S., Wozney, K. & Broughton, R. (1989). Factors influencing drinking behaviours in alcoholic panickers and non-panickers. *Behaviour Research and Therapy, 27*, 167–71.

Noyes, R., Clancy, J., Garvey, M. & Anderson, D. (1987). Is agoraphobia a variant of panic disorder or a separate illness? *Journal of Anxiety Disorders, 1*, 3–13.

Nuechterlein, K. H. & Dawson, M. E. (1984). Information processing and attentional functioning in the developmental course of schizophrenic disorders. *Schizophrenia Bulletin, 10*, 160–203.

Ontiveros, A., Fontaine, R. & Elie, R. (1991). Refractory depression: The addition of lithium to fluoxetine or desipramine. *Acta Psychiatrica Scandinavica, 83*, 188–92.

Orne, M. T., Dinges, D. F. & Orne, E. C. (1984). On the differential diagnosis of multiple personality in a forensic case. *International Journal of Clinical and Experimental Hypnosis, 32*, 118–69.

Ost, I. (1987). Applied relaxation: Description of a coping technique and review of controlled studies. *Behaviour Research and Therapy, 26*, 13–22.

Owens, D., Johnstone, E. C., Crow, T. J., Frith, C. D., Jagoe, J. R. & Kreel, L. (1985). Lateral ventricular size in schizophrenia: Relationship to the disease process and its clinical manifestation. *Psychological Medicine*, *15*, 27–41.

Ozonoff, S, Pennington, B. & Rogers, S. (1991). Executive function deficits in high-functioning autistic individuals: Relationship to theory of mind. *Journal of Child Psychology and Psychiatry, 32(7)*, 1081–1106.

Parikh, R., Lipsey, J., Robinson, R. & Price, T. (1988). A two-year longitudinal study of poststroke mood disorders: Prognostic factors related to one and two year outcome. *International Journal of Psychiatry in Medicine*, *18*, 45–56.

Parnas, J., Schulsinger, F., Teasdale, T. W., Schulsinger, H., Feldman, P. M. & Mednick, S. A. (1982). Perinatal complications and clinical outcome within the schizophrenia spectrum. *British Journal of Psychology*, *140*, 416–20.

Patel, C. (1987). *Fighting heart disease*. London: Dorling Kindersley.

Patterson, G. R., Dishion, T. J. & Bank, L. (1984). Family interaction: A process model of deviancy training. *Aggressive Behavior*, *10*, 253–67.

Paul, G. (1979). Outcome of systematic desensitization. In C. M. Franks (ed.), *Behaviour therapy: Appraisal and status*. New York: McGraw-Hill.

Petit, M. & Dollfus, S. (1986). Facteurs biochimiques de resistance aux antidepresseurs. *L'Encephale*, *12*, 207–15.

Petti, T. A. (1978). Depression in hospitalized psychiatry patients: Approaches to measuring depression. *Journal of the American Academy of Child Psychiatry*, *22*, 11–21.

Philipp, M., Maier, W. & Delmo, C. (1991a). The concept of major depression: I. Descriptive comparison of six competing operational definitions including ICD-10 and DSM-III-R. *European Archives of Psychiatry and Clinical Neuroscience*, *240*, 258–65.

Philipp, M., Maier, W. & Delmo, C. (1991b). The concept of major depression: II. Agreement between six competing operational definitions in 600 psychiatric inpatients. *European Archives of Psychiatry and Clinical Neuroscience*, *240*, 266–71.

Poirier, M. & Benkelfat, C. (1986). Bonnes et mauvaises associations therapeutiques dans le traitement des depressions resistantes. *L'Encephale*, *12*, 225–30.

Polich, J. (1991). P300 in clinical applications: Meaning, method and measurement. *American Journal of EEG Technology*, *31*, 201–31.

Pols, R. G. & Hawks, D. V. (1987). *Is there a safe level of daily consumption of alcohol for men and women? Recommendations regarding responsible drinking behaviour*. Canberra: Australian Government Publishing Service.

Pope, H., McElroy, S. & Nixon, R. (1988). Possible synergism between fluoxetine and lithium in refractory depression. *American Journal of Psychiatry*, *145*, 1292–94.

Popkin, M., Tucker, G. & Caine, E. (1989). The fate of organic mental disorders in DSM-IV: A progress report. *Psychosomatics*, *30*, 438-41.

Price, L., Charney, D. & Heninger, G. (1985). Efficacy of lithium-tranylcypromine treatment in refractory depression. *American Journal of Psychiatry*, *142*, 619–23.

Price, L., Charney, D. & Heninger, G. (1987). Reserpine augmentation of desipramine in refractory depression: Clinical and neurobiological effects. *Psychopharmacology, 92*, 431–37.

Prior, M. R. (1979). Cognitive abilities and disabilities in infantile autism: A review. *Journal of Abnormal Child Psychology, 7*, 357–80.

Prior, M. R. (1984). Developing concepts of childhood autism: The influence of experimental cognitive research. *Journal of Consulting and Clinical Psychology, 52*, 4–16.

Prior, M. & Griffin, M. (1985). *Hyperactivity: Diagnosis and management.* London: William Heinemann Medical Books.

Prior, M. & Hoffmann, W. (1990). Brief report: Neuropsychological testing of autistic children through an exploration with frontal lobe tests. *Journal of Autism and Developmental Disorders, 20(4)*, 581–90.

Prior, M. & Sanson, A. (1978). A follow-up study of autistic children in Victoria. *Australian Autism Review, 4*, 20-23.

Prior, M., Tress, B., Hoffmann, W. & Boldt, D. (1984). A computed tomographic study of children with classic autism. *Archives of Neurology, 41(5)*, 482.

Prior, M. & Werry, J. (1986). Autism, schizophrenia and allied disorders. In H. Quay & J. Werry (eds), *Psychopathological disorders of childhood* (3rd ed.). New York: John Wiley & Sons, pp. 156–210.

Pritchard, W. S. (1981). Psychophysiology of P300. *Psychological Bulletin, 89*, 506–40.

Pritchard, W. S. (1986). Cognitive event-related potential correlates of schizophrenia. *Psychological Bulletin, 100*, 43–66.

Prochaska, J. O. & DiClemente C. C. (1984). Self-change processes, self-efficacy and decisional balance across five stages of smoking cessation. In P. F. Anderson, L. E. Mortenson & L. E. Epstein (eds), *Advance in cancer control.* New York: Alan R. Liss, Inc.

Prochaska, J. O. & DiClemente C. C. (1986). Toward a comprehensive model of change. In W. R. Miller & N. Heather (eds), *Treating addictive behaviors: Processes of change.* New York: Plenum Press, pp. 3–27.

Putnam, F. W. (1989). *Diagnosis and treatment of MPD.* New York: Guildford.

Putnam, F. W., Guroff, J. J., Silberman, E. K., Barban, L. & Post, R. M. (1986). The clinical phenomenology of multiple personality disorder: Review of 100 recent cases. *Journal of Clinical Psychiatry, 57*, 285–93.

Quay, H. C. (1979). Classification. In H. C. Quay & J. S. Werry (eds), *Psychopathological disorders of childhood* (2nd ed.). New York: John Wiley & Sons.

Quay, H. C. & Petersen, D. R. (1983). *The revised behavior problem checklist.* Miami, Fla.: University of Miami.

Queiroz, L. O., Motta, M. A., Madi, M. B., Sossai, D. L. & Boren, J. J. (1981). A functional analysis of obsessive-compulsive problems with related therapeutic problems. *Behaviour Research and Therapy, 19*, 377–88.

Rachman, S. (1984). The experimental analysis of agoraphobia. *Behaviour Research and Therapy, 22*, 631–40.

Rachman, S. J. (1991). Neo-conditioning and the classical theory of fear acquisition. *Clinical Psychology Review, 11*, 155–75.

Rachman, S. J. & Hodgson, R. J. (1980). *Obsessions and compulsions*. Englewood, N.J.: Prentice Hall.

Ramaekers, G. (1991). Functions of the corpus callosum in adults. In G. Ramaekers & C. Njiokiktjien (eds), *The child's corpus callosum: Pediatric behavioural neurology*, vol. 3. Amsterdam: Suyi Publications, pp. 40–77.

Rapee, R. (1985). A case of panic disorder treated with breathing retraining. *Journal of Behavior and Experimental Psychiatry, 16*, 63–65.

Rapee, R., Mattick, R. & Murrell, E. (1986). Predictors of agoraphobic avoidance: An exploratory analysis. *Journal of Anxiety Disorder*, 2, 203–17.

Rapee, R. M. & Murrell, E. (1988). Predictors of agoraphobic avoidance. *Journal of Anxiety Disorders*, 2, 203–17.

Rapoport, J. L. (1986). Antidepressants in childhood attention deficit disorder and obsessive compulsive disorder. *Psychosomatics, 27(11)*, 30–36.

Rapoport, J. L. (1989). *Obsessive-compulsive disorder in children and adolescents*. Washington D.C.: American Psychiatric Press Inc.

Rasmussen, S. A. & Tsuang, M. T. (1986). Clinical characteristics and family history in DSM-III obsessive-compulsive disorder. *American Journal of Psychiatry, 143*, 317–22.

Rathus, S. A. (1973). A 30 item schedule for assessing assertive behavior. *Behavior Therapy, 4*, 398–406.

Raw, M. (1986). Smoking cessation strategies. In W. R. Miller & N. Heather (eds), *Treating addictive behaviors: Processes of change*. New York: Plenum Press, pp. 279–87.

Regier, D. A., Farmer, M. E., Rae, D. S., Locke, B. Z., Keith, S. J., Judd, L. L. & Goodwin, F. K. (1990). Comorbidity of mental disorders with alcohol and other drug abuse: Results from the epidemiologic catchment area (ECA) study. *Journal of the American Medical Association, 264*, 2511-18.

Reiss, S., Peterson, R., Gursky, D. & McNally, R. (1986). Anxiety sensitivity, anxiety frequency, and the prediction of fearfullness. *Behavior Research and Therapy, 24*, 1–8.

Riddle, M. A., Scahill, L., King, R., Hardin, M. T., Towbin, K. E., Ort, S. I., Leckman, J. & Cohen, D. J. (1990). Obsessive compulsive disorder in children and adolescents. *Journal of the American Academy of Child and Adolescent Psychiatry, 29(5)*, 766–72.

Riley, A. J. & Riley, E.J . (1978). A controlled study to evaluate directed masturbation in the management of primary orgasmic failure in women. *British Journal of Psychiatry, 133*, 404–9.

Rimland, B. (1965). *Infantile autism* (2nd ed). New York: Appleton-Century-Crofts.

Rimland, B. (1971). The differentiation of childhood psychoses: An analysis of checklists for 2218 psychotic children. *Journal of Autism and Childhood Schizophrenia, 1(2)*, 161–74.

Rimm, D. & Masters, J. (1979). *Behavior therapy.* New York: Academic Press.

Risser, N. L. & Belcher, D. W. (1990). Adding spirometry, carbon monoxide, and pulmonary symptom results to smoking cessation counselling: A randomised trial. *Journal of General and Internal Medicine*, *5*, 16–22.
Robins, L.N. (1966). *Deviant children grown up*. Baltimore: The Williams & Wilkins Company.
Robins, L. N. (1978). Sturdy childhood predictors of adult antisocial behaviour: Replications from longitudinal studies. *Psychological Medicine*, *8*, 611–22.
Robins, L. N. (1979). Follow-up studies. In H. C. Quay & J. S. Werry (eds), *Psychopathological disorders of childhood* (2nd ed.). New York: John Wiley & Sons.
Robins, L. N. (1981). Epidemiological approaches to natural history research. *American Academy of Child Psychiatry*, *20*, 566–80.
Rosen, R. C. & Beck, J. G. (1988). Patterns of sexual arousal: Psychophysiological processes and clinical applications. New York: Guilford Press.
Rosenbaum, M. (1980). The role of the term schizophrenia in the decline of the diagnosis of multiple personality. *Archives of General Psychiatry*, *37*, 1383–85.
Ross C. A. (1989). *Multiple personality disorder: Diagnosis, clinical features and treatment*. New York: John Wiley & Sons.
Ross, D. & Ross, S. (1976). Hyperactivity: Current issues, research and theory (2nd ed). New York: John Wiley & Sons.
Rothenberg, A. (1990). Adolescence and eating disorder: The obsessive compulsive syndrome. *Psychiatric Clinics of North America*, *13(3)*, 469–88.
Russell, G. F. M. (1973). The management of anorexia nervosa. *Symposium of Anorexia Nervosa and Obesity: Royal College of Physicians of Edinburgh*, *42*.
Rutter, M. (1982). Syndromes attributed to minimal brain dysfunction in childhood. *Journal of Psychiatry*, *139*, 21–32.
Rutter, M. (1983). Cognitive deficits in the pathogenesis of autism. *Journal of Child Psychology & Psychiatry*, *27(2)*, 513–31.
Rutter, M. (1989a). Annotation: Child psychiatric disorders in ICD-10. *Journal of Child Psychology & Psychiatry*, *30(4)*, 499–513.
Rutter, M. (1989b). Attention deficit disorder/hyperkinetic syndrome: Conceptual and research issues regarding diagnosis and classification. In T. Sagrolden & T. Archer (eds), *Attention deficit disorder: Clinical and basic research*. Hillsdale, N.J.: Erlbaum.
Rutter, M., Bolton, P., Harrington, R., Le Couteur, A., Macdonald, H. & Simonoff, E. (1990). Genetic factors in child psychiatric disorders — II: Empirical Findings. *Journal of Child Psychology and Psychiatry*, *31(1)*, 39–83.
Rutter, M., Cox, A., Tupling, C., Berger, M. & Yule, W. (1975). Attainment and adjustment in two geographical areas: The prevalence of psychiatric disorder. *British Journal of Psychiatry*, *126*, 493–509.
Rutter, M. & Giller, H. (1983). *Juvenile delinquency: Trends and perspectives*. Middlesex, England: Penguin Books.
Rutter, M., MacDonald, H., Le Couteur, A., Harrington, R., Bolton, P. & Bailey, A. (1990). Genetic factors in child psychiatric disorders: Empirical findings. *Journal of Child Psychology and Psychiatry*, *31*, 39–83.
Rutter, M. & Quinton, D. (1984). Parental psychiatric disorder: Effects on children. *Psychological Medicine*, *14*, 853–80.

Saitoh, O., Niwa, S., Hiramatsu, K., Kameyama, T., Rymar, K. & Itoh, K. (1984). Abnormalities in late positive components of event-related potentials may reflect a genetic predisposition to schizophrenia. *Biological Psychiatry, 19*, 293–303.

Sandberg, S. T., Wieselberg, M. & Shaffer, D. (1980). Hyperkinetic and conduct problem children in a primary school population: Some epidemiological considerations. *Journal of Child Psychology and Psychiatry, 21*, 293–310.

Sanders, G. L. & Cairns, K. V. (1987). Loss of sexual spontaneity. *Medical Aspects of Human Sexuality, 21* 37–43.

Sanders, M. R. & Dadds, M. R. (1982). The effects of planned activities and child management training in parent training: An analysis of setting generalization. *Behavior Therapy, 13*, 452–61.

Sanders, M. R. & Dadds, M. R. (1992). *Behavioral family intervention*. New York: Pergamon Press.

Sarbin, T. R. & Coe, W. C. (1979). Hypnosis and psychopathology: Replacing old myths with fresh metaphors. *Journal of Abnormal Psychology, 88*, 506–25.

Schneider, K. (1959). *Clinical Psychopathology.* (Trans. M. W. Hamilton.) London: Grune & Stratton.

Schover, L. R. & Lo Piccolo, J. (1982). Treatment effectiveness for dysfunctions of sexual desire. *Journal of Sex and Marital Therapy, 8*, 179–97.

Schreiner-Engel, P. & Schiavi, R. C. (1986). Lifetime psychopathology in individuals with low sexual desire. *Journal of Nervous Mental Disorders, 174*, 646–51.

Schulsinger, F. (1980). Biological psychopathology. *Annual Review of Psychology, 31*, 583–606.

Schulsinger, F., Parnas, J., Petersen, E. T., Schulsinger, H., Teasdate, T. W., Mednick, S. A., Moller, L. & Silverton, L. (1984). Cerebral ventricular size in the offspring of schizophrenia mothers. *Archives of General Psychiatry, 41*, 602–6.

Schwartz, S. (1981). Language coding abilities in infantile autism. *Applied Psycholinguistics, 2*, 25–31.

Schwartz, S. (1982). Is there a schizophrenic language? *The Behavioral and Brain Sciences, 5*, 579–626.

Schwartz, S. & Johnson, J. H. (1985). *Psychopathology of childhood* (2nd ed.). Elmsford, N.Y.: Pergamon Press.

Seligman, M. (1970). On the generality of the laws of learning. *Psychological Review, 77*, 406–18.

Selyé, H. (1976). *The stress of life* (rev. ed.). New York: McGraw-Hill.

Shah, A. & Wing, L. (1986). Cognitive impairments affecting social behaviour in autism. In E. Schopler & G. Mosibov (eds), *Social Behaviour in Autism*. New York: Plenum, pp. 153–169.

Shakow, D. (1962). Segmental set: A theory of the formal psychological deficit in schizophrenia. *Archives of General Psychiatry, 6*, 1–17.

Shantz, C. U. (1983). Social cognition. In P. H. Mussen (ed.), *Handbook of child psychology: Cognitive development* (4th ed.), vol. III. New York: Wiley & Sons, pp. 495–555.

Share, D. L. & Schwartz, S. (1988). A note on the distinction between attention deficit disorder and reading disability: Are there group-specific cognitive deficits? *Brain & Language, 34*, 350–52.

Shaywitz, S. E. & Shaywitz, B. A. (1989). Critical issues in attention deficit disorder. In T. Sagrolden & T. Archer (eds), *Attention deficit disorder: Clinical and basic research*. Hillsdale, N.J.: Lawrence Erlbaum Associates.

Shea, M., Pilkonis, P., Beckham, E., Collins, J., Elkin, I., Sotsky, S., & Docherty, J. (1990). Personality disorders and treatment outcome in the NIMH treatment of depression collaborative research program. *American Journal of Psychiatry, 147*, 711–18.

Sheehan, D. (1982). Current concepts of psychiatry: Panic attacks and phobiae. *New England Journal of Medicine, 307*, 156–58.

Sher, K. J., Mann, B. & Frost, R. O. (1984). Cognitive deficits in compulsive checkers: Further explorations. *Behaviour Research and Therapy, 22*, 493–502.

Siegman, A. W., Dembroski, T. M. & Ringel, N. (1987). Components of hostility and the severity of coronary artery disease. *Psychosomatic Medicine, 49*, 127–35.

Simons, R. F. (1982). Physical anhedonia and future psychopathology: An electrocortical continuity? *Psychophysiology, 19*, 433–41.

Sims, A. (1988). *Symptoms in the mind: An introduction to descriptive psychotherapy*. London: Balliere Tundall.

Smith, J. & Birchwood, M. (1987). Education for families with schizophrenic relatives. *British Journal of Psychiatry, 150*, 645–52.

Southworth, S. & Kirsch, I. (1988). The role of expectancy in exposure-generated fear reduction in agoraphobia. *Behaviour Research and Therapy, 26*, 113–20.

Spanier, G. B. (1976). Measuring dyadic adjustment. *Journal of Marriage and the Family, 38*, 15–28.

Spanos, N. P., Weekes, J. R. & Bertrand, L. D. (1985). Multiple personality: A social psychological perspective. *Journal of Abnormal Psychology, 94*, 362–76.

Spence, S. H. (1985). Group versus individual treatment of primary and secondary female orgasmic dysfunction. *Behaviour Research and Therapy, 23*, 539–48.

Spence, S. H. (1991). *Psychosexual therapy: A cognitive-behavioural approach*. London: Chapman & Hall.

Spielberger, C. D., Gorsuch, R. L. & Lushene, R. E., (1970). *STAI Manual*. Palo Alto: Consulting Psychologists Press.

Spitzer, R. L., Endicott, J. & Robins, E. (1978). Research diagnostic criteria: Rationale and reliability. *Archives of General Psychiatry, 35*, 773–82.

Steinberg, M., Howland, F. & Cicchetti, D. (1986). *The structured clinical interview for DSM-III-R dissociative disorders: A preliminary report on proceedings of the Third International Conference on Multiple Personality/Dissociative States*. Chicago: Rush-Presbyterian-St. Lukes Medical Center.

Stephens, D. A., Astrup, C., Carpenter, W. T., Jr., Shaffer, J. W. & Goldberg, J. (1982). A comparison of nine systems to diagnose schizophrenia. *Psychiatry Research, 6*, 127–43.

Stephens, J. (1978). Long-term prognosis and follow-up in schizophrenia. *Schizophrenia Bulletin, 4*, 25–30.

Stevens, B. C. (1973). Evaluation of rehabilitation for psychotic patients in the community. *Acta Psychiatrica Scandinavica, 46*, 136–40.

Stoller, L. & McNally, R. (1991). Cognitive bias in symptomatic and recovered agoraphobics. *Behaviour Research and Therapy, 29*, 539–45.

Strang, J. & Farrell, M. (1991). *Hepatitis*. London: Institute for the Study of Drug Dependence.

Strauss, A. & Lehtinen L. E. (1947). *Psychopathology and education of the brain injured child*. New York: Grune & Stratton.

Stress Working Party (1988). Stress and cardiovascular disease: A report from the National Heart Foundation of Australia. *Medical Journal of Australia, 148*, 510–14.

Strober, M. & Yager, J. (1985). A developmental perspective on the treatment of anorexia nervosa in adolescents. In D. M. Garner & P. E. Garfinkel (eds), *Handbook of psychotherapy for anorexia nervosa and bulimia*. New York: Guilford Press.

Swedo, S. E., Rapoport, J. L., Leonard, H., Lenane, M. & Cheslow, D. (1989). Obsessive compulsive disorder in children and adolescents: Clinical phenomenology of 70 consecutive cases. *Archives of General Psychiatry, 46(4)*, 335–41.

Szatmari, P., Bartolucci, C. & Bremner, R. (1983). Aspergers syndrome and autism comparisons on early history and outcome. *Developmental Medicine & Child Neuropsychology, 31*, 709–20.

Tanaghow, A., Lewis, J. & Jones, G. (1989). Anterior tumour of the corpus callosum with atypical depression. *British Journal of Psychiatry, 155*, 854–56.

Tantam, D. (1991). Asperger syndrome in adulthood. In U. Frith (ed.), *Autism and Asperger syndrome*. Cambridge: Cambridge University Press.

Targum, S., Greenberg, R., Harmon, R., Kessler, K., Salerian, A. & Fram, D. (1984). Thyroid hormone and the TRH stimulation test in refractory depression. *Journal of Clinical Psychiatry, 45*, 345–46.

Tarrier, N. & Barrowclough, C. (1990). Family interventions for schizophrenia. *Behavior Modification, 14(4)*, 408–40.

Tarrier, N., Barrowclough, C., Porceddu, K. & Watts, S. (1988). The assessment of psychophysiological reactivity to the expressed emotion of the relatives of schizophrenic families. *British Journal of Psychiatry, 152*, 618–24.

Task Force on DSM-IV. (1991). *DSM-IV options book: Work in progress — 9/1/91*. Washington, D.C.: American Psychiatric Association.

Teasedale, G. & Jennett, B. (1974). Assessment of coma and impaired consciousness: A practical scale. *Lancet, 2*, 81–84.

Thigpen, C. H. & Cleckley, H. M. (1957). *The three faces of Eve*. New York: McGraw-Hill.

Thyer, B., Himle, J. & Fischer, F. (1988). Is parental death a selective precursor to either panic disorder or agoraphobia? A test of the separation anxiety hypothesis. *Journal of Anxiety Disorders, 2*, 333–38.

Tinbergen, N. (1951). *The study of instinct*. Oxford: Clarendon Press.

Torgersen, S. (1983). Genetic factors in anxiety disorders. *Archives of General Psychiatry, 140*, 1085–89.

Touyz, S. W., Beumont, P.J.V & Dunn, S. M. (1987). Behaviour therapy in the management of patients with anorexia nervosa: A lenient flexible approach. *Psychotherapy and Psychosomatics, 48*, 151–56.

Touyz, S. W., Beumont, P.J.V., Glaun, D., Phillips, T. & Cowie, I. (1984). A comparison of lenient and strict operant conditioning programmes in refeeding patients with anorexia nervosa. *British Journal of Psychiatry, 144*, 517–20.

Turner, S., Toone, B. & Brett-Jones, A. (1986). Computersied tomography scans in early schizophrenia — preliminary findings. *Psychological Medicine, 16(1)*, 219–25.

Van Krevelen, D. (1971). Early infantile autism and autistic psychopathy. *Journal of Autism and Childhood Schizophrenia, 1*, 82–86.

Vandereycken, W. (1987). The management of patients with anorexia nervosa and bulimia — basic principles and guidelines. In P. J. V. Beumont, G. D. Burrows & R. C. Casper (eds), *Handbook of eating disorders. Part 1. Anorexia and bulimia nervosa*. Amsterdam: Elsevier, pp. 235–54.

Venables, J. F. (1930). Anorexia nervosa, study of the pathogenesis of nine cases. *Guys Hospital Report, 80*, 213.

Venables, P. H. (1964). Performance and level of activation in schizophrenics and normals. *British Journal of Psychology, 55*, 207–18.

Venables, P. H. (1978). Cognitive disorder. In J. K. Wing (ed.), *Schizophrenia: Toward a new synthesis*. London: Academic Press, pp. 117-37.

Wakefield, J. C. (1987). The semantics of success: Do masturbation exercises lead to partner orgasm? *Journal of Sex and Marital Therapy, 13*, 3–14.

Wallace, D. H. & Barbach, L. G. (1974). Preorgasmic group treatment. *Journal of Sex and Marital Therapy, 1*, 146–54.

Ward, C., Beck, A., Mendelson, M., Mock, J. & Erbaugh, J. (1962). The psychiatric nomenclature. *Archives of General Psychiatry, 7*, 198–205.

Ward, J., Darke, S., Hall, W. & Mattick, R. (1992). Methadone maintenance and the human immunodeficiency virus: Current issues in treatment and research. *British Journal of Addiction, 87*, 447–53.

Ward, J., Mattick, R. P. & Hall, W. (1992). *Key issues in methadone maintenance therapy: A research perspective*. Sydney: University of New South Wales Press.

Ward, P. B., Catts, S. V., Armstrong, M. A. & McConaghy, N. (1984). P300 and psychiatric vulnerability in university students. *Annals of the New York Academy of Sciences, 425*, 645–52.

Ward, P. B., Catts, S. V., Fox, A. M., Michie, P. T. & McConaghy, N. (1991). Auditory selective attention and event-related potentials in schizophrenia. *British Journal of Psychiatry, 158*, 534–39.

Ward, P. B., Catts, S. W. & McConaghy, N. (in press). P300 and conceptual loosening in normals: An event-related potential correlate of 'thought disorder'?

Waterhouse, L. & Fein, D. (1984). Developmental trends in cognitive skills for children diagnosed as autistic and schizophrenic. *Child Development, 55*, 236–48.

Watson, J. & Rayner, R. (1920). Conditioned emotional reactions. *Journal of Experimental Psychology, 3*, 1–14.

Wechsler, D. (1967). *Wechsler Preschool and Primary Scale of Intelligence*. New York: Psychological Corporation.

Wechsler, D. (1974). *WISC-R manual: Wechsler Intelligence Scale for Children* (rev.) New York: Psychological Corporation.

Weekes, C. (1977). *Simple effective treatment*. London: Angus & Robertson.

Weiss, G., Minde, K., Wherry, J. S., Douglas, V. & Nemeth, E. (1971). Studies on the hyperactive child: VIII. Five year follow-up. *Archives of General Psychiatry, 24*, 409–14.

Weissman, A. & Beck, A. (1978). *Development and validation of the Dysfunctional Attitude Scale: A preliminary investigation*. Paper presented at the annual meeting of the American Educational Research Association, Toronto, Canada.

Welkowitz, L. A., Bond, R. N. & Anderson, L. T. (1989). Social skills and initial response to behaviour therapy for obsessive compulsive disorder. *Phobia Practice and Research Journal, 2(2)*, 67–86.

West, D. J. (1982). *Delinquency: Its roots, careers and prospects*. London: Heinemann.

West, D. J. & Farrington, D. P. (1977). *The delinquent way of life*. London: Heinemann.

Wilcox, D. & Hager, R. (1980). Toward realistic expectations for orgasmic response in women. *Journal of Sex Research, 16*, 162–79.

Williams, C. A. & Forehand, R. (1984). An examination of predictor variables for child compliance and noncompliance. *Journal of Abnormal Child Psychology, 12*, 491–504.

Williams, G. (1987). Erectile dysfunction: Diagnosis and treatment. *British Journal of Urology, 60*, 1–5.

Williams J. M. et al. (1989). *Cognitive psychology and emotional disorders*. New York: John Wiley & Sons.

Williams, S., Turner, S. & Peer, D. (1985). Guided mastery and performance desensitization treatment for severe agoraphobia. *Journal of Consulting and Clinical Psychology, 53*, 237–47.

Williams, S. & Watson, N. (1985). Perceived danger and perceived self-efficacy as cognitive determinants of agoraphobic behaviour. *Behaviour Research and Therapy, 16*, 136–46.

Williams, S. & Zane, G. (1989). Guided mastery and stimulus exposure treatments for severe performance anxiety in agoraphobia. *Behavior Research and Therapy, 27*, 237–45.

Wilson, A. J., Touyz, S. W., Dunn, S. M. & Beumont, P. J. V. (1989). The Eating Behaviour Rating Scale (EBRS): A measure of eating pathology in anorexia nervosa. *International Journal of Eating Disorders, 8 (5)*, 583–92.

Wilson, P., Spence, S. H. & Kavanagh, D. J. (1989). *Cognitive behavioural interviewing for adult disorders*. London: Routledge.

Wing, J. K. (1988). The concept of negative symptoms. *British Journal of Psychiatry, 155* (Supp. 7), 10–14.

Wing, J. K. & Brown, G. W. (1970). *Institutionalism and schizophrenia*. Cambridge: Cambridge University Press.

Wing, L. (1981). Language, social and cognitive impairments in autism and severe mental retardation. *Journal of Autism and Developmental Disorders, 11(1)*, 31–44.

Wing, L. (1987). The continuum of autistic characteristics. In E. Schopler & G. Mesibov (eds), *Diagnosis and assessment of autism*. New York: Plenum.
Wing, L. (1991). The relationship between Asperger's syndrome and Kanner's autism. In U. Frith (ed.), *Autism and Asperger syndrome*. Cambridge: Cambridge University Press, pp. 93–121.
Wing, L. & Gould, J. (1979). Severe impairments of social interaction and associated abnormalities in children: Epidemiology and classification. *Journal of Autism and Development Disorders*, *9*, 11–29.
Witelson, S. F. (1985). On hemispheric specialisation and cerebral plasticity from birth: Mark II. In C. T. Best (ed.), *Hemispheric function and collaboration in the child*. Orlando, Fla.: Academic Press, pp. 33–85.
Wolf, M. M., Braukmann, C. J. & Ramp, K. A. (1987). Serious delinquent behaviour as part of a significantly handicapping condition: Cures and supportive environments. *Journal of Applied Behaviour Analysis*, *20*, 347–59.
World Health Organization. (1992). *International classification of diseases and related health problems* (10th ed.). Geneva: World Health Organization.
Wynne, L. C., Ryckoff, I. M., Day, J. & Hirsch, S. I. (1958). Pseudo-mutuality in the family relations of schizophrenics. *Psychiatry*, *21*, 205–20.

Zilbergeld, B. (1978). *Men and sex*. London: Fontana.
Zimmer, D. (1987). Does marital therapy enhance the effectiveness of the treatment for sexual dysfunction? *Journal of Sex and Marital Therapy*, *13*, 193–209.
Zitrin, C. (1981). Combined pharmacological and psychological treatment of phobias. In M. MavissaKalian & D. Barlow (eds), *Phobia: Psychological and pharmacological treatments*. New York: Guilford.
Zubin, J. & Spring, B. (1977). Vulnerability — a new view of schizophrenia. *Journal of Abnormal Psychology*, *86*, 103–26.
Zuckerman, M. (1974). The sensation seeking motive. In B. Maher (ed.), *Progress in experimental personality research*, vol. 7. New York: Academic Press.

